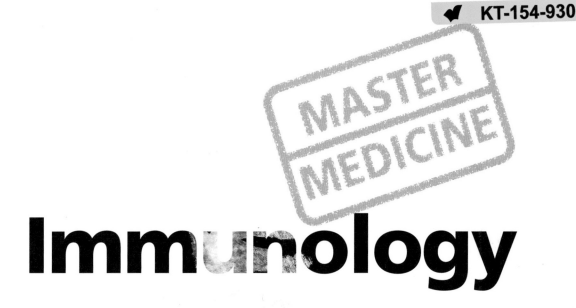

Immunology

Commissioning Editor: Timothy Horne
Development Editor: Barbara Simmons
Project Manager: Emma Riley
Design Direction: George Ajayi

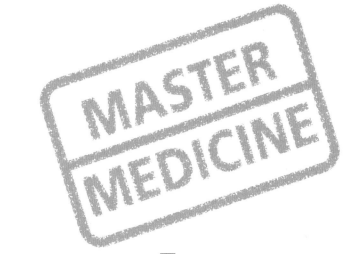

Immunology

A core text with self-assessment

J. DAVID M. EDGAR

BSc FRCP FRCPath
Consultant Immunologist and
Head of the Regional Immunology Service
The Royal Hospitals
Belfast
Northern Ireland

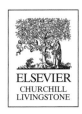

ELSEVIER
CHURCHILL
LIVINGSTONE

EDINBURGH LONDON NEW YORK OXFORD PHILADELPHIA ST LOUIS SYDNEY TORONTO 2006

ELSEVIER
CHURCHILL LIVINGSTONE

An imprint of Elsevier Limited

First edition 2006

ISBN 0443 072795

British Library Cataloguing in Publication Data
A catalogue record for this book is available from the British Library

Library of Congress Cataloguing in Publication Data
A catalog record for this book is available from the Library of Congress

Notice

Neither the Publisher nor the Author assumes any responsibility for any loss or injury and/or damage to persons or property arising out of or related to any use of the material contained in this book. It is the responsibility of the treating practitioner, relying on independent expertise and knowledge of the patient, to determine the best treatment and method of application for the patient.

The Publisher

Working together to grow
libraries in developing countries

www.elsevier.com | www.bookaid.org | www.sabre.org

ELSEVIER   BOOK AID International   Sabre Foundation

ELSEVIER   your source for books, journals and multimedia in the health sciences

www.elsevierhealth.com

The publisher's policy is to use paper manufactured from sustainable forests

Printed in China

Acknowledgements

I would like to thank Barbara Simmons at Elsevier and Jane Ward, freelance copy-editor, for their guidance and encouragement which was invaluable. A number of colleagues gave freely of their time to comment on particular chapters and I am grateful to Alistair Crockard, David Comer, Frank Jones, Gary Wright, Pascal McKeown, Patrick Bell and Paul Jackson for their helpful advice. I am, however, most grateful to Orla, Olivia, Phoebe and Charlie for their support and understanding throughout the writing of this book.

Using this book

Clinical immunology is a relatively new medical specialty that encompasses the diagnosis and management of immunodeficiency, allergy and autoimmune diseases. In the UK, clinical immunology services are provided on a regional or subregional basis usually from a centre with a specialist immunology laboratory service. In addition to direct patient care, clinical immunologists have an important role in directing the provision of laboratory services and providing advice to colleagues on the appropriate investigation of their patients.

Layout of the book

Understanding immunological disorders does require some familiarity with basic immunology. For that reason, it has been necessary to include a chapter on basic immunological science and a second on mechanisms of inflammation, both acute and chronic. These chapters are not intended to be a full account of current knowledge of basic immunology; there are many detailed scientific texts available that serve that purpose. Rather, they are intended to remind the reader of the key elements of the immune response and how these interact together. They should provide a frame of reference for the description of clinical conditions that are described in the rest of the book.

The subsequent chapters deal with immunisation, immunodeficiency, allergy, autoimmune disease, inflammatory arthritis and connective tissue diseases, vasculitis, immune-based therapies, lymphoproliferative diseases, transplantation and the use of the immunology laboratory. This is a very wide spectrum of disease and one would not expect an individual immunologist to deal with all these clinical conditions. However, all of these conditions have an immunological basis, and aspects of their diagnosis, management or complications do give rise to important clinical questions.

The aim of this book is to provide the core knowledge of clinical immunology that would be expected from a new medical graduate. I have tried to address the most immunological common questions posed, for example

How do I diagnose allergy?

When should I suspect an immunodeficiency?

What blood tests should I use and when?

Inevitably, some areas have been included that would be considered rare in most doctors' clinical experience, such as primary immunodeficiency. These details have, however, been included because of their clinical importance and the fact that these disorders commonly go unrecognised for many years. Consequently, it is very important to raise awareness of these disorders in the doctors of the future. The purpose of the book is not to teach all aspects of immunology to the level expected of an expert but rather to address the common clinical challenges that arise in everyday practice and to indicate that there are specialists who can help when things get complicated!

Approaching examinations

The most important preparation for any examination is a carefully planned programme of study throughout the course. Self-assessment can help to identify your own personal strengths and weaknesses and can guide you in necessary revision or further study.

Examinations are an inevitable part of the process of studying medicine, as for any other discipline. Like most other aspects of education, styles of examination change with time. While in the past examinations commonly consisted of essay questions followed by a viva, current trends in examination are to have objective, structured examinations that test the whole breadth of the curriculum and can be demonstrated to be reliable assessments of knowledge and its application. The most common examination assessment methods currently are multiple choice questions (MCQ), short notes, essays, data interpretation, objective structured clinical examinations (OSCE) and viva. In preparation for an examination, it is essential to know what types of question you will encounter and how your answers will be marked. It is also a very good idea to practise answering those types of question under 'practice examination' conditions. Candidates are often surprised by how tiring a 3 hour examination can be and many people find they need to bring in a snack to keep them going.

Once you are in the examination room, it is essential to plan your time carefully. You must identify how many questions of each type you have to answer and allocate a fixed amount of time for each. Do not be tempted to spend longer than you should on one question, just because it may be a favourite topic. You are unlikely to gain significant extra marks but will lose out in other questions for which you have inadequate time. Try to factor in a small amount of time for reviewing questions at the end of the examination to ensure that you have not misread all or part of a question or made an 'obvious' mistake.

Self-assessment

Each chapter has a set of self-assessment questions that may take the form of MCQs, short notes, data interpretation or case histories. This material may be used before or after reading the relevant chapter depending on whether you wish to assess your existing knowledge or how much you have recalled and understood from the chapter. In approaching examinations, self-assessment should confirm your knowledge and, therefore, increase your confidence.

Multiple choice questions

The majority of the self-assessment material is in the MCQ form as this is the most common form of examination question. MCQs test factual recall and are, therefore, a good means of assessing a student's knowledge of a subject area. They are usually of one of two types: either multiple true/false or one best answer/best of five. Multiple true/false questions are the traditional type of MCQ. In these questions an initial statement (the stem) is made, for example 'Which of the following are features of Addison's disease?' followed by five statements that are typically unrelated to one another (i.e. they may individually relate to diagnosis, aetiology, clinical features, treatment, etc.). Any number of the statements may be true or false. It is essential to read the stem carefully, often several times if you are unsure of exactly what is being asked. 'Little' words, such as only, never, rarely, commonly and always, are very important and can significantly influence how you answer such a question. The expression 'may occur' has a very different meaning in this context than does 'characteristic'. The latter may mean a feature that should be there and the absence of which would make you question the appropriateness of a diagnosis. The former simply means that a feature may (or may not) be present in the particular condition. You should make sure that you know what marking system is used before undertaking an MCQ examination. In examinations comprising traditional MCQ, there are often negative marks assigned to incorrect answers and, therefore, candidates are usually advised only to answer those questions about which they are certain. 'Guessing' the answers is a very risky approach as you may gather significant negative marks.

Increasingly, MCQs are being developed in the one best answer/best of five format. These types of question have a traditional stem statement followed by five options, only one of which is correct. Usually, the five options will be related (i.e. they will all concern one of area such as diagnosis, investigation, treatment, prognosis, etc.). Where possible, the stem will be a short clinical scenario, for example 'A 55-year-old man is admitted to hospital with a chest infection. Which one of the following antibiotics would be the most appropriate first line therapy?'. This type of MCQ, therefore, differs from the traditional format in that candidates are asked to compare five similar answers and choose the 'best' or most appropriate one. Consequently, this type of MCQ does test more than just factual recall. By asking candidates to compare five similar options, an element of judgement can be assessed. The use of clinical scenarios in the stem means that the MCQ can be tailored toward actual clinical practice rather than recall of textbook knowledge, which may seem remote from the bedside. In this book, both formats of MCQ are used: how do you know which type you are answering? The key is to read the stem carefully and look for the clue 'Which one of the following ...'.

Short notes

Short notes do appear in a number of examinations. They are also a test of factual knowledge, but do not in general attract negative marks. Most short note questions require you to identify four or five key points about the subject and write the core facts only. In answering short notes, time management is critical. Do not be tempted to write more than the core facts.

Essays

Essays are gradually disappearing from most examinations. They were popular in the past because examining bodies felt that they tested more than just factual recall. The essay gave an opportunity for the candidate to offer opinions and a critical evaluation of different aspects of a subject. It is, however, difficult to standardise essay questions and fair comparison of different candidates' answers can be difficult. Most essay questions currently set tend to be structured in two or three sections to overcome some of these difficulties. Often the percentage marks allocated to each section will be indicated. In answering such questions, you need to allocate time carefully and write a structured plan. The plan should have a logical theme. Examiners do take note of such plans, particularly if time constraints have limited the candidate's ability to complete the actual essay.

Data interpretation

Data interpretation questions test more than factual recall. They assess the understanding of basic principles, normal values and pattern recognition. You should look at all the data provided and each piece of information must be evaluated. Data interpretation questions should be answerable by a logical approach. In answering the question, you should establish a list of possible options and then 'test' each of these against the data provided. Which one fits the data best? Do any of the data exclude one of your options? This type of question usually does not include negative marking. As for short notes, however, it is very important not to spend too much time on any one difficult question. You can come back to it at the end of the examination.

Objective structured clinical examinations

OSCEs provide a platform for covering a large number of diverse clinical topics in a totally structured format so that students can be assessed objectively. These examinations are very time-consuming and laborious to design and set up but, ultimately, are more objective and, therefore, more fair to the students. The OSCE generally utilises a range of examination formats, including picture cards, slides, data, radiographs, electrocardiographs, etc., as well as practical sessions that may test history taking, practical demonstrations and clinical skills. Marks are weighted such that the clinical hands-on and practical stations are given priority. Virtually anything can be written into an OSCE format! However, all questions are organised into set stations with a finite time interval, generally lasting from 4 to 6 minutes. Hence, the number of questions asked on a particular topic must be focused but limited. The majority of OSCE questions will generally cover the core issues and, unless one's knowledge is threadbare across a wide range of topics, it is very difficult to fail an OSCE. Very few questions would be particularly difficult and these would be included to identify the distinction candidates.

Viva

The viva can seem a very daunting challenge although these days it is usually reserved for two categories of students: those who have done well and may be awarded a distinction and those who are on the borderline of pass/fail. Usually there are two examiners, who will take turns in asking questions. You should answer their questions as succinctly as possible. You can influence the course of the viva by mentioning subjects about which you are confident. Examiners do like to ask supplementary questions on issues you may raise. Try not to 'wander off' the subject and avoid mentioning areas about which you know very little. Do not be afraid to ask for clarification if you are not sure what the examiner is asking and, if you genuinely do not know something, then do not be afraid to say so. Examiners generally appreciate honesty. The general rule in a pass/fail viva is that the examiners will wish to assess whether you are 'safe to practise'. In that respect, they will often ask you to describe how you would respond to a particular clinical situation. You should answer to the best of your ability; however, if you feel something is outside your knowledge or clinical competence, you should say so and indicate from whom you would seek advice.

Conclusion

Preparation for examinations is an important part of the learning process and we hope that the advice given here is helpful. Learning is, however, more concerned with understanding basic principles and their application to real clinical situations. We hope that you will find this book stimulates your interest in clinical immunology.

Chapter overview

This chapter gives an account of the basic components of the normal function of the human immune system. It describes the multiple cellular and soluble components that make up the immune system, how these are subclassified and how they interact together to generate an effective immune response. The aim of this chapter is to provide sufficient basic science for an understanding of the common clinical issues that are addressed in the subsequent chapters. It is not intended as a comprehensive account of the immense complexity of the human immune system. There are, however, many excellent basic science texts currently available to which the reader is referred.

1.1 Introduction

Learning objectives

You should:
- understand the difference between the innate and adaptive immune systems
- be familiar with the key cellular and soluble components of each
- understand how the two systems interact in the generation of an immune response
- understand the principles of immunological specificity and memory.

The human immune system comprises multiple physical, chemical and cellular components that, in com-bination, protect the individual from infection by many types of microorganism. Traditionally, these components are classified as **innate** or **adaptive**. The innate system components provide a constant level of protection while the adaptive immune system recognises and provides microorganism specific protection and has a long-lasting immunological memory. Hence the adaptive immune system is so named because it is capable of specifically responding to the multitude of potential pathogens in the external environment.

While we describe the individual components of the immune system individually and classify them into innate and adaptive systems, it should be clear that these individual elements work closely together to protect the body from infection and provide long-lasting immunity to microorganisms already encountered.

1.2 Innate system

Learning objectives

You should:
- be familiar with the cellular and soluble components of the innate system
- understand the classical and 'alternate complement' pathways
- understand bacterial killing by phagocytes.

Physical and chemical defences

Intact skin and mucous membranes are essential to protect us from infection. Mucous membranes are usually bathed in secretions and, within these secretions, enzymes (e.g. lysozyme in tears) or acids (e.g. hydrochloric acid in gastric secretions) provide additional antimicrobial protection. The interferons (interferons α, β and γ) are a family of molecules that have antiviral actions and provide an important line of innate defence. Patients with severe burns, and skin loss, who become prone to severe and life-threatening infections, exemplify the importance of physical protection in immune defence. These defences are illustrated in Figure 1.

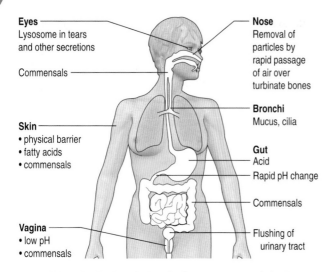

Eyes
Lysosome in tears and other secretions

Commensals

Nose
Removal of particles by rapid passage of air over turbinate bones

Bronchi
Mucus, cilia

Skin
• physical barrier
• fatty acids
• commensals

Gut
Acid
Rapid pH change

Commensals

Vagina
• low pH
• commensals

Flushing of urinary tract

Fig. 1 The physical and chemical components of the innate immune system.

Complement

The complement system is a series of 26 proteins circulating in the bloodstream. They form a cascade of **proenzymes**, the activation of each catalysing the activation of subsequent downstream components. Complement has a number of crucial functions in the immune response including

• disposal of immune complexes
• chemotaxis
• activation of mast cells (via anaphylotoxins)
• lysis of infected cells.

The classical pathway

The complement cascade is divided into two activation pathways (classical and alternate) that lead to the cleavage and activation of C3 (Fig. 2) and a final common lytic pathway that leads to the formation of the membrane attack complex (MAC) (Fig. 3).

The classical pathway is activated by the formation of immune complexes (soluble antigen–antibody combinations) and has an important role in solubilising and disposing of these complexes. The components of the classical pathway are activated in the following sequence: C1, then C4 followed by C2. Activation involves the cleavage of each molecule in turn; this forms an enzyme complex that activates the next molecule and releases molecular fragments, which have other important properties. The formation of the classical pathway C3 convertase (C4b2a) results in cleavage of C3 and the initiation of the terminal pathway. The cleavage products include C4a and C2a, which are chemoattractants for phagocytes and cause degranulation of mast cells (anaphylotoxins). Thus, activation of the classical pathway recruits other inflammatory cells to the area of activation.

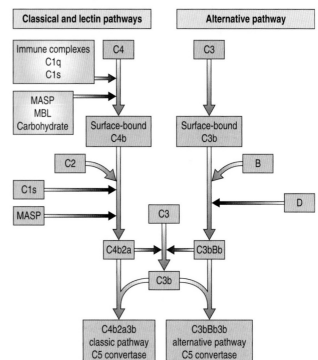

Fig. 2 The classical, lectin and alternate pathways of complement activation. The three pathways converge at the cleavage of C3 and the formation of a C5 convertase, which triggers the final lytic pathway. MASP, mannose-binding lectin-associated serine protease; MBL, mannose-binding lectin.

A further mechanism of classical pathway activation is known as the lectin pathway. Mannan-binding lectin (MBL; also known as mannan-binding protein (MBP)) binds directly to cell-surface components (terminal mannose groups). This binding activates two serine proteases, MASP1 and MASP2 (mannan-binding lectin-associated serine proteases) and the enzyme complex generated will activate C4 directly in the absence of antibody.

In two clinical conditions, cryoglobulinaemia (Ch. 11) and C1 inhibitor deficiency (Ch. 4), there is inefficient activation of the classical pathway, with limited formation of the C3 convertase. Measurement of complement levels in serum from such patients will, therefore, typically indicate low levels of C4 with relative preservation of C3.

The alternate pathway

The alternate pathway is thought to be a more primitive mechanism of complement activation and consists of components factor B, factor D and properdin (Fig. 2). These components are not activated by exposure to immune complexes but by exposure to endotoxin or polysaccharide, which form part of bacterial cell walls. They also form an alternate C3 convertase (C3bBb) that

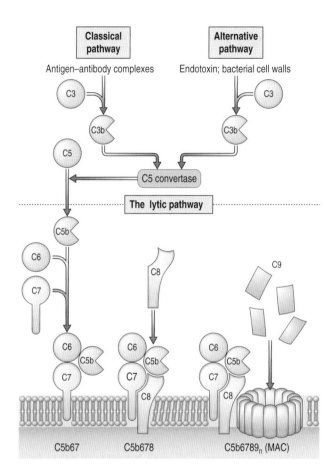

Fig. 3 The final lytic pathway of complement, leading to the pore-forming membrane attack complex (MAC).

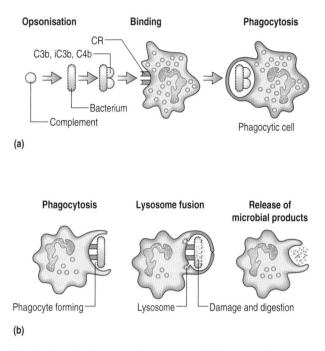

(a)

(b)

Fig. 4 Opsonisation and phagocytosis. (a) Opsonisation of microorganisms with complement or antibody molecules enhances the specific binding of the microorganism via complement or Fc receptors on the phagocyte cell surface. (b) The phases of phagocytosis and killing of a microorganism.

leads to activation of the terminal pathway. While the two pathways are described as distinct, they are linked through their activation of C3 and both are likely to be activated in most inflammatory situations.

Phagocytic cells

If microorganisms are successful in breaching the body's physical defences, they are targeted by phagocytic cells, whose purpose is to engulf and destroy them. These phagocytic cells include polymorphonuclear cells (PMN: neutrophils, eosinophils and basophils) and macrophages/monocytes. The process of phagocytosis and bacterial killing is indicated schematically in Figure 4. The phagocytic cell recognition of the bacterium is enhanced if it is opsonised (see above), in which case there is specific recognition and binding of C3b by phagocytic cell membrane receptors. The cell membrane then engulfs the bacterium forming a **phagosome**. The phagosome then fuses with **lysosomes**, which release toxic enzymes causing bacterial killing in the **phagolysosome**. Some bacteria (e.g. pneumococci) can resist phagocytosis by virtue of their capsules, while others (e.g. staphylococci) release toxins that destroy phago-

cytes. Although some microorganisms can survive within phagocytic cells (e.g. mycobacteria), giving rise to chronic infection, most are killed in the phagolysosome by a combination of acid pH, oxygen metabolites (e.g. hydrogen peroxide) and various cytotoxic proteins. However, not all killing is intracellular and macrophages or polymorphonuclear cells can secrete toxic molecules in order to kill large targets, e.g. worms (helminths).

1.3 Adaptive system

Learning objectives

You should:
- be familiar with the key cellular and soluble components of the adaptive system and how they contribute to immunological specificity and memory
- be able to identify primary and secondary lymphoid organs
- understand the role of the HLA (human leukocyte antigen) system in cell–cell interactions
- understand the role of B cells in antibody production
- understand the T cell subsets and their roles
- understand antigen processing and presentation.

Development of the adaptive system

Lymphocytes originate from stem cells in the bone marrow and eventually mature into B, T and natural killer (NK) cells. B lymphocytes are responsible for antibody production, while T cells have antiviral, antifungal and immunoregulatory functions. B cells complete their maturation in the bone marrow, but T cells require passage through the thymus, where they complete their maturation and education process. During this passage T cells learn to identify 'self-antigens'; any autoreactive T cells are either allowed to die (by apoptosis) or are rendered non-reactive (tolerant).

Anatomy of the adaptive system

The major lymphoid organs are classified as **primary** or **secondary** (Fig. 5). The bone marrow and thymus are referred to as primary lymphoid organs. These are the primary sites for the maturation of lymphoid stem cells into mature B and T cells, respectively. It is, therefore, in the primary lymphoid organs that lymphocytes develop their repertoire of specific antigen receptors (cell-surface immunoglobulin molecules and T cell receptors) that enable them to respond to antigenic challenge throughout life. It is also within the primary lymphoid organs that lymphocytes are deleted or rendered unreactive (**anergic**) if they are autoreactive and, therefore, potentially harmful to the host.

Cellular and antibody responses are generated within the secondary lymphoid organs. The secondary lymphoid organs include

- lymph nodes

- the spleen
- Peyer's patches
- tonsils and adenoids.

These are strategically located to encounter micro-organisms entering the body through external tissues, blood, gut and upper airway, respectively. The spleen responds to blood-borne antigen. Regional lymph nodes respond to antigen in the tissues from which the lymph drains. Mucosal associated lymphoid tissue responds to antigen encountered at the mucosal sites. The structure of secondary lymphoid tissue is exemplified by the lymph node (Fig. 6). Lymph drains to the node, enters the subcapsular sinus and travels through the trabecular structure toward the medulla. The cortex is primarily a B cell region and the cells are organised into primary and secondary follicles. The paracortex is primarily a T cell area. The medulla contains both B and T cells and most of the plasma cells, which secrete large amounts of antibody molecules into the efferent lymph. The physical proximity of B and T cells in the architecture is essential for the close cellular interaction and antigen presentation that will allow responses to be generated. A characteristic of mature lymphocytes is their ability to 'traffic' from peripheral blood into the tissues and secondary lymphoid organs. This property allows lymphocytes to encounter antigen in almost all physical locations. The individual blood supply for each node with specialised high endothelial venules allows lymphocytes from remote regions to enter the lymph node at the paracortex. Both lymphocytes and antibody leave via the efferent lymphatic vessel.

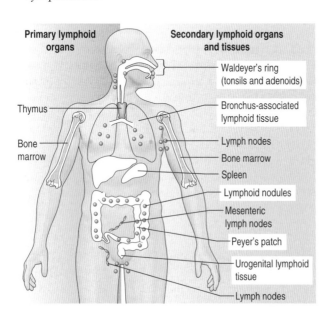

Fig. 5 The distribution of primary and secondary lymphoid tissue throughout the body.

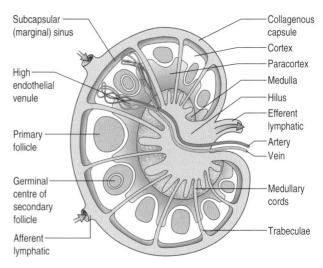

Fig. 6 Structure of a regional lymph node.

Mucosal immune system

The lymphoid tissues of the gut, genitourinary tract, breast and lungs behave, to a certain extent, autonomously and are termed the 'mucosal immune system'. B cells (largely IgA secreting) and T cells recirculate selectively throughout the mucosal immune system. This transfer of cells between mucosal sites ensures that antigen exposure at any one mucosal site will facilitate protective immunity at other locations.

The human leukocyte antigen systems

An understanding of the mammalian major histocompatibility complex (MHC), which is known in humans as the human leukocyte antigen (HLA) system, is fundamental to understanding adaptive immune responses. The HLA system is the major determinant of transplant rejection response; however, its physiological role is to control cell–cell interactions particularly within the immune system. The HLA genes lie on the short arm of chromosome 6 and are grouped in two major sets referred to as class I and class II (Fig. 7). Each set contains three genetic loci that have a large number of alleles coding for HLA antigens. The genes for some complement components and cytokines also lie within the same region (in the class III region), but their products are quite unrelated to class I and class II molecules. Class I and II antigens are central to antigen presentation and the generation of an effective immune response.

Class I molecules consist of a large α-chain, and a small β-chain known as β_2-microglobulin. The gene for β_2-microglobulin is on a different chromosome and shows no sequence variability. Class I antigens (i.e. alleles at the A, B and C loci) are expressed on all nucleated cells (two from each locus on diploid cells). Therefore on diploid cells there are usually six different class I antigens expressed: two each of HLA-A, HLA-B and HLA-C.

Class II HLA molecules are two-chain (α and β) structures; both chains are encoded in the HLA locus and are polymorphic. Class II antigens (alleles at the DP, DQ and DR loci) are expressed on a more limited range of cells: classical antigen-presenting cells (APC), B lymphocytes and activated T lymphocytes. Similar to class I expression, there are usually six different class II molecules expressed at the cell surface: two each of HLA-DP, HLA-DQ and HLA-DR.

Knowledge of the HLA alleles expressed by an individual is clearly essential for most organ transplantation. Additionally, particular HLA types are also known to be associated with certain diseases. In a few clinical conditions the HLA association is so strong as to be helpful in diagnosis, for example HLA B27 and ankylosing spondylitis.

Cytokines

Cytokines are a series of low-molecular-weight proteins that are essential in cell–cell communication. They were originally recognised as molecules that mediated signalling between white blood cells and were, therefore, termed 'interleukins'. This name persists for many cytokines and is abbreviated to IL, giving IL-1, IL-2, IL-3, etc. The recognition that these molecules functioned in the interaction of a much greater range of cells led to the more generic term cytokine being adopted. Cytokines act through binding to specific cell-surface receptors and this binding initiates a range of intracellular signalling pathways that ultimately affect nuclear functions such as gene transcription. In this way, cytokines may activate specific cellular functions or indeed reduce/suppress certain cellular activities. Cytokines will, therefore, influence cells that express the relevent surface receptor. In general, cytokines act on cells adjacent within the microenvironment and this is known as **paracrine** activity. Some cytokines will also act on the cell that produced the cytokine (**autocrine** activity) and occasionally on cells distant within the body (**endocrine** activity). Examples of the latter two include IL-2 activating the producing T cell via the CD25 receptor (autocrine) and IL-1 acting on the hypothalamus to cause fever and somnolence (endocrine).

The major cytokines, their actions and potential clinical importance are summarised in Table 1.

Lymphocytes

Peripheral blood normally contains 70–90% T cells, 5–10% B cells and approximately 1–10% natural killer cells. Lymphocytes are the major effector cells of the adaptive immune response. Microscopically, they are small round cells with relatively large nuclei; however, an understanding of their function and interactions

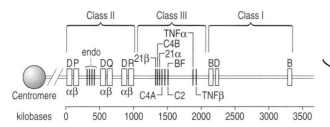

Fig. 7 Organisation of the major histocompatibility complex (MHC or HLA) on the short arm of chromosome 6. Regions I and II code for the class I and II molecules. Region III codes for complement proteins C2 and C4, factor B, factor F, 21β- and 21α-hydroxylase, and tumour necrosis factor (TNF) α and β.

Table 1 The major cytokines, their sources and actions

Cytokine	Source	Actions
Tumour necrosis factor α and β	Macrophages	Antitumour, antiviral, vascular damage, polymorphonuclear neutrophil activation, bone resorption, induces interleukin-1, etc.
Interferon-α	Macrophages	Antiviral
Interferon-β	Fibroblasts	Antiviral
Interferon-γ	T cells	Antiviral, activates macrophages, increases mycobactericidal activity
Interleukin-2	T cells	Activates T, B and natural killer cells
Interleukin-5	T cells, mast cells	Eosinophil growth and activation
Interleukin-6	T cells, fibroblasts, antigen-presenting cells, hepatocytes	B cell growth and differentiation, induces acute phase response
Interleukin-8	T cells, monocytes	Neutrophil activation and chemotaxis
Granulocyte–macrophage colony-stimulating factor	Macrophages	Granulocyte growth and maturation

depends on knowledge of at least some of their microscopic cell-surface receptors. These include members of the HLA system, T and B cell antigen receptors and other cell-surface receptors classified as **CD antigens** (Table 2).

B cells and antibodies

The main function of B cells is antibody production, but immunological 'help' from T cells is required for the majority of antibody responses. Most B cell responses are, therefore, termed 'T-dependent'. Some polymeric antigens do, however, stimulate B cells directly and these are termed T-independent antigens (e.g. bacterial capsular polysaccharides).

For T-dependent responses, B cells are triggered to proliferate by interaction between their surface immunoglobulin and the antigen, but they require additional signals from T helper cells in order to differentiate into plasma cells and secrete antibody. These signals consist of non-antigen-specific cytokines (particularly IL-4 and IL-6) and cell–cell signalling. The interaction of these cell-surface molecules is essential in facilitating effective B cell antibody production. One example is the interaction between gp39 (CD40 ligand (CD40L)) on T cells with CD40 on B cells, which is required for B cells to 'switch' from IgM to IgG production during an immune response.

During T-dependent responses, some proliferating B lymphocytes are retained in germinal centres instead of differentiating 'terminally' into plasma cells. These are the memory B cells.

B cells produce antibody molecules of five classes: IgD, IgA, IgE, IgM and IgG, which have different structures and function. Antibody has a primary role in combating microorganisms free in the blood or tissue spaces, primarily viruses in their extracellular stage and many bacteria. The antibody or immunoglobulin molecule has a basic four-chain structure, which is exemplified in antibodies of the IgG class (Fig. 8). The N-terminal end of the heavy and light chains is the variable region, which is responsible for antigen binding (fraction antigen bindin (Fab)). The three constant sequence domains of the heavy chain (CH_1, CH_2, CH_3)

Table 2 Major CD markers and lymphocyte subpopulations

CD marker	Population identified
CD3	All T cells
CD4	T helper cells
CD8	T cytotoxic cells
CD19	B cells
CD16/CD56	Natural killer cells
HLA-DR	All B cells, activated T cells
CD25 (interleukin-2 receptor)	Activated T cells

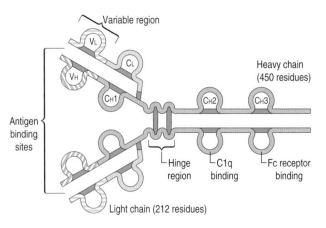

Fig. 8 The basic structure of IgG_1. The N terminal end of the heavy and light chains is the variable region responsible for antigen binding (Fab). The Fc region is responsible for complement (C1q) activation and binding to cell surfaces via Fc receptors.

and the single constant domain of the light chain (CL) make up the fraction constant (Fc) region, which is responsible for complement activation and binding to cell surfaces via Fc receptors. This C-terminal portion determines the class of antibody and is responsible for many of the biological functions of the molecule. The major role of antibody molecules is to bind to microorganisms via the Fab portion, enhancing phagocytosis, as phagocytes possess Fc receptors. This process of coating microorganisms with antibody is known as **opsonisation**. The basic, four-chain structure is preserved in all five classes of immunoglobulin; however, each class has certain characteristics that serve specific functions.

IgG. These molecules are involved in the activation of complement, attachment to phagocytic cells, passage into the tissues and transport across the placenta. The four IgG subclasses (IgG$_1$, IgG$_2$, IgG$_3$ and IgG$_4$) vary somewhat in these functions (Table 3).

IgM. These large molecules with a pentameric structure are mainly confined to the bloodstream and are very efficient at activating complement and agglutinating foreign material because of the 10 antigen-combining sites per pentameric complex.

IgA. These molecules form the predominant immunoglobulin class secreted at mucosal sites. The molecules have a dimeric structure and are protected from proteolytic damage by a special polypeptide: the secretary chain (Sc). The secretary chain is produced by the mucosal epithelial cells and acts as a receptor-transporter, binding to and taking the antibody into external sites. IgA can, therefore, survive proteolytic attack in secretions of the eyes, lungs, nose, gut and urinary tract.

IgE. The IgE molecule attaches via its Fc region to receptors on mast cells. When two bound IgE molecules are cross-linked by antigen, intracellular signalling results in release of mediators from mast cell granules and the clinical features of acute allergy.

IgD. These molecules are found mainly on B cell membranes and act as antigen receptors. The soluble form is not thought to have a significant physiological role.

Antibody diversity

In order to protect the individual from the entire range of potential environmental pathogens, it is estimated that the immune system must be able to produce antibody molecules with approximately 10^8 different antigenic specificities. This diversity is achieved by a combination of mechanisms that includes the association of molecular chains and the rearrangement of genes within the B cell.

- Each heavy chain can be associated with either a kappa or a lambda light chain.
- Antibody molecule chains are encoded by genes giving rise to three (light chain: V, J, C) or four (heavy chain: V, D, J, C) different families. The combination of different V–D–J–C gene products to create a single chain produces a huge range of potential sequence diversity in the final molecule.
- During the multiple recombination necessary to create an antibody molecule, there is potential for even a single amino acid residue change to alter the final antigen specificity significantly.
- During the life of a B cell, point mutations may occur within the variable regions (**somatic mutation**), resulting in a change of binding affinity of the antibody molecule. Increased affinity for antigen confers a selective advantage to any B cell, whereas lower affinity molecules are less likely to compete successfully for antigen and those B cells will not be stimulated. This phenomenon is termed **affinity maturation**.

After gene rearrangement, and the production of an antibody molecule of a certain specificity, this remains the antigen-binding specificity of that B cell and any daughter cells. The maintenance of a unique antigenic specificity through generations of B cells is the molecular basis of immunological memory. The heavy chain C gene can, however, change to allow class switching (e.g. IgM–IgG) during the immune response, as occurs in moving from a primary to a secondary response.

T cells

The major effector role of T cells is the elimination of viruses, fungi and protozoa, but they also act as

Table 3 Immunoglobulin classes and their properties

Class and subclass	Structure	Major functions	
		Complement activation	Opsonisation
IgG			
IgG$_1$	Monomer	+	+
IgG$_2$	Monomer	+	
IgG$_3$	Monomer	+	+
IgG$_4$	Monomer		+
IgM	Pentamer	+	
IgA		Mucosal protection	
IgA$_1$	Dimer		
IgA$_2$	Dimer		
IgE	Monomer	Mast cell activation	
IgD	Cell surface bound	Antigen binding	

coordinators of the overall adaptive immune response. B and T lymphocytes are impossible to distinguish by light microscopy and, therefore, more sophisticated techniques are needed (e.g. flow cytometry) that can identify cell-type-specific surface antigens (CD antigens: Table 2). It is helpful to remember some of the more common CD numbers as these are important in describing primary immunodeficiency states and lymphoproliferative diseases. All T cells bear the CD3 antigen, which is associated on the cell surface with the T cell receptor (TCR). The two major T cells subsets are defined by the additional expression of either CD4 or CD8.

CD8+ T cells

The CD8+ T cell is also known as a **cytotoxic T cell**; these cells are responsible for killing abnormal host cells (e.g. virally infected, malignantly transformed or transplanted cells). Cytotoxic T cells destroy target cells by several mechanisms including cell membrane interactions (such as that of the Fas antigen (CD95) with its ligand) and the release of cytotoxic substances: perforins, granzymes and other cytokines.

CD4+ T cells

The CD4+ T cell is also known as a **helper T cell** (Th); these cells provide signals and cytokines that are essential for effective B cell activation and antibody production and generation of effective cytotoxic T cell responses. There are two subtypes: Th1 and Th2.

The T cell receptor

The TCR (Fig. 9) is a two-chain (α and β or γ and δ) molecule that recognises linear fragments of small foreign peptides in combination with molecules of the HLA system. The T cell only recognises antigenic fragments when they are *presented* in association with the appropriate HLA class I or II molecule. The TCR is structurally similar to antibody molecules and belongs to the immunoglobulin supergene family of molecules. The TCR-associated CD4 or CD8 molecules determine whether the individual T cell recognises antigen in association with class I or class II molecules. The CD4+ T cells are *restricted to* recognition of antigenic fragments in association with class II molecules, while CD8+ T cells are *restricted* to recognising antigenic fragments in association with class I molecules. As class I molecules are expressed on all nucleated cells of the body, CD8+ T cells can identify intracellular antigen at any site. CD4+ cells can only be stimulated by specialised or activated cells that express HLA class II.

Antigen processing and presentation

The process of stimulation of lymphocytes by antigenic fragments is known as antigen presentation and is undertaken by a limited range of cells (Fig. 10). The APCs include macrophages, dendritic cells of the spleen and lymph nodes, Langerhans' cells of the skin and B cells. Antigenic fragments are presented to T cells in specialised **antigen-binding grooves** in HLA class I and class II molecules:

- class I molecules present peptides that are endogenously synthesised, e.g. viral proteins synthesised in an infected cell
- class II molecules present peptides from external proteins, e.g. extracellular microorganisms that have been engulfed and degraded to peptides by the APC.

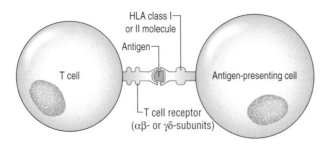

Fig. 9 T cell antigen recognition. The T cell receptor only recognises antigenic fragments when they are presented in association with the appropriate HLA class I or II molecule.

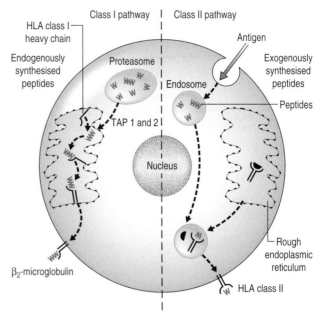

Fig. 10 The two distinct pathways for the processing and presentation of endogenous (class I) and of exogenous (class II) antigens. Class II heavy chains combine with β_2-microglobulin in the endoplasmic reticulum in the presence of antigenic peptides.

There are distinct intracellular pathways involved for class I and class II presentation. Class II molecules are synthesised within the rough endoplasmic reticulum (RER) and, bound to a second molecule called the invariant chain, are transported to the endosomal compartment. There the invariant chain is replaced by antigenic fragment and the complex is transported to the cell surface. Class I molecules are also synthesised in the RER and are initially anchored on the inner surface of this organelle. Peptide fragments generated in cytoplasmic proteasomes are transported into the RER by specialised transporter proteins (transporters of antigenic peptides) TAP-1 and TAP-2. The peptide fragments then bind to the class I molecule and this complex associates with β_2-microglobulin before being transported to the cell surface.

Activation of T helper cells

Activation of CD4$^+$ T cells is dependent on a series of costimulatory signals (cell–cell surface binding and soluble cytokines) (Fig. 11). In addition to TCR recognition of the HLA/antigenic fragment, the CD4 molecule binds to a non-polymorphic region of the HLA class II molecule. Several other adhesion molecule pairs (leukocyte function-related antigen (LFA) 1 and intercellular adhesion molecule (ICAM) 1; CD2 and LFA-3) link together, strengthening the cellular adhesion. The interaction of the T cell-surface molecule CD28 with B7 molecules on APCs is believed to be crucial to T cell activation, as is the secretion by the APC of IL-1. The result of these 'positive signals' is the generation of gene transcription factors, such as NFAT (nuclear factor of activated T cells), which switch on genes (e.g. the gene for IL-2) within the T cell nucleus. Once IL-2

is secreted, it acts on both the responding and the neighbouring cells.

In contrast to CD28, a molecule termed CTLA4 appears to be crucial in *downregulating* the T cell immune response. CTLA4 appears on T cells late in their activation and also binds to B7 molecules, but this binding delivers a negative signal to 'switch off' responding T cells.

Regulation of immune responses

Both T and B cells are activated by recognition of specific antigens. Effective removal/degradation of antigen by a combination of mechanisms is, therefore, an important physiological endpoint for an immune response. However, the immune system has several additional mechanisms that regulate the nature and intensity of the immune response.

Apoptosis

Apoptosis (programmed cell death) is now recognised as an important regulatory mechanism for the disposal of immune cells that have completed their function. Failure of apoptosis in the rare condition *autoimmune lymphoproliferative syndrome* results in diffuse lymph node enlargement and autoimmune disease.

Anti-idiotype antibodies

Anti-idiotype antibodies are antibodies directed against the V region of the Fab portion (idiotype) of other antibody molecules and may block or modulate antibody function.

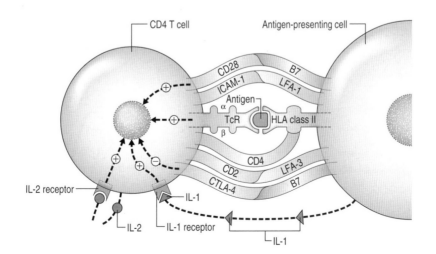

Fig. 11 Activation of CD4$^+$ T cells. In addition to antigen recognition via the T cell receptor (TCR), a range of cell surface molecules and soluble cytokines deliver additional positive (+) or negative (–) signals. Interleukin (IL) 2 secretion activates both the secreting T cell (autocrine) and its near neighbours (paracrine).

T suppressor cells

T suppressor cells have not been identified in humans, although research continues to determine whether such a discrete population exists. There is, however, good evidence that the pattern of cytokines that CD4+ T cells secrete preferentially induces either a cellular or antibody response. The differentiation of CD4+ T cells subsets according to the pattern of cytokines they secrete is known as the Th1/Th2 model.

The T helper 1 / T helper 2 model

Prior to activation, most CD4+ T cells are Th0 (i.e. they have the potential of secreting a wide range of cytokines). After activation, however, there is a preferential commitment towards either a Th1 or Th2 pattern (Fig. 12). The Th1 cytokines are IL-2, IL-12 and interferon-γ, inducing a cellular immune response, while Th2 cytokines are IL-4, IL-5, IL-6 and IL-10, inducing an antibody response. There is mutual suppression between these two dominant patterns of cytokine secretion such that, once a response has become committed in either direction, this pattern will tend to be maintained. This differentiation of T cells may, therefore, explain the concept of suppression of the immune response seen in certain situations. It is also important in understanding the influence of the immune response on the pattern of clinical diseases such as leprosy (see hypersensitivity; Ch. 2).

Primary and secondary antibody responses

The outcome of an effective adaptive immune response is the generation of long-term protective immunity to specific organisms. This is most commonly confirmed by the presence of high titres of antigen-specific IgG in serum. The generation of long-term antibody (humoral) immunity has two distinct phases (Fig. 13), which are the end result of the cellular interactions described above.

On first exposure to an antigen, a B cell with a complementary surface immunoglobulin molecule binds to and is stimulated to proliferate by the antigen and by local production of Th2 cytokines such as IL-4, IL-5 and IL-6. The B cell proliferates and divides, creating a clone of identical daughter cells all of which synthesise identical immunoglobulin molecules. This *primary* antibody response is characterised by the production of IgM; however, as B cells interact with CD40L-expressing T cells, they *switch* to IgG production. In parallel with this, a population of memory B cells is produced. Thus a primary antibody response is characterised by an interval of approximately 5 days between antigen exposure and measurable antigen-specific IgM in the bloodstream. In contrast, on subsequent exposure to the same antigen, there exists an already expanded clone of specific IgG-producing B cells and memory B cells ready to respond. This is demonstrable as the *secondary* antibody response, which has a much shorter interval between antigen exposure and the detection of antigen-specific immunoglobulin in the bloodstream and a quantitatively greater immunoglobulin response dominated by IgG (Fig. 13). An effective immune response to an infection or immu-

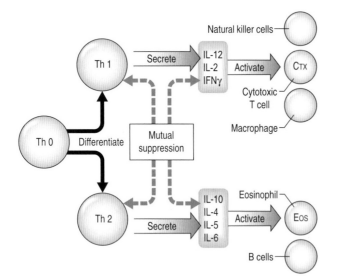

Fig. 12 T cells differentiate along two major axes depending on their pattern of cytokine secretion to give T helper (Th) 1 cells, which tend to promote cellular responses, and Th2 cells, which tend to promote antibody production and IgE-mediated responses. Th1 cells exert a suppressive effect on Th2 and vice versa. The distinction between these subsets is not absolute in humans.

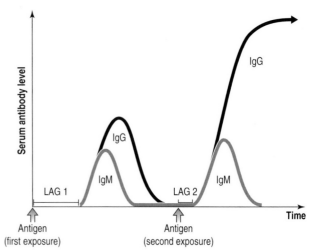

Fig. 13 Primary and secondary antibody responses typify the adaptive immune response to antigen. Memory cells induced in the primary response become rapidly activated upon re-exposure to the same antigen.

nisation can thus produce very effective long-term immunity with high levels of antigen-specific IgG circulating in the blood ready to interact with the microorganism should it be encountered.

1.4 Adaptive response to microorganisms

Learning objectives

You should:
- understand how the different systems interact to respond to an infection
- be aware of the different response required for an intracellular infection
- understand the methods used by infecting organisms to evade the host defences.

The basic components of the immune system have been described, but in order to put this in to a clinical context, we will discuss how these components interact to respond to bacteria, viruses and fungi. Infection can be considered as an imbalance between the microorganism's virulence factors and the host's defence mechanisms. If there is a particularly virulent organism (e.g. a new variant of the influenza virus), many otherwise healthy individuals will be infected and a pandemic may result. In contrast, organisms with low virulence, which do not cause illness in healthy individuals, may cause severe illness in those with deficient immune systems (e.g. *Pneumocystis carinii* pneumonia in primary and secondary immunodeficiencies; Ch. 4). It is, therefore, useful to think about which components of the immune system are particularly responsible for the response to different microorganisms.

Bacterial infection

Once the physical and chemical barriers have been overcome, the major innate response to bacterial infection is mediated via the complement and mononuclear phagocyte systems. The alternate complement pathway is activated by bacterial cell wall products, leading to lysis of the microorganism. Phagocytic cells engulf and kill bacteria. The adaptive response to extracellular bacteria is via the antibody system, which generates specific antibody to neutralise bacteria and their toxins and cause opsonisation. This, in turn, activates the complement system via the classical pathway. Intracellular bacteria are 'protected' from antibody-mediated mechanisms and, therefore, T cell-mediated response is important for those organisms, including mycobacteria, salmonella, etc.

Viral infection

The innate response to viruses can also include neutralisation by the complement system (e.g. Epstein–Barr virus can activate the classical pathway leading to viral lysis) but specific engulfment and killing is via macrophages rather than polymorphonuclear phagocytes (Fig. 14). Interferons provide both resistance to viral infection and inhibition of viral replication.

While the antibody system is important in neutralising viruses in their *extracellular* or *viraemic* phases, the major adaptive response is T cell mediated. Viral proteins are specifically expressed at the cell surface in the context of HLA class I molecules and these are recognised by the TCR on cytotoxic T cells, resulting in cellular death. In addition, the Th1 and Th2 subsets release a range of cytokines that have specific antiviral actions and also potentiate other aspects of the immune response.

Fungal infection

Fungi may cause superficial or deep infections, the latter usually only in the immunocompromised. Fungi such as *Candida albicans* are ubiquitous and the factors that usually allow infection by this fungus are disturbances in the normal microflora, pH, temperature and mucosal turnover at mucosal sites (vaginal/oral). The use of systemic antibiotics or corticosteroids often predisposes to such infection. Experience from immunodeficiency states, both primary and secondary, indicates that T cell immunity is dominant in protection from fungal infection.

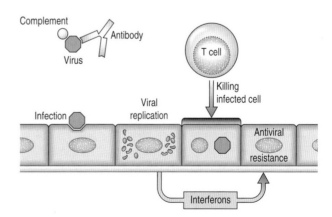

Fig. 14 Response to viral infections can be either via the innate system, with neutralisation by the complement system (e.g. Epstein–Barr virus can activate the classical pathway leading to viral lysis) or via specific engulfment and killing by macrophages. Interferons provide both resistance to viral infection and inhibit viral replication.

15

Parasitic infection

Protozoa

Protozoal infections, including malaria, leishmaniasis, trypanosomiasis and toxoplasmosis, are caused by microorganisms with complex life cycles and many individual strategies to avoid or evade the immune response. In general terms, activation of macrophages is an important early component of the response and the resulting release of cytokines including IL-1 and IL-6 accounts for symptoms of fever and the acute phase response. Antibody responses are present; however, as many of these organisms are intracellular for at least part of their life cycle, antibody may be relatively ineffective against infection. T cell responses are thought to be important in at least some of these conditions, including leishmaniasis, in which limited cutaneous forms are identified in contrast to the systemic or visceral disease. There are many immunological similarities to the response to *Mycobacterium leprae* (Ch. 2).

Helminths

The immunological response to helminth infection includes increased IgE production, eosinophilia and mastocytosis. These responses are mediated by the Th2 subset. It is known that parasite-specific IgE can bind to the helminth and lead to local activation of mast cells, with release of damaging mediators locally causing inflammation. Smooth muscle contraction induced by mast cell mediators may assist expulsion of helminths from the body. Eosinophils also act locally by releasing major basic protein and eosinophil cationic protein, which damages the helminth cell wall.

Self-assessment: questions

Multiple choice questions

1. Regarding antibody molecules:
   a. There are three isotypes of human immunoglobulin
   b. Serum IgG comprises two subclasses, IgG_1 and IgG_2
   c. The body produces more IgA per day than any other isotype
   d. IgG is the most concentrated isotype in serum
   e. IgG exists in serum as a pentameric structure

2. Lymphocytes:
   a. Recognise foreign antigen
   b. Have phagocytic functions
   c. Are not found in the skin
   d. Are not found in healthy gut mucosa
   e. Have characteristically small nuclei

3. Antigen-presenting cells:
   a. All express MHC class II molecules on their surface
   b. Have phagocytic functions
   c. Are present in the skin
   d. Secrete interleukin-2
   e. Stimulate T cells

4. T cells:
   a. Have an important role in immunoglobulin synthesis
   b. Possess surface immunoglobulin molecules
   c. Recognise whole/native antigen
   d. Recognise small fragments of antigen
   e. Secrete interleukin-2 when activated

5. The functions of the complement system include:
   a. Antibody production
   b. Opsonisation of bacteria
   c. Mast cell degranulation
   d. Solubilisation of immune complexes
   e. Lysis of cells

6. The classical pathway of complement activation:
   a. Is stimulated by bacterial cell walls
   b. Consists of components C5-9
   c. Results in the formation of immune complexes
   d. Assists in the disposal of immune complexes
   e. May result in anaphylactoid reactions

7. Which of the following statements about cytokines are correct?
   a. They are high-molecular-weight proteins
   b. They typically act on cells in the immediate vicinity of the producing cell
   c. They do not stimulate the producing cell
   d. They have specific, non-overlapping functions
   e. They directly stimulate specific nuclear receptors

8. $CD4^+$ T cells are:
   a. cytotoxic to virally infected cells
   b. only stimulated by cells expressing MHC class I molecules
   c. the most common T cells in peripheral blood
   d. antigen-presenting cells
   e. only present in secondary lymphoid organs

9. The T cell receptor:
   a. Is an immunoglobulin molecule
   b. Is linked to the CD3 molecule
   c. Binds specifically to intracellular adhesion molecule 1
   d. Binds antigen in soluble form
   e. Initiates intracellular signalling

10. The secondary immune response:
    a. Occurs primarily in the bone marrow
    b. Usually occurs 3 days after first antigen exposure
    c. Is dominated by production of IgG
    d. Involves antibody production from pre-B cells
    e. Is dominated by production of IgM

Short note questions

Write short notes on:
1. Compare and contrast the innate and the adaptive immune systems.
2. The immunoglobulin molecule, its structure and function.
3. T cell subsets and their function.
4. The pathways of antigen presentation for endogenous and exogenous antigens.

Self-assessment: answers

Multiple choice answers

1. a. **False.** There are five isotypes of human immunoglobulin (IgM, IgA, IgG, IgD and IgE). IgD is not routinely detected in serum but functions as a cells surface receptor on early B cells.
   b. **False.** IgG has four subclasses.
   c. **True.** The body produces more IgA per day than of any other isotype. There is approximately 3 g per day produced in the gastrointestinal tract.
   d. **True.** IgG is the most concentrated isotype in serum.
   e. **False.** IgM not IgG exists as a pentamer in serum.

2. a. **True.** Lymphocytes recognise antigen through specialised cell-surface receptors: T cell receptor on T cells, surface immunoglobulin on B cells.
   b. **False.** They are not phagocytic but become activated upon binding specific antigen.
   c. **False.** Lymphocytes are found throughout the body.
   d. **False.** Lymphocytes have very important functions at mucosal sites where there is a high antigenic load to be encountered (the mucosal immune system).
   e. **False.** Microscopically, the nuclei of lymphocytes are relatively large.

3. a. **True.** MHC class II molecules are essential for the presentation of antigenic peptides to T cells and are therefore expressed on all 'professional' antigen-presenting cells.
   b. **True.** 'Professional' antigen-presenting cells, e.g. macrophages, are phagocytic and break down antigen into small peptide fragments before presenting these to T cells.
   c. **True.** Specialised antigen-presenting cells exist throughout the body. In the skin they are known as Langerhans' cells.
   d. **True.** Secretion of interleukin-1 occurs during antigen presentation.
   e. **True.** Antigen presentation causes activation of T cells.

4. a. **True.** T cells provide essential 'help' to B cells to induce and maintain immunoglobulin synthesis.
   b. **False.** T cells do not express surface immunoglobulin molecules.
   c. **False.** T cells do not recognise whole/native antigen.
   d. **True.** T cells recognise small fragments of antigen via the T cell receptor.
   e. **True.** T cells secrete interleukin-2 when activated.

5. a. **True.** Complement does influence antibody production as hypocomplementaemic animals and some complement-deficient patients have been shown to have impaired antibody responses.
   b. **True.** Opsonisation of bacteria is a major function of complement proteins.
   c. **True.** Mast cell degranulation is mediated by anaphylotoxins produced by the cleavage of complement proteins.
   d. **True.** Solubilisation of immune complexes is an important function of early classical pathway components.
   e. **True.** Mediated by the terminal component, the membrane attack complex.

6. a. **False.** It is stimulated by immune complexes.
   b. **False.** It comprises components C1, C4, C2.
   c. **False.** It is involved in the removal of immune complexes. Immune complexes are formed by antibody molecules binding to antigen.
   d. **True.** It solubilises immune complexes and facilitates their disposal.
   e. **True.** Complement activation may cause anaphylactoid reactions by direct activation of mast cells via anaphylotoxins.

7. a. **False.** They are low-molecular-weight proteins.
   b. **True.** Most actions are in the local microenvironment.
   c. **False.** They can stimulate the producing cell (autocrine activity).
   d. **False.** The functions of many cytokines overlap with others.
   e. **False.** They act through cell-surface receptors.

8. a. **False.** They are not cytotoxic.
   b. **False.** They are stimulated by cells expressing MHC class II.
   c. **True.** CD4$^+$ T cells usually account for approximately 60% of circulating T cells in peripheral blood.

d. **False.** They are not antigen-presenting cells.

e. **False.** CD4+ cells are widely distributed in the body.

9. a. **False.** Although it is an immunoglobulin-like molecule.

   b. **True.** It is linked to the CD3 molecule and this is functionally important.

   c. **False.** It does not bind specifically to intracellular adhesion molecule 1.

   d. **False.** The T cell receptor expresses antigenic fragments, not whole/native antigen.

   e. **True.** Binding of the T cell receptor is the first step in antigen-specific signalling.

10. a. **False.** The secondary immune response is not primarily a function of the bone marrow.

    b. **False.** The secondary response does not occur after first antigen exposure.

    c. **True.** It is dominated by production of IgG.

    d. **False.** Antibody production is from mature B cells and plasma cells.

    e. **False.** It is not dominated by production of IgM.

Short note answers

1. Dividing the components of the immune system into innate and adaptive elements assists us in understanding their function. It also reflects the development of the immune system in higher animals. Initially describe the characteristics that define and differentiate the innate from the adaptive systems. It is crucial to discuss the characteristics of specificity and memory in the responses. List the major components of both systems and highlight those components that may in different circumstances function in both an innate and adaptive way (e.g. macrophages). Describe how the two systems interact in preventing infection by a range of microorganisms.

2. It would be essential to draw a schematic diagram of an antibody molecule to answer this question. The four-chain structure of an IgG molecule should be drawn, indicating the heavy and light chains and those regions where the amino acid sequence is constant and those where it is variable. The functions associated with particular regions should also be highlighted (antigen binding, complement activation, Fc receptor binding). The different structures and functions of IgA, IgM, IgD and IgE should also be indicated.

3. T cells should be defined in terms of their origin from bone marrow stem cells and maturation through the thymus. They should be described in terms of their surface expression of the T cell receptor and the pan T cell marker CD3. There should be further classification of the T helper (Th) and T cytotoxic subsets and their respective expression of CD4 and CD8 antigens. It would be important to discuss the differing functions of the CD4+ and CD8+ subsets in terms of their interaction with B cells and direct cytotoxic action on host cells bearing foreign antigens. In this context, you should also discuss the subdivision of CD4+ cells into Th1 and Th2 subsets defined by their predominant pattern of cytokine secretion.

4. It would be important to define endogenous (from within) and exogenous (from without) antigens and to give examples, such as self-antigen, viral protein or malignant antigens as endogenous, and fragments from the breakdown of microorganisms as exogenous. There should be a description of the two major antigen processing and presentation pathways, ideally with a schematic diagram. This should indicate that endogenous antigens are chiefly presented in the context of HLA class I molecules while exogenous antigens are presented by HLA class II antigens. It would be relevant to highlight that these molecules present to the CD8+ and CD4+ subpopulations of T cells and indeed that the CD8 and CD4 molecules directly bind to the HLA class I and class II molecules during antigen presentation. This is directly relevent to the differing function of the major T cell subsets and this aspect should also be discussed.

2 Inflammation and hypersensitivity

Chapter overview

Inflammation is a protective response that involves the interaction of a number of cellular and molecular components. These interacting elements must be coordinated and controlled in order to deliver an appropriate response to injury or infection. Acute inflammation is characterised by four cardinal physical signs: **rubor** (redness), **calor** (heat), **tumour** (swelling) and **dolor** (pain). It occurs rapidly after injury and is caused chiefly by components of the innate immune system. The purpose of acute inflammation is the localisation and eradication of any infective agent or the healing of injury; inflammatory responses, however, can also harm normal tissue and, therefore, these responses must be controlled in both their intensity and extent to prevent inappropriate inflammation and potential inflammatory disease.

Furthermore, some microorganisms have developed very effective strategies to evade the inflammatory response. Infection with these agents can lead to chronic inflammation because there is continued immunological activation, but a failure to eradicate the microorganism.

In addition to a simple division of inflammation into acute and chronic forms, there are four types of immunological hypersensitivity (types I–IV) described in which specific immunological mechanisms result in harmful effects and often clinical disease. This chapter will describe and explain both acute and chronic inflammation, the classification of hypersensitivity and how these mechanisms relate to human disease.

2.1 Acute and chronic inflammation

Learning objectives

You should:
- understand how the innate immune response causes the four cardinal signs of inflammation
- understand how the cellular and soluble elements interact to generate acute inflammation
- know why inflammatory responses are targeted and limited
- understand how chronic inflammation can occur.

Inflammation describes the body's response to infection or damage and it involves a much greater range of cell types and mediators than the narrow range described in the generation of an adaptive immune response. Inflammation should either be self-limiting or responsive to appropriate therapy; however, if therapy fails, a chronic inflammatory process may ensue, leading to inflammatory disease. It is recognised that the immune system can cause tissue damage in a number of stereotypical ways and these have been classified into four types of hypersensitivity. Each type of hypersensitivity involves different cells, molecules and target antigens and results in different clinical manifestations. In some clinical conditions, more than one mechanism may occur in the same disease process.

Acute inflammation

The previous chapter described the individual elements of the immune system that are involved in an effective immune response, chiefly antigen-presenting cells and lymphocytes. However, in addition to those responses, the invasion of the body by microorganisms is associated with other effects including local inflammation and a systemic **acute phase response**. The classical definition of acute inflammation is the occurrence of *local redness, heat, swelling* and *pain*; this is seen when an immunogen is injected into the skin. Underlying this microscopically is an invasion of the tissues by polymorphonuclear neutrophils, macrophages and later lymphocytes and an increase in vascular permeability,

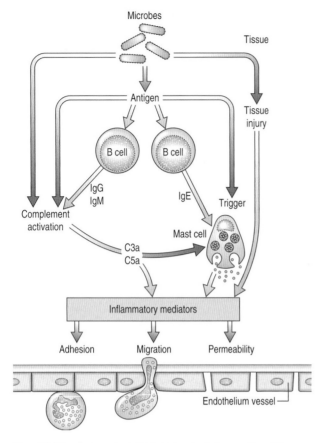

Fig. 15 The immune system in acute inflammation. The interactions of a range of innate and adaptive components contribute to acute inflammatory processes.

causing fluid exudation (Fig. 15). There may also be local tissue effects including increased glandular mucus production and tissue remodelling mediated by fibroblasts and endothelial cells, ultimately causing scar formation. A systemic element with increased synthesis of **acute phase proteins** is also common. The mechanisms underlying the local acute inflammatory changes can be classified as

* release of preformed mediators from tissues and immune cells
* activation of soluble reaction cascades
* synthesis of new inflammatory mediators.

Release of preformed mediators

Release of preformed mediators is one of the first tissue responses to injury. The immediate aggregation of platelets that accompanies blood vessel damage is associated with release of **serotonin** (5-hydroxytryptamine), which promotes vasoconstriction, further platelet aggregation and the formation of a platelet plug.

Other preformed mediators released include histamine, heparin, lysosomal enzymes and proteases, neu-

trophil chemotactic factor and eosinophil chemotactic factor. These factors subsequently induce vasodilatation, increasing blood flow to the site of injury, and recruit specific inflammatory cells to the area. This release of mediators, their effect on surrounding blood vessels and smooth muscle and the attraction of certain types of white blood cell to the area are crucial to the early inflammatory response.

Activation of soluble reaction cascades

Vascular endothelial cell damage activates plasma clotting factor XII (Hageman factor), which, in turn, activates the fibrin, fibrinolytic and kinin cascades (Figs 16 and 17):

* the fibrin cascade results in the conversion of prothrombin to thrombin (resulting in platelet aggregation) and subsequently fibrinogen to fibrin (resulting in clot formation)
* the counterbalancing fibrinolytic cascade causes the conversion of plasminogen to plasmin, which breaks down clots and releases other inflammatory mediators
* the kinin cascade converts prekallikrein to kallikrein, which, in turn, converts kininogen to bradykinin (resulting in vasodilatation, increased vascular permeability and pain induction).

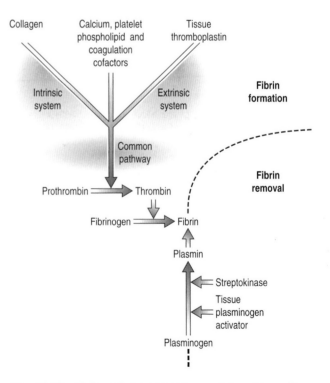

Fig. 16 The fibrin and plasmin pathways interact to maintain a balance in clot formation and breakdown.

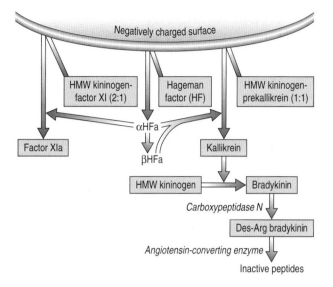

Fig. 17 The kinin pathway generates important mediators (e.g. bradykinin) that contribute to vasodilatation. HMW, high molecular weight.

The effects of these three cascades are essential for controlled acute inflammation: clot formation limits blood loss and acts as a barrier to infection. Fibrinolysis limits the degree of clot formation, preventing inappropriate thrombus formation and vascular obstruction, and it allows the release of inflammatory mediators from cells trapped in the clot. Bradykinin causes increased blood flow, with increased delivery of inflammatory cells and exudation of mediators into the area of damaged tissue. Note that angiotensin-converting enzyme is an important factor in the degradation of bradykinin. The drugs that inhibit this enzyme (known as ACE inhibitors or ACEI) are used in the treatment of hypertension but can be associated with the side effect of angioedema, which is probably caused by excessive accumulation of bradykinin.

The complement cascade

The complement pathways are described in Chapter 1, and activation of complement is crucial to the acute inflammatory process. Release of complement cleavage products is particularly important in coordinating inflammatory activity and the final formation of the membrane attack complex provides a mechanism for killing targeted cells.

Activation of both the alternative (e.g. by binding to foreign antigen) and classical (e.g. by binding to immune complexes) pathways results in the cleavage of C3 to C3b and C3a. Deposition of C3b onto bacterial cell walls (opsonisation) allows phagocytes to bind

to the bacterium, via specific C3b receptors, and commence the process of phagocytosis.

C3a along with C5a are termed **anaphylotoxins** and they stimulate platelet aggregation, degranulation of mast cells, basophils and eosinophils. Additionally, C5a is a chemoattractant that recruits inflammatory cells (neutrophils and macrophages) into the affected area, activates neutrophils and increases vascular permeability to allow their entry into the tissues.

Ultimately, the assembly of the terminal complement pathway components C5-C9 into the membrane attack complex causes pore formation in the cell wall and lysis of the target cell.

Release of newly formed mediators

Damage to phospholipid cell walls causes release of arachidonic acid, which is subsequently metabolised via the lipooxygenase and cyclooxygenase pathways (Fig. 18). This tends to occur somewhat later (4–6 hours after injury) in the reaction.

The lipooxygenase pathway generates *leukotrienes* (LTB4, LTC4 and LTD4), chemotactic and activating factors (the previously described 'slow reactive substance of anaphylaxis (SRS-A)' is a mixture of leukotrienes LTC4 and LTD4). The cyclooxygenase pathways generates **prostaglandins** including **prostacyclin** (prostaglandin I_2), and **thromboxanes**. The physiological effects of early and late phase mediators are summarised in Table 4.

Acute phase response

Acute inflammation is associated with the production of proinflammatory cytokines including IL-1, IL-6 and

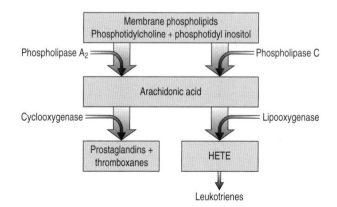

Fig. 18 Arachidonic acid metabolism is mediated by two distinct pathways, catalysed by lipooxygenase and cyclooxygenase, which generate distinct sets of late mediators of inflammation. HETE, hydroxyeicosatetraenoic acid.

Table 4 The physiological effects of early- and late-phase mediators in type I hypersensitivity reactions

Mediators	Effect
Preformed (early)	
Histamine	Vasodilatation increased, vascular permeability, bronchoconstriction
Heparin	Anticoagulation
Lysosomal enzymes	Proteolysis
Neutrophil chemotactic factor	Chemotaxis of neutrophils
Eosinophil chemotactic factor	Chemotaxis of eosinophils
Newly synthesised (late)	
Leukotrienes LTC4, LTD4	Vasodilatation
Leukotriene LTB4	Bronchoconstriction, chemotaxis
Prostaglandins, thromboxanes	Vasodilatation, platelet activation, bronchoconstriction
Platelet-activating factor	Platelet activation

IL-8. These cytokines stimulate the liver to produce a series of proteins that are collectively known as the acute phase proteins, including α_1-antitrypsin, complement components (C3 and C4), C-reactive protein (CRP), fibrinogen and haptoglobins. These have a range of functions including enzyme inhibition (α_1-antitrypsin), opsonisation (CRP binds to the C polysaccharide of *Streptococcus pneumoniae*), scavenging (haptoglobins), etc. In clinical terms, measurement of acute phase proteins is useful to assess the degree of inflammation in an individual and also to assess the response to therapy. Measurements of serum CRP are particularly useful in this respect as it has a short half life (approximately 6 hours) and a response to therapy (e.g. commencement of antibiotics) should be quickly reflected in a falling CRP level.

Chronic inflammation

The purpose of an acute inflammatory response is the eradication of the agent or microorganism that triggered the initial response. In some circumstances that eradication is ineffective or incomplete and a phase of chronic inflammation ensues. The nature of chronic inflammatory damage is dependent on the triggering agent, the affected site and the dominant immune response. There are separate chapters on autoimmune disease, and connective tissue disease and vasculitis, but the following section details the basic immunological classification system of hypersensitivity reactions, in which immune responses may cause tissue damage.

2.2 Hypersensitivity

Learning objectives

You should:
- be aware that different components of the adaptive immune system can cause the four types of hypersensitivity reaction
- understand the classification of hypersensitivity reactions
- know that each type of hypersensitivity can result in clinical disease.

The term **hypersensitivity** describes antigen-specific immune reactions that are either inappropriate or excessive and result in harm to the host. Gell and Coombs classified hypersensitivity reactions into four different types based on their underlying immunological mechanisms and clinical manifestations (Table 5). The term hypersensitivity is often used interchangeably with **allergy** (meaning altered reactivity); however, allergy is best reserved for type I hypersensitivity.

Type I hypersensitivity reactions commonly occur against apparently innocuous environmental antigens (allergens), whereas types II, III and possibly IV reactions may occur against environmental (commonly infectious) agents or self-antigens in the course of autoimmune disease.

Multiple factors determine whether a hypersensitive rather than a normal immunological response occurs, including the genetic make-up of the individual, the physical and chemical properties of the antigen and its

Table 5 Gell and Coombs' classification of hypersensitivity reactions

Type of reaction	Effector mechanism	Clinical disorders
I	IgE mast cells	Allergic rhinitis, urticaria, angioedema
II	IgG directed at cell surface antigens	Transfusion reactions, acute graft rejection, Graves' disease, myasthenia gravis, Goodpasture's syndrome
III	Immune complexes	Cryoglobulinaemia, systemic lupus erythematosus, poststreptococcal glomerulonephritis
IV	CD4 lymphocytes	Delayed type hypersensitivity, contact eczema, granulomatous reactions

mode of delivery into the individual. Hypersensitivity reactions are not mutually exclusive and a particular disease may, therefore, involve more than one hypersensitivity mechanism in its pathogenesis. An understanding of the four types of hypersensitivity, therefore, helps to explain the immunopathogenesis of many conditions and in the following section these will be illustrated with specific clinical examples.

Type I hypersensitivity

Type I hypersensitivity reactions are the immunological basis for clinical allergy. The antigens involved are commonly referred to as **allergens** in the context of type I hypersensitivity. The term **atopic** is used to describe patients who suffer from the clinical triad of: **allergic, rhinitis, eczema** and **asthma**.

Type I reactions typically occur within minutes of exposure to allergen and involve the interaction of **allergen**, **allergen-specific IgE** and tissue **mast cells**. Before a type I response can occur, the immune system must previously have encountered the antigen and stimulated B cells to produce antigen/allergen-specific IgE. IgE is normally present in very low concentrations in the serum but total IgE levels are increased in patients with parasitic infections, in most atopic patients, as well as in many apparently healthy individuals. A high total serum IgE does not, however, cause an allergic response; there must be an elevation of allergen-specific IgE. Mast cells found in the mucosa of the airways and gut as well as in connective tissues bind IgE via specialised surface receptors for the Fc portion of IgE molecules (Fig. 19).

On re-exposure to allergen, the IgE molecules on the surface of the mast cell bind allergen via their available antigen-binding (Fab) portion and become cross-linked. This initiates a series of intracellular signals that results in the release of the mast cell's cytosolic granular contents into the surrounding microenvironment. It is the release of these preformed, and later newly synthesised, mediators, some of which are also involved in acute inflammation, that causes the clinical manifestations of allergic disease (see Ch. 5). It is important to note that mast cells can also be activated via the complement receptors and by some drugs.

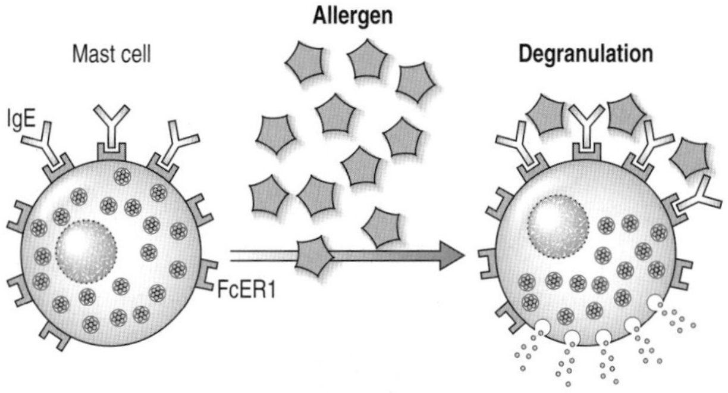

Type II hypersensitivity

Type II hypersensitivity reactions are also mediated by antibody, but in contrast to type I reactions the antibodies involved are either of the IgG or IgM class. A characteristic of type II reactions is that the antibody response is directed against antigens that are expressed on cell surfaces, not against soluble antigens. The pathogenic antibodies in these reactions bind to antigens on cell surfaces via their Fab portion. These bound antibodies, therefore, act as a focus for further cellular and complement-mediated damage to specific cell types or organs (Fig. 20).

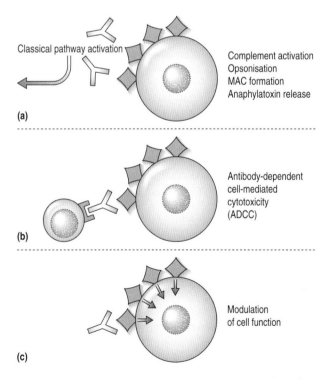

Fig. 20 Type II hypersensitivity involves the interaction of antibody with cell-bound antigen. This may have several consequences including (a) activation of the complement cascade, (b) recruitment of cytotoxic cells or (c) modulation of cellular function.

Fig. 19 Type I (immediate) hypersensitivity involves the interaction of allergen-specific IgE, mast cells bearing receptors for the Fc portion of IgE (FcER1) and allergen. Release of preformed mediators shown here is followed 4–6 hours later by release of newly formed mediators.

Activation of the complement system

Activation of the complement system has been described above, but in the context of type II reactions, the binding of antibody to specific cell-surface antigens focuses the activation of complement on that cell/organ. This results in cell- or organ-specific damage via the effects of C3b deposition, the anaphylatoxins and the membrane attack complex.

Antibody-dependent cell-mediated cytotoxicity

The direct interaction of the Fc portion of the bound antibody with Fc receptor-bearing cells (natural killer cells, platelets, phagocytes) allows these cells to engage the target tissues, focusing their damaging effects onto the antigen-expressing cellular membrane. This is antibody-dependent cell-mediated cytotoxicity.

Antibody-mediated modulation of cellular function

Antibody binding to specific cell-surface receptors can, in some circumstances, lead to a modulation of the cell's function; this is particularly important in some forms of thyroid disease (see below).

Complement activation and antibody-dependent cell-mediated cytotoxicity are part of the immune system's normal response to infection. A normal response causes damage to cells bearing foreign (e.g. microbial or tumour) antigens. Type II reactions are abnormal, however, in two key respects:

- they may be directed against an individual's own cellular antigens
- the response causes damage to the individual's own cells disproportionate to the potential hazard of the antigen concerned.

Clinical examples of type II hypersensitivity

Typical examples of type II hypersensitivity include transfusion reactions, autoimmune haemolytic anaemia, hyperacute graft rejection, Goodpasture's syndrome and Graves' disease. Transfusion reactions and hyperacute graft rejections involve the recognition of truly foreign antigens and ought to be preventable conditions with adequate blood grouping, tissue typing and cross-matching. In autoimmune haemolytic anaemia, the antibody is directed against 'self' blood group antigens, for example the Rhesus system (Ch. 6).

Goodpasture's syndrome is characterised by auto-antibodies to glomerular basement membrane, which also bind to pulmonary basement membrane. The resultant type II hypersensitivity reaction and inflammation at these two sites can cause acute renal failure and severe pulmonary haemorrhage.

Graves' disease is a good illustration of how antibody recognition of a cell-surface antigen may result in modulation of cell function. The autoantibodies in this case are directed against the receptor for thyroid-stimulating hormone. The result is that the antibody mimics the effect of thyroid-stimulating hormone and causes the gland to secrete an excess of thyroxine, resulting in clinical hyperthyroidism. In this condition, treatment is directed towards reducing the thyroid gland response using either antithyroid drugs or surgical resection.

Type III hypersensitivity

Type III reactions are also antibody mediated but, in contrast to type II reactions, the antigenic targets of type III reactions are soluble and not bound to the cell membrane. The combination of soluble antigen and specific antibody, of IgG or IgM class, results in the formation of **immune complexes**. These immune complexes circulate in the bloodstream and, consequently, the damage caused is not limited to one particular cell type or organ but may occur at remote sites throughout the body.

Immune complexes are formed during normal antibody responses as a means of assisting antigen disposal. These immune complexes are quickly cleared by the monocyte/macrophage system, in particular by the phagocytes of the liver, the Kupffer cells. When immune complexes persist, either in the circulation or as deposits within tissues, they activate a number of inflammatory pathways and the response becomes *hypersensitive*.

Antigens that cause immune complex formation may be either *exogenous* (infectious or environmental agents) or *endogenous* (self-antigens in autoimmune responses). Two classic examples of type III reactions demonstrate the effector mechanisms involved.

The **Arthus reaction** occurs in experimental animals that have been repeatedly immunised with antigen, resulting in high levels of antigen-specific IgG. A subsequent intradermal injection of antigen causes the rapid local accumulation of immune complexes and a reaction, which peaks approximately 6–24 hours later. The immune complexes cause local complement activation, with recruitment of polymorphonuclear phagocytes to the perivascular area. The release of lysosomal enzymes from polymorphonuclear phagocytes causes vascular damage, resulting in oedema and haemorrhage. This is seen as a raised reddened area at the injection site. The Arthus reaction is, therefore, a tissue-localised type III hypersensitivity reaction.

Serum sickness is a condition that was seen in the pre-antibiotic era when patients were treated with injections of antibody raised in other animal species, e.g. horses. It was characterised by urticaria, arthralgia (joint pain) and glomerulonephritis (inflammation of the renal glomeruli). Approximately 1 week after injection, antibody forms that reacts with the persisting antigen to form immune complexes in the circulation (Fig. 21). This causes complement activation by the classical pathway and the appearance of the typical clinical features. Immunofluorescent examination of renal biopsies from affected individuals demonstrates deposition of immune complexes and complement components within glomeruli and small blood vessels; the symptoms persist as long as immune complexes are detectable in the circulation. Repeated injections of antigen cause persistence of the immune complexes and the serum sickness syndrome. Serum therapy is rarely, if ever, undertaken now; however, immune complex formation does occur both in acute and chronic infection and in autoimmune and malignant disease. A number of factors, including complex size, duration of antigen exposure, host response and local tissue factors, determine where and when immune complexes persist and cause hypersensitive reactions.

Complex size

Large immune complexes generally activate complement efficiently and become coated with complement fragments (e.g. C3b). This enables blood cells, which bear the complement receptor 1 (C3b receptor, CR1), to bind the immune complexes via C3b and transport them to the liver for degradation by Kupffer cells. Small immune complexes are also cleared by the reticuloendothelial system, although this pathway deals less efficiently with intermediate-sized immune complexes. Consequently, intermediate-sized immune complexes are most likely to persist and cause type III hypersensitivity.

Duration of antigen exposure

Chronic antigen exposure allows continuous immune complex formation, analogous to the serum sickness model where repeated injections of antigen were administered. Clinical examples of conditions in which chronic antigen exposure is believed to be important in generating a type III response include infections (e.g. hepatitis B virus infection, bacterial endocarditis) and autoimmune conditions (e.g. systemic lupus erythematosus).

Host response

Host responses are also considered important in both the production of immune complexes and in the failure to remove them from the circulation. Individuals who preferentially produce low-affinity antibody favour the production of small/intermediate immune complexes, which are difficult to clear. In addition, individuals deficient in the early components of the classical pathway, C2 and C4, have an increased incidence of diseases mediated by immune complexes (Ch. 7). This results from their reduced ability to cleave C3 via the classical pathway and, therefore, their diminished ability to coat circulating immune complexes effectively with C3b to facilitate their disposal.

Local tissue factors

Local tissue factors are also important in determining where immune complexes are deposited and hence at which anatomical sites inflammation is focused. Haemodynamic factors such as *blood pressure, turbulence* and *filtration* affect immune complex deposition. High blood pressure and increased glomerular filtration rate contribute to immune complex accumulation in the renal glomerulus. Turbulence occurs particularly at sites of vessel bifurcation and increases immune complex deposition at these sites. Furthermore, physicochemical properties of the antigen or immune complex, including particle size, electrostatic charge and degree of glycosylation of complexes, will also influence their ultimate tissue destination.

Clinical examples of type III hypersensitivity

Classical examples of human disease involving type III hypersensitivity are immune complex-mediated glomerulonephritis, systemic lupus erythematosus and

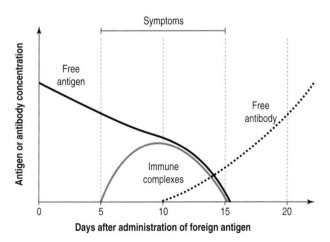

Fig. 21 Experimental serum sickness demonstrates the formation of immune complexes typical of type III reactions.

extrinsic allergic alveolitis. In immune complex-mediated glomerulonephritis, the nature of the glomerular damage is greatly influenced by the type of immune complex involved and its rate of deposition. With rapidly deposited immune complexes, a proliferative response is likely (e.g. poststreptococcal glomerulonephritis), whereas with slower deposition, membranous glomerulonephritis occurs (e.g. in hepatitis B infection or malignant disease).

In extrinsic allergic alveolitis, the patient has preformed IgG antibody to inhaled allergen and develops an Arthus type reaction within the alveoli upon reexposure. The clinical features of acute alveolitis usually occur about 6 hours after exposure, corresponding to immune complex formation and recruitment of the damaging effector mechanisms, including complement and polymorphonuclear phagocytes.

Type IV hypersensitivity

Type IV hypersensitivity reactions differ from types I–III in that the primary immunological effectors in type IV reactions are cells — mainly lymphocytes and monocytes — and not antibody molecules as in types I–III. Type IV responses are also referred to as **delayed-type hypersensitivity** as the reactions occur 12 hours or more following exposure to antigen (Table 6). They are further classified into three subtypes based on the time of peak response, their clinical manifestations, and the cell types and sites of the body involved (Fig. 22). The common feature is the involvement of T lymphocytes (particularly the $CD4^+$ T helper subset), and antigen-presenting cells.

Contact hypersensitivity

Contact hypersensitivity is caused by low-molecular-weight antigens, which alone are incapable of eliciting an immune response. They stimulate the immune system by binding to normal body proteins and in this form are described as **haptens**. The most common example is probably **nickel hypersensitivity** where patients develop an eczematous reaction to nickel contained in costume jewellery, watches, trouser buttons, etc. The rash that appears is typically eczematous but is usually limited to areas of skin that are in direct con-

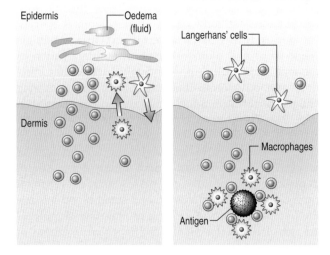

Fig. 22 The anatomical sites of contact (epidermal) and tuberculin-type (dermal) hypersensitivity.

tact with the metal. The immunological mechanism of the reaction is well defined and is divided into **sensitisation** and **elicitation** phases (Figs 23 and 24). Nickel (or another low-molecular-weight hapten) is absorbed

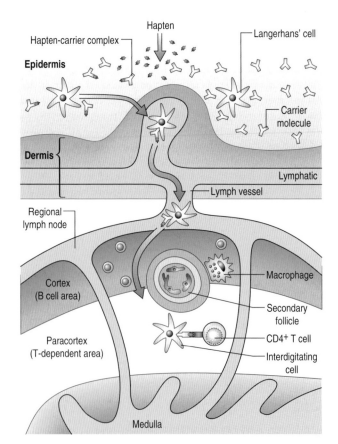

Fig. 23 Sensitisation to low-molecular-weight molecules (haptens), e.g. nickel in contact hypersensitivity.

Table 6 Peak response times for the three forms of type IV hypersensitivity reactions

Type IV reaction	Peak response
Contact	48–72 hours
Tuberculin	48–72 hours
Granulomatous	21–28 days

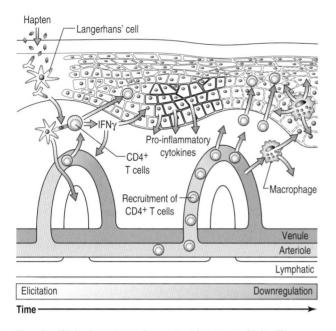

Fig. 24 Elicitation phase in contact hypersensitivity. The Langerhans' cells present the hapten to CD4⁺ T cells, which release interferon-γ (IFNγ). This, in turn, causes the release of pro-inflammatory cytokines, and the recruitment of macrophages.

directly through the skin and is taken up in the epidermis by **Langerhans' cells**, which are antigen-presenting cells, related to dendritic cells. Langerhans' cells migrate from the skin to the paracortical regions of local lymph nodes where the antigen is presented to T cells, stimulating the development of memory T cells. This results in the sensitisation of the individual to the allergen. In the elicitation phase, cutaneously absorbed antigen is presented to the memory T cells in the dermis, causing the secretion of cytokines such as interferon-γ and tumour necrosis factor-α. These soluble mediators induce keratinocytes to express MHC class II molecules and the adhesion molecule ICAM-1, which is also induced on dermal endothelial cells. These two factors contribute to the recruitment of further lymphocytes and macrophages to the inflamed area, and within 24 hours, lymphocytes enter the epidermis. By 48 hours, the epidermis contains lymphocytes and macrophages and is oedematous; this causes the clinical appearance of an eczematous rash. This immunological process is mimicked during the **patch test**, which is commonly used by dermatologists in the investigation of contact hypersensitivity.

Tuberculin hypersensitivity

In contrast to contact hypersensitivity, tuberculin hypersensitivity is a phenomenon that chiefly occurs in the dermis. Koch observed that when patients suffering

from tuberculosis were given an intradermal injection of tuberculin (an antigen derived from *Mycobacterium tuberculosis*) they suffered both a local and a systemic reaction. The local skin reaction is characterised by an area of induration and swelling, and this response is now recognised as being mediated by sensitised lymphocytes.

This type IV reaction is used clinically as a means of determining the sensitisation status of individuals in tests for tuberculosis and leprosy. The **Mantoux test** and **Lepromin test** involve the intradermal injection of *M. tuberculosis* and *M. leprae* extracts, respectively. These are useful models to explain the tuberculin reaction.

Following the intradermal injection of antigen, lymphocytes begin to accumulate around blood vessels at about 12 hours and this accumulation peaks at approximately 48 hours. There is a predominance of CD4⁺ T cells, with a CD4⁺:CD8⁺ cell ratio of approximately 2:1. Macrophages accumulate in the dermis simultaneously with lymphocytes and there is migration of some Langerhans' cells from the epidermis. These cells are focused at the site of foreign antigen in the dermis and cause inflammation; however, the response is usually self-limiting, as antigen is progressively removed by these immune cells. Both contact sensitivity and the tuberculin reaction may be contrasted with a type III Arthus reaction in that they do not involve antibody, complement activation or recruitment of neutrophils and other polymorphonuclear cells.

Granulomatous hypersensitivity

Where antigen persists, however, the initial tuberculin response may develop into a granulomatous hypersensitivity, which is the most severe form of type IV hypersensitivity and clinically the most important. **Granulomas** are collections of macrophages, some of which coalesce to form **giant cells**, surrounded by a cuff of small lymphocytes. The macrophages often have the appearance of epithelial cells, and are known as **epithelioid** cells. Granulomas are formed when the immune system fails to remove foreign antigen, which then persists, usually within macrophages.

Normal antigen presentation is associated with production of the cytokine IL-1 by antigen-presenting cells, causing the activation of T cells, which in turn produce IL-2 and express the IL-2 receptor on their cell membrane. These events contribute to the proliferation of T cells and induction of the cellular response. High levels of IL-1 have been demonstrated in early granulomatous lesions, suggesting that macrophage production of this cytokine is an important early event in recruitment of cells for granuloma formation. The activated T cells are predominantly of the T helper 1 phenotype (Th1; see Ch. 1); that is, they preferentially produce interferon-γ and IL-2. They are, therefore, potent activators of monocytes/macrophages and of other T cells and hence contribute to the accumulation of the cells necessary for granuloma formation. In the later stages of experimental lesions, tumour necrosis factor-α production appears to predominate over IL-1, suggesting that there may be initial cellular recruitment followed by a maintenance phase, which may be partially defined in terms of local cytokine production.

Clinical conditions associated with granuloma formation include **tuberculosis**, **leprosy**, **schistosomiasis**, **leishmaniasis** and **sarcoidosis**. In pulmonary tuberculosis, much of the lung damage is caused by granuloma formation. Reactivation of disease, which is often seen in later life, is associated with an age-related reduction in memory T cell function, allowing renewed mycobacterial growth.

Leprosy is an excellent example of how the immune status of an individual determines the clinical phenotype of disease. There are two major forms of leprosy, **tuberculoid** and **lepromatous**. Tuberculoid disease is largely asymptomatic and is characterised by hypopigmented (pale) areas of the skin, which histologically appear as typical granulomatous lesions with few detectable mycobacteria. These patients have potent type IV hypersensitivity responses to *M. leprae,* the CD4+ T cell population being predominantly of the Th1 phenotype. This results in the more effective clearance of organisms. In lepromatous leprosy, there are widespread skin lesions containing numerous bacilli but few lymphocytes. These patients have a predominant Th2 phenotypic response to the organism (Th2 cells secrete IL-4, IL-5 and IL-10) and no clear granuloma formation. Consequently *M. leprae* is able to proliferate and disseminate more freely in lepromatous leprosy and the patient suffers the systemic effects of the infection. Host hypersensitivity may, therefore, be advantageous under certain circumstances.

Self-assessment: questions

Multiple choice questions

1. Acute phase proteins include:
   a. Interleukin-1
   b. Interleukin-6
   c. C-reactive protein
   d. C3
   e. Fibrinogen

2. Which of the following are cardinal signs of inflammation?
   a. Increased pulse rate
   b. Increased respiratory rate
   c. Localised swelling
   d. Erythema
   e. Rash

3. Which of the following soluble mediators causes swelling?
   a. C1 inhibitor
   b. C3
   c. C2 kinin
   d. C4
   e. C3b

4. Which of the following statements are true regarding hypersensitivity reactions?
   a. Type II hypersensitivity reactions involve antibody, complement and cells
   b. Type III hypersensitivity reactions are a major cause of asthma
   c. Type IV reactions are exemplified in lepromatous leprosy
   d. Type II reactions may have profound metabolic consequences
   e. Type I reactions are associated with increased total serum IgE

5. The atopic syndrome:
   a. Is diagnosed by a high serum IgE level
   b. Is characterised by reactions to many dietary components
   c. Is inherited as an autosomal dominant with incomplete penetrance
   d. May be reliably diagnosed using patch tests
   e. May be associated with immuno-deficiency

6. In tuberculoid leprosy, the most important cells involved in granuloma formation are:
   a. B cells
   b. Mast cells
   c. Neutrophils
   d. Natural killer cells
   e. T cells

7. Which of the following are direct activators of mast cells?
   a. IgG
   b. Morphine
   c. C3a
   d. IgA
   e. IgM

8. Which are the common sites for immune complex deposition?
   a. Renal glomeruli
   b. Abdominal aorta
   c. Synovial joints
   d. Liver
   e. Small intestine

9. Which of the following clinical conditions are associated with significant immune complex formation?
   a. Chronic active hepatitis
   b. Coeliac disease
   c. Systemic lupus erythematosus
   d. Rheumatoid arthritis
   e. Farmer's lung

10. Why are steroids used to treat acute asthmatic attacks?
    a. To suppress IgE production
    b. To prevent histamine release
    c. To suppress arachidonic acid metabolism
    d. To block IgE binding to mast cells
    e. To suppress autoantibody production

Short note questions

Write short notes on:
1. The acute phase response.
2. Mast cells.
3. Type II hypersensitivity.
4. Immune complex formation.

Self-assessment: answers

Multiple choice answers

1. a. **False.** Interleukin-1 is a cytokine.
   b. **False.** Interleukin-6 is a cytokine.
   c. **True.** Measurement of C-reactive protein is of value in identifying the presence and severity of an acute phase response. Because of its short half life (6 hours), it is also valuable for monitoring response to therapy.
   d. **True.** C3 is activated to C3a, which along with C5a, is an anaphylatoxin, stimulating platelet aggregation, degranulation of mast cells, basophils and eosinophils.
   e. **True.** The acute phase proteins include α_1-antitrypsin, complement components (C3 and C4), C-reactive protein, fibrinogen and haptoglobins.

2. a. **False.** Increased pulse rate is not a sign of inflammation but it may occur in fever, which can occur at the same time as inflammation.
   b. **False.**
   c. **True.** Localised swelling, erythema, heat and malaise are the cardinal signs of inflammation (tumour, rubor, calor and dolor).
   d. **True.** See c.
   e. **False.** Rash does occur in contact hypersensitivity.

3. a. **False.** Deficiency of C1 inhibitor is associated with recurrent swelling.
   b. **False.**
   c. **True.** C2 kinin is a complement component derived from C2a that, along with bradykinin, is an important mediator in angioedema.
   d. **False.** C4 is an acute phase protein.
   e. **False.** C3b is a complement fragment that coats large immune complexes enabling them to be removed.

4. a. **True.** Type II hypersensitivity reactions involve antibody, complement and cells.
   b. **False.** Type I reactions are involved in eczema and asthma.
   c. **False.** Type IV reactions are weak in lepromatous leprosy, which is associated with a high mycobacterial load.
   d. **True.** Type II reactions may have profound metabolic consequences when the antigenic target is a hormone receptor, for example antibodies against thyroid-stimulating hormone receptor in Graves' disease.
   e. **True.** Raised total serum IgE is a common finding in the atopic individual; however, it is not a

specific marker of type I hypersensitivity. Raised allergen-specific IgE is a useful diagnostic test.

5. a. **False.** The atopic syndrome is a clinical triad of eczema, rhinitis and asthma; while a high serum IgE may be used as a marker of atopy in research studies, it is not a component of the syndrome.
   b. **False.** True food allergy may occur in atopic individuals as well as non-atopics. Reactions to multiple dietary components would not be typical of food allergy and would require critical evaluation (Ch. 5).
   c. **True.** Atopy is not an inherited disorder.
   d. **False.** Patch tests are appropriate for type IV hypersensitivity reactions.
   e. **True.** There is said to be an increase in atopy in some antibody-deficiency syndromes.

6. a. **False.** These patients have type IV hypersensitivity responses to *M. leprae* involving CD4$^+$ T cells predominantly of the Th1 phenotype.
   b. **False.**
   c. **False.** Neutrophils are involved in inflammation.
   d. **False.** Natural killer cells are involved in antibody-dependent cell-mediated cytotoxicity.
   e. **True.** Granuloma formation is characterised by organised clusters of macrophages and monocytes with surrounding lymphocytes, mainly T cells. Cells may merge, forming giant cells.

7. a. **False.** IgG, IgA and IgM do not directly activate mast cells, with the exception of rare forms of autoimmune urticaria (see Ch. 5).
   b. **True.** Morphine directly stimulates mast cells; hence anaphylactoid reactions can occur on administration of opiates.
   c. **True.** C3a acts via specific receptors on the mast cells surface.
   d. **False.** See a.
   e. **False.** See a.

8. a. **True.** Renal glomeruli are a common site for immune complex deposition.
   b. **False.** However, small blood vessels and sites of vessel branching are other typical sites.
   c. **True.** Synovial joints are also a common site of deposition.
   d. **False.** The Kupffer cells in the liver are crucial in disposal of immune complexes but are not a typical site for damage mediated by immune complexes.
   e. **False.**

9. a. **False.** Chronic active hepatitis is associated with autoantibodies against liver antigens.

b. **False.** Coeliac disease is associated with antibodies against dietary components and endomysial sheath.

c. **True.** Systemic lupus erythematosus is typically associated with immune complex formation, causing a range of symptoms including renal, joint and vascular disease.

d. **True.** Rheumatoid arthritis is also associated with the formation of rheumatoid factors in a significant number of patients. These immune complexes can cause subcutaneous nodules, joint and vascular disease.

e. **True.** Immune complex formation is an essential component of the pathogenesis of farmer's lung. This is a form of extrinsic allergic alveolitis; inhalation of fungal spores (*Micropolyspora faenii*) by patients with pre-formed IgG antibodies results in fever and an inflammatory alveolar reaction some 6–10 hours later.

10. a. **False.** The absolute level of IgE in serum does not relate to clinical severity of allergic disease.

b. **False.** Steroids do not prevent histamine release.

c. **True.** Suppression of arachidonic acid metabolism prevents the generation of late-phase mediators from mast cells and the deterioration in asthma control 4–6 hours after initiation of treatment.

d. **False.** Steroids do not prevent IgE binding to mast cells.

e. **False.** Autoantibody production is not relevant to this condition.

Short note answers

1. You would be expected to define the acute phase response as an increase in serum levels of a series of acute phase proteins (including complement proteins, fibrinogen, haptoglobins, fibrinogen, etc.). You should describe the factors that trigger an acute phase response (infection, trauma) and define the underlying immunological mechanisms of the process, in particular describing the key cytokines that initiate the changes. A description of the function of the different acute phase proteins would be helpful in setting this in the context of acute inflammation. It would also be helpful to describe the potential clinical benefit in measurement of acute phase proteins in clinical practice.

2. An initial description of mast cells with a schematic diagram should indicate the key structural features that underlie the physiological function of mast cells. This should certainly include the abundance of cytoplasmic granules and their key constituents and also the cell-surface receptors for IgE molecules and complement components. A description of the processes that lead to activation of mast cells is essential and should include IgE-mediated and non-IgE-mediated pathways. The difference between early and late phase activation of mast cells should be discussed, comparing and contrasting the mediator release that characterises both phases. The effects of the preformed and newly synthesised mediators on tissues should be described and this should be related to clinical symptoms and signs where possible. Additional description of the two main breakdown pathways for arachidonic acid would be desirable as it would allow discussion of pharmacological aspects of the management of acute allergic reactions including the use of steroids as well as the mechanisms of, for example, salicylate hypersensitivity.

3. Short notes on type II hypersensitivy provide an opportunity to discuss the mechanism underlying a wide range of clinical conditions. It is essential to initially describe and define type II reactions as being mediated by IgG antibodies directed at cell-bound antigen, thus differentiating them from type III reactions, which involve the formation of immune complexes. Discussion should then focus on the different immunological mechanisms that are activated by IgG binding via its Fab portion to cells. This should include activation of the complement system, attraction of inflammatory cells, particularly neutrophils to the area and the development of antibody-mediated cytotoxicity. Having established the inflammatory mechanisms that are activated by a type II response, it then would be desirable to highlight a number of clinical conditions in which these mechanisms are known to be central to disease pathogenesis. A number of examples are discussed in the chapter including blood transfusion reactions, Goodpasture's syndrome and autoimmune thyroid disease.

4. As for the other short notes, an initial definition is important and in this example it should include the specific binding of an antibody molecule to antigen via its Fab portion. Immune complex formation should be described as part of the normal physiological disposal of foreign antigens. It would be helpful to discuss the role of the complement pathways in this process and also the function of the reticuloendothelial system in the process. You

should then discuss abnormal or pathological immune complex formation. This should include the factors that predispose to abnormal immune complex production, e.g. excess or abnormal antigen production, disorders of antibody production and abnormalities of the normal disposal mechanisms of complement and the phagocytic systems. Discussion of experimental models of serum sickness and its typical clinical features would be valuable and this could be related to the clinical features of human diseases known to be associated with immune complex formation.

3 Immunisation

Chapter overview

This chapter deals with the basic immunological and practical aspects of immunisation with particular reference to the current UK immunisation schedule. It also describes the classification of different types of immunisation and gives examples of a number of different types of vaccine in common usage. The recognition of common side effects as well as some current controversies in connection with immunisation is discussed.

3.1 Introduction

Learning objectives

You should:
- be aware of the immunological principles underlying immunisation
- understand the indications for immunisation in adults and children.

The principles of immunisation were established by Edward Jenner, an 18th century English physician who demonstrated that the deliberate infection of a child with cowpox (vaccinia) protected the child from subsequent infection by the lethal disease smallpox (variola). It is from this early work with vaccinia that the terms **vaccine** and **vaccination** were derived and these remain in common usage despite the fact that *immunisation* is the preferred terminology.

Widespread immunisation of children has been responsible for the virtual eradication of certain diseases in the developed world that formerly caused epidemics and pandemics. The incidence of diphtheria, tetanus, pertussis, poliomyelitis, measles, mumps, rubella and *Haemophilus influenzae* B meningitis, which all caused significant mortality and long-term morbidity, have been significantly reduced by mass immunisation in the UK. This progress has been mirrored worldwide with smallpox being officially declared eradicated in 1980. It is expected that both poliomyelitis and measles could be similarly eradicated with continuation of current immunisation programmes. However, at present, measles remains a major cause of death in children under 5 years of age in the third world.

Immunisation is, therefore, the method by which we protect children and adults from subsequent infection with a specific organism by the (usually) parenteral administration of either a related organism or a non-viable component of the organism. Immunisation is successful because it exploits the specificity and memory of the immune system to induce long-lasting immunity. Administration of a first dose usually induces a primary antibody response, while subsequent booster doses induce a secondary response, mimicking the normal protective antibody response to microorganisms (Ch. 1). Vaccines differ in their ability to induce long-term immunity. Some (e.g. for mumps, measles and rubella (MMR)) require two doses whereas others (e.g. tetanus toxoid) require a primary course of three injections with subsequent booster doses to maintain protective immunity.

3.2 Principles of immunisation

Learning objectives

You should:
- understand the difference between active and passive immunisation
- understand the difference between live attenuated and inactivated vaccines.

Type of vaccine

Vaccines take one of several forms (Table 7).

Live vaccines are viable microorganisms (bacteria/viruses) that are administered parenterally/orally and proliferate within the body. This proliferation stimulates a protective immune response but the microorganisms have been altered in such a way as to prevent them causing disease. **Inactivated vaccines** are usually whole organisms that have been treated to prevent their proliferation (killed vaccines). Because they do not proliferate, they induce a less-potent immune response and, therefore, a series of injections is usually required to induce protective immunity. **Subunit vaccines** comprise one element of the microorganism (e.g. capsular polysaccharide) and these also usually require a series of injections. **Detoxified exotoxins** induce immunity against the disease-causing toxin and also require a series of doses to induce immunity. Examples of live attenuated vaccines include oral poliomyelitis (OPV/Sabin type), MMR, varicella zoster and bacille Calmette–Guérin (BCG) vaccines. Oral polio vaccine has been replaced in the UK by a new inactivated vaccine (IPV), which is a component of several combination vaccines. BCG is derived from *Mycobacterium bovis* but induces immunity to a range of mycobacterial species including *Mycobacterium tuberculosis*. Inactivated vaccines that contain whole organisms include pertussis, typhoid, inactivated poliomyelitis (IPV/Salk type); influenza and pneumococcal vaccines contain only immunising components/subunits of the organism. Vaccines such as tetanus and diphtheria contain toxoid (i.e. toxin inactivated by formaldehyde). **Conjugated vaccines** are those in which a component of the infectious agent, usually a polysaccharide, is linked to a protein to enhance the immune response. This is particularly important in children under 2 years of age, who respond poorly to polysaccharide antigens. Examples of conjugated vaccines include *H. influenzae* B (Hib), meningitis C and the recently introduced poly-valent (seven valent) conjugated pneumococcal vaccine (Prevenar).

Live vaccines are contraindicated in patients with significant immunodeficiency as even these attenuated forms may induce disease in patients with impaired immunity.

Recently, a range of combination vaccines have been introduced in the UK to reduce the number of injections required to complete the primary immunisation schedule and to increase immunisation uptake. These combination vaccines include:

- diphtheria, tetanus, acellular pertussis, inactivated polio and Hib (DTaP/IPV/Hib)
- diphtheria, tetanus, acellular pertussis, inactivated polio (DTaP/IPV)
- diphtheria, tetanus, inactivated polio (Td/IPV).

The current UK schedule for childhood vaccination is indicated in Table 8.

Active immunisation

Active immunisation involves the administration of an antigen (either live attenuated or inactivated organisms or their products) that induces an immune response in the recipient resulting in protective immunity. This is the principle that underlies the majority of routinely administered immunisation.

The programme of active immunisation of children aims to produce benefits for both the individual and the wider community by production of

- protective antibody
- antigen-specific T cells
- immunological memory, to sustain levels of the above
- herd immunity.

Herd immunity refers to the concept that the natural spread of disease is prevented if a sufficiently high

Table 7 Immunisation against infectious disease

Vaccine	Type of vaccine	Dose regimen
Tuberculosis (BCG)	Live attenuated	Single dose
DTaP/IPV/Hib	Combination inactivated	Three doses
DTaP/IPV	Combination inactivated	Booster doses
Hepatitis B	Monoclonal hepatitis B surface antigen (subunit)	Three doses
Influenza	Inactivated viral particles	Single dose
MMR	Live attenuated	Single dose
MenC	Conjugated subunit (capsular polysaccharide)	Single dose
Pneumovax II	Unconjugated subunit (23-valent capsular polysaccharide)	Single dose
Polio (Prevenar)	Conjugated subunit (7-valent polysaccharide)	One–three doses

BCG, bacille Calmette–Guérin; D, diphtheria; T, tetanus; aP, acellular pertussis; IPV, inactivated polio; Hib, Haemophilus influenzae type B; MMR, measles, mumps, rubella; MenC, meningococci group C.

Table 8 UK schedule of immunisation

Vaccine	Age	Notes
Diphtheria, tetanus, pertussis, polio and *Haemophilus influenzae* type B (DTaP/IPV/Hib)	One dose at three ages: 2, 3 and 4 months	One injection
Meningitis C	One dose at three ages: 2, 3 and 4 months	One injection
Measles, mumps, rubella (MMR)	12–15 months	One injection
Diphtheria, tetanus, pertussis, polio (DTaP/IPV)	3–5 years	One injection
Bacille Calmette–Guérin (BCG)	10–14 years (or infancy in certain areas)	Skin test at 10–14 years then vaccinate if needed
Booster tetanus, polio (T/IPV)	13–18 years	One injection

percentage of the population are immunised and protected from infection. It is expected that 75–90% of the population must be immunised to achieve this for most infectious diseases.

Passive immunisation

Passive immunisation is the process of administering protective antibodies (either hyperimmune serum or pooled immunoglobulin) to an individual in order to help them to eradicate an organism. Passive immunisation provides short-term protection from specific pathogens (e.g. herpes zoster or rabies) but it does not induce long-term immunity (immunological memory) as there is no stimulation of endogenous antibody or T cell production.

In the context of antibody-deficiency syndromes (Chs 4 and 9), regular intravenous immunoglobulin (ivIg) infusions (pooled immunoglobulin) every 3 weeks provide long-term passive immunity and protection from infection by a wide range of organisms.

3.3 Adverse reactions to immunisation

Learning objectives

You should:
- be aware of the potential adverse reactions to immunisation
- understand how to deal with an anaphylactic reaction
- know the contraindications to immunisation in adults and children.

Mass immunisation has produced great benefits for both society and individuals in dramatically reducing the incidence of infectious diseases and preventing their long-term complications. There have, however,

been a number of occasions when adverse publicity regarding a particular vaccine has resulted in understandable public anxiety and a decreased uptake of the vaccine. In the 1970s, this phenomenon was observed in respect of pertussis immunisation. There were reports of neurological damage occurring after pertussis immunisation and there was a fall in uptake of immunisation to approximately 30% of the UK population. This was well below the level required to protect the community and the rate of pertussis infection increased dramatically, with a significant number of childhood deaths and cases of serious neurological damage resulting from the naturally acquired infection. After these reports, the National Childhood Encephalopathy Study was established to ascertain if there was a link between pertussis immunisation and encephalopathy. After 3 years of study, it was concluded that if there was a link, the risk was too small to be demonstrated statistically. This example demonstrated that vaccine-related risk was very much less than the risk of the natural infection.

In the UK in the late 1990s, concern was raised about a possible link between MMR vaccination and autistic spectrum disorder and also with inflammatory bowel disease. The overwhelming body of scientific and medical opinion worldwide is that no such links exist, yet despite this, public concern persists and MMR uptake levels remain below the desired level. There is, therefore, an ongoing task in providing factual, evidence-based advice to parents in respect of the benefits and risks of vaccination to enable them to make informed decisions.

Risks of immunisation

All vaccines are subjected to extensive safety and efficacy testing before they are licensed for use; however, there are rare occasions when adverse reactions may occur following immunisations. These may be considered as immediate or late reactions.

Immediate reactions

Anaphylaxis occurs rarely following immunisation. The clinical features are described in detail in Chapter 5. Based on experience of the introduction of MMR vaccination in the UK in 1994, the frequency of anaphylaxis after immunisation with MMR is estimated at 1:100 000. It is, however, impossible to predict which children may be particularly susceptible to anaphylaxis following vaccination and, therefore, it is an imperative that appropriately trained staff and facilities are available to treat anaphylactic reactions should they occur. Adults or children should also be observed following immunisation to ensure they are clinically well before being discharged home. There is no universally accepted time period for observation; indeed anaphylactic reactions may occur up to 72 hours after immunisation. In general, however, most clinicians would recommend observation for 30–60 minutes after immunisation.

Differential diagnosis of collapse following immunisation

Anaphylactic reactions are the most serious adverse events that can occur and are potentially fatal; however, it is important to differentiate anaphylaxis from the much more common occurrence of fainting attacks (syncope) or other causes including seizures/convulsions.

Syncope occurs commonly after injections in both adults and adolescents, but it is rare in very young children. The management of syncope is for the patient to lie down supine with elevation of the legs to assist maintenance of central blood pressure. The patient usually regains consciousness in 1–2 minutes. If a young child collapses after immunisation and a central (carotid) pulse cannot be felt, the attack should be presumed to be an anaphylactic reaction and emergency treatment

instituted. Table 9 compares and contrasts the major clinical features of anaphylactic reactions and syncope.

Other types of 'reaction'

Children commonly suffer from febrile illnesses and unexplained rashes at the ages when they receive the bulk of their immunisations and, therefore, many such episodes will occur coincidentally associated in time with vaccination. It is common for rashes, fevers or local injection site reactions to be reported after immunisation; most of these are mild and self-limiting. It can, however, be very difficult to be certain if a reaction is causally related to immunisation even when there is a close association in time. There are some typical reactions that do occur: for example, a morbilliform rash 5–10 days after measles immunisation or parotid swelling 3 weeks after mumps immunisation. Fever occurring with 3 days of measles immunisation is unlikely to have been caused by the vaccine and is more likely to result from intercurrent infection.

In general, the risk of serious illness following natural infection far outweighs those of any adverse reaction to immunisation.

Controversies in immunisation

Egg allergy

It was previously considered that egg allergy was a contraindication to vaccination with MMR; however, this is no longer the case. Several large studies have shown that patients with egg allergy, including those with positive skin tests and a history of anaphylactic reactions following ingestion of egg, are at no greater risk of adverse reaction to MMR than children who are not egg allergic. The UK Department of Health advice is, therefore, that egg allergy is not a con-

Table 9 The major clinical features of anaphylactic reactions and syncope

	Anaphylactic reaction	Syncope ('fainting')
Timing	0–72 hours (although the majority will be immediate)	0–1 hour
Symptoms	None/'sense of impending doom', retrosternal tightness	None/anxiety, nausea, blurred vision, dizziness, hyperventilation, paraesthesia, carpopedal spasm
General signs	Pallor, apnoea	Sweating, weakness, hyperventilation
Skin	Pallor, urticaria, angioedema: affecting face, lips, tongue or peripheries	Pallor
Cardiovascular	Hypotension, tachycardia, weak/absent central pulse	Hypotension, bradycardia, preserved central pulse
Respiratory	Difficulty breathing, hoarse voice, stridor, acute bronchospasm, audible wheeze/'silent chest'	Initial hyperventilation
Neurological	Prolonged hypotension may trigger secondary generalised seizure	Transient jerking/eye rolling may be observed

traindication to MMR immunisation. There is some published evidence, chiefly from Japan, that gelatine allergy may cause adverse reactions to MMR (in which gelatine is a stabilising agent). Children with a history suggestive of gelatine allergy should, therefore, be fully assessed by an appropriately trained paediatrician or immunologist/allergist prior to MMR immunisation. As mentioned below, egg allergy is a contraindication to immunisation with influenza or yellow fever vaccine.

Oral polio vaccine and the immunocompromised patient

Oral polio vaccine (Sabin) has been replaced in the UK schedule of immunisation by inactivated polio vaccine. It is still worth mentioning a specific issue related to oral polio vaccine (OPV) for areas where it may still be in use: it should not be given to immuno-compromised children/adults or members of their household. This is because the live attenuated virus is excreted in faeces and could, therefore, infect close contacts with immune deficiency. Inactivated polio vaccine (Salk type) should be administered in such cases.

MMR and the immunocompromised

Close contacts of immunocompromised patients (but not the patients themselves) should be given MMR. In this situation, the live attenuated virus is not excreted and, therefore, it poses no threat to the immunocom-promised individual.

Convulsions

Where there is a close family or personal history of febrile convulsions, advice on pyrexia prevention should be given prior to immunisation.

Inflammatory bowel disease and autism

A personal or family history of inflammatory bowel disease or of autistic spectrum disorder does not con-traindicate any immunisation. There is no evidence of a link between measles vaccination and the later development of inflammatory bowel disease. Similarly, there is no convincing link between MMR vaccination and the development of autism.

Contraindications to immunisation

There are occasions when an individual should either not receive certain specified immunisations or have such immunisations postponed.

Acute illness (upper respiratory tract infection, diarrhoea, otitis media). Only unwell individuals with a fever of > 38°C should have their immunisations post-poned. They should be rebooked for 1 week later.

Previous adverse reaction. If a previous immunisation has resulted in a severe local (extensive area of red-ness or induration at the site of injection) or gen-eral reaction (anaphylactic reaction, bronchospasm, laryngeal oedema, fever > 39.5°C within 72 hours, prolonged unresponsiveness, inconsolable scream-ing for > 4 hours, convulsions or encephalopathy within 72 hours), then specialist advice should be sought.

Pregnant women. Live vaccines should not be given to pregnant women because of the risk of harm to the fetus. There may be specific circumstances (e.g. for-eign travel) where specialist advice is necessary.

Anaphylactic reaction to egg. A definite history of ana-phylactic reaction to egg is a contraindication to influenza and yellow fever vaccines. However, egg allergy is not a contraindication to MMR immuni-sation.

Live vaccines and immunodeficiency. Immunodeficient patients may develop vaccine-related disease after administration of live vaccines. These are, therefore, contraindicated for patients who:

- are within 6 months of having received chemotherapy/radiotherapy for malignant dis-ease
- have received an organ transplant and are tak-ing immunosuppressive treatment
- have received a bone marrow transplant within the previous 6 months
- have received prednisolone (at daily doses of 2 mg/kg for at least 1 week or 1 mg/kg for at least 1 month) within the previous 3 months (children)
- have received a daily dose of 40 mg for more than 1 week (adults)
- may have received lower doses of corticosteroids but had this combined with other immunosup-pressive agents.
- have primary or secondary immunodeficiency affecting the cell-mediated system.

Misconceptions regarding immunisation

There are a number of circumstances or conditions that are often misconstrued as a contraindication to immu-nisation, some of the more common of these are a his-tory of

- atopy: asthma, eczema and rhinitis
- stable neurological conditions, e.g. Down's syndrome, cerebral palsy

- prematurity
- current antibiotic or topical steroid therapy
- 'replacement' steroid therapy
- previous pertussis, measles, rubella or mumps infection
- neonatal jaundice
- recent surgery
- underweight or past the age recommended by the schedule
- child being breast-fed or mother being pregnant.

These are not contraindications to routine immunisation.

3.4 Adult immunisation

Learning objectives

You should:
- understand the indications for immunisation in adults
- be aware of the particular problems of asplenic patients
- be aware of current advice in your locality.

Indications for adult immunisation

Indications for adult immunisation are under regular review and this section refers to the current advice in the UK. Adults who have not previously been immunised should be given a full course of a combined preparation containing inactivated polio vaccine. The latter should usually be repeated at 10-year intervals to maintain protective immunity. Oral polio vaccine is now only available for use during outbreaks. Some adults are regarded as at 'high risk' of certain infections and additional immunisation is, therefore, recommended for them. Guidance in the UK in 2004 for administration of influenza and pneumococcal vaccines is indicated in Box 1.

Foreign travel

Advice regarding necessary immunisation for foreign travel depends on the country to be visited and the vaccination history of the individual concerned. Such advice is regularly updated and is beyond the scope of this chapter. Table 10 gives some general indications. Advice should be sought from the appropriate local authorities.

Asplenic patients

The spleen is an important site of antibody production and, therefore, removal of the spleen is an important cause of secondary immunodeficiency (Ch. 4). The most common reason for an absent spleen is surgical removal following abdominal trauma or as part of the treatment for lymphoproliferative disease or autoimmune thrombocytopenia. Occasionally, individuals have a congenitally absent spleen and patients with sickle cell or coeliac disease may also have a degree of splenic hypofunction. Irrespective of the cause, patients without a spleen or with impaired splenic function are at increased risk of infection by encapsulated bacteria, such as *Streptococcus pneumoniae* and *H. influenzae,* and a number of protozoal infections, including babesiosis and falciparum malaria. This is because the spleen is important in the generation of antibody responses to polysaccharides and these responses are crucial to the protection of the individual from these organisms. If splenectomy is planned, it is, therefore, important to ensure prior immunisation with pneumococcal

Table 10 Immunisation for international travel

Infection	High-risk areas	Route of transmission	Immunisation comment
Cholera	Africa, Asia, Middle East	Contaminated water/food	Immunisation is ineffective
Hepatitis A	Outside northern Europe, North America, Japan, Australasia	Contaminated water/food	Inactivated vaccine, single dose effective
Hepatitis B	Outside northern Europe, North America, Japan, Australasia	Sexual contact, needlestick injuries	Especially important for healthcare workers; recombinant subunit vaccine: 3 doses over 6 months required
Meningococcal infection	Africa, Saudi Arabia	Direct contact; high risk at Hajj and Umrah pilgrimages (Saudi Arabia)	Tetravalent vaccine protects against serotypes A, C, W135 and Y (this is additional to the meningitis C vaccine)
Typhoid	Outside northern Europe, North America, Japan, Australasia	Contaminated water/food	Typhoid vaccine should be given, but is not a substitute for careful food and water hygiene

Box 1 Indications for influenza and pneumococcal vaccine in adults

Influenza vaccine
Indications are:
- chronic respiratory disease (includes asthma)
- chronic heart disease
- chronic renal failure
- diabetes mellitus
- immunodeficiency from either disease or treatment
- asplenia or splenic dysfunction.

Pneumococcal vaccine
Pneumococcal vaccination is indicated in the above conditions and in addition:
- homozygous sickle cell disease
- coeliac disease
- immunodeficiency caused by disease or treatment, *including* human immunodeficiency virus (HIV)
- chronic liver disease including cirrhosis
- prior to cochlear implant surgery and in unimmunised patients with cochlear implants
- prior to splenectomy or chemotherapy.

Varicella-zoster vaccine
Varicella-zoster vaccine is recommended for seronegative healthcare workers in direct contact with patients.

(Pneumovax II), HiB and meningococcal (Meningivac) vaccines. Specific antibody levels to each should be measured before and 4 weeks after immunisation to ensure a satisfactory response. Long-term follow up is advised, with regular measurement of specific antibody levels. While 'normal' and 'protective' levels of antibodies specific to these organisms are difficult to define with certainty, nominal values are quoted by reference laboratories and if levels fall into the suboptimal range, repeat immunisation should be considered. In clinical practice, splenectomy is often undertaken as an emergency and is, therefore, unplanned. In those circumstances, triple immunisation (as above) should be undertaken as soon as possible afterwards, accepting that the antibody response is likely to be less effective than in a planned, presplenectomy approach.

A major clinical concern in asplenic patients is the occurrence of overwhelming pneumococcal septicaemic illness (OPSI). This condition is characterised by its sudden onset and rapidly fatal outcome if not recognised and treated early. It is estimated that there is a 1–2% risk of death from pneumococcal septicaemic illness in the first 15 years following splenectomy. For this reason, lifelong antibiotic prophylaxis (adult dose: penicillin V 250 mg twice daily) is recommended.

Self-assessment: questions

Multiple choice questions

1. When a baby receives his first dose of diphtheria, tetanus, acellular pertussis, inactivated polio and *Haemophilus influenzae* B (DTaP/IPV/Hib) vaccine, the resulting immune response:
   a. Does not involve the innate immune system
   b. Results from B cells acting independently of other cells to produce antibody
   c. Is dependent on memory cells
   d. Is predominantly generated in the spleen
   e. Is characterised by IgM production after approximately 5 days

2. After a baby has received his second dose of diphtheria, tetanus, acellular pertussis, inactivated polio and *Haemophilus influenzae* B (DTaP/IPV/Hib) vaccine, the resulting immune response:
   a. Does not involve the innate immune system
   b. B cells act independently of other cells to produce antibody
   c. Competition for antigen is an important feature
   d. The time delay until IgM production is approximately 3 days
   e. The IgG response persists for up to 1 month

3. A 17-year-old male with non-Hodgkin's lymphoma requires splenectomy for haemolytic anaemia. Which one of the following immunisations is it most important to undertake before surgery?
   a. Bacille Calmette–Guérin (BCG)
   b. Measles
   c. Pertussis
   d. Pneumovax (pneumococci)
   e. Tetanus toxoid

4. Which of the following vaccines is 'live'?
   a. Tetanus
   b. Pneumovax
   c. Influenza
   d. Measles, mumps, rubella (MMR)
   e. Bacille Calmette–Guérin (BCG)

5. Which of the following immunisations is contraindicated in a child with egg allergy?
   a. *Haemophilus influenzae* type B (HiB)
   b. Influenza
   c. Measles, mumps, rubella (MMR)
   d. Polio
   e. Yellow fever

Case history questions

History 1

> A mother brings her baby daughter to the vaccination clinic for her second set of diphtheria, tetanus, acellular pertussis, inactivated polio and *Haemophilus influenzae* B (DTaP/IPV/Hib) immunisations. Her baby is well but she reports to the nurse that after her first set of immunisations, the baby was up crying for most of the night. What advice would you give?

1. Reassure her and proceed with vaccination.
2. Delay vaccination for a month.
3. Proceed with vaccination and prescribe oral paracetamol for the next 24 hours.
4. Proceed with tetanus and pertussis only.
5. Proceed with diphtheria and tetanus only.

History 2

> A 6-month-old child attends for her primary immunisation course. Her mother has delayed attending because she has atopic eczema and she was worried by media reports of vaccine problems in allergic children. On further enquiry you identify that the child was breast-fed until 3 months of age, when she transferred to formula bottle feeds. She is taking some semisolid foods including pureed food and scrambled egg. Her elder brother has nut allergy. What advice would you give?

1. Proceed with normal immunisation schedule.
2. Delay immunisation until after 1 year of age.
3. Immunise with diphtheria, tetanus, acellular pertussis (DTaP) but omit vaccination for meningitis C.
4. Immunise with diphtheria, tetanus and inactivated polio (TT/IPV) but omit acellular pertussis.
5. Delay immunisation until eczema has resolved.

History 3

A mother reports that her baby boy developed a rash 6 days after measles, mumps, rubella (MMR) vaccination. He had a raised temperature and was very tired. She is worried because she has heard from a friend that this might be a sign of egg allergy and she has read in the paper that MMR can cause autism. What advice would you give?

1. Reassure regarding allergy but agree to refer to a paediatric neurologist for assessment.
2. Agree to send a test for egg allergy and refer to a paediatric neurologist.
3. Reassure regarding autism, but send test for egg allergy.
4. Reassure that this is a normal response to MMR.
5. Ensure that the child does not receive a booster MMR.

History 4

A 32-year-old man attends your practice for advice regarding immunisation. He has recently been diagnosed positive for human immunodeficiency virus (HIV) and is keen to boost his immunity to maximum levels. A recent CD4$^+$ cell count was 0.3×10^9/l (normal range, 0.5–1.5×10^9/l). What advice do you give?

1. Repeat primary immunisation course.
2. No additional vaccines.
3. Pneumovax only.
4. Pneumovax and influenza vaccines.
5. Pneumovax, influenza and measles, mumps, rubella (MMR).

Self-assessment: answers

Multiple choice answers

1. a. **False.** Antigen-presenting cells are involved and these are part of the innate immune system.
   b. **False.** B cells do not act independently; in the majority of responses they require 'help' from appropriately activated CD4$^+$ T cells.
   c. **False.** The first immunisation elicits a primary response and, therefore, memory cells are not involved.
   d. **False.** The main response is in regional lymph nodes.
   e. **True.** The characteristic 'lag period' is 5 days in a primary response and the major initial/isotype produced is IgM.

2. a. **False.** Antigen-presenting cells are part of the innate immune system.
   b. **False.** B cells do not act independently; in the majority of responses they require 'help' from appropriately activated CD4$^+$ T cells.
   c. **True.** Competition for antigen in the lymph nodes means that antibodies of higher affinity have a selective advantage and this is part of the process of affinity maturation.
   d. **True.** The 'lag period' is shorter in a secondary antibody response.
   e. **False.** For most antigens, IgG production should be sustained for much longer than 1 month.

3. a. **False.** Response to this vaccine is not impaired by splenectomy.
   b. **False.** Response to this vaccine is not impaired by splenectomy.
   c. **False.** Response to this vaccine is not impaired by splenectomy.
   d. **True.** Responses to polysaccharide antigens such as pneumococcal capsular polysaccharide are predominantly generated in the spleen. It is important to maximise protection against pneumococci before splenectomy.
   e. **False.** Response to this vaccine is not impaired by splenectomy.

4. a. **False.** Tetanus vaccine is a modified toxin or 'toxoid'.
   b. **False.** Pneumovax comprises capsular polysaccharides.
   c. **False.** Influenza is a subunit vaccine.

   d. **True.** Measles, mumps, rubella (MMR) is a live vaccine.
   e. **True.** Bacille Calmette–Guérin (BCG) is a live attenuated strain of *Mycobacterium bovis*.

5. a. **False.**
   b. **True.** Influenza vaccine may contain traces of egg protein.
   c. **False.** Despite the common misconception, MMR is not contraindicated in patients allergic to egg.
   d. **False.**
   e. **True.** Yellow fever vaccine may contain traces of egg protein.

Case history answers

History 1

1. No; inconsolable crying for more than 4 hours after immunisation is a contraindication to repeat immunisation.
2. No.
3. No.
4. No; pertussis is the vaccine one would wish to avoid in this case.
5. Yes; diphtheria and tetanus immunisation should proceed.

History 2

1. Yes; the history indicates that while the mother is concerned about allergies, there is no contraindication to normal immunisation.
2. Delay in immunisation is not indicated and would incur an increased risk of infection on the child.
3. There is no indication in this case to avoid vaccination for meningitis C.
4. There are no indications to omit pertussis (acellular pertussis vaccine) in this case.
5. Eczema is not a contraindication to immunisation.

History 3

1. This is not an indication for neurological assessment.
2. This is not an indication to test for egg allergy or a referral to a paediatric neurologist.

3. The mother should be reassured regarding autism and, as in 2, this is not an indication to test for egg allergy.
4. This is the correct approach; the woman should be advised to use paracetamol to control the temperature and ensure adequate fluid intake until symptoms resolve (usually in 2–3 days).
5. This is not a significant adverse reaction and so the child can receive the booster.

History 4

1. The primary immunisation course should not be repeated because it includes live vaccines, which are contraindicated in a patient with HIV and significant immunodeficiency (CD4$^+$ cell count $0.1 \times 10^9/l$). These include bacille Calmette–Guérin (BCG) and measles, mumps, rubella (MMR).
2. No, as immunisation is indicated to boost immunity.
3. Pneumovax alone would not be adequate.
4. Pneumovax and influenza vaccines are the correct choice.
5. This combination would not be given. While MMR is thought to be safe and indicated in the early stages of HIV infection, it is contraindicated in those with significant immunodeficiency.

Immunodeficiency

Chapter overview

Defects in immunity may arise at any age. Primary immunodeficiencies may be the result of single gene defects, usually presenting in childhood, or may be of multifactorial aetiology and present at any age. Secondary immunodeficiency may be caused by a wide range of factors including malnutrition, medical disorders, drug therapy or specifically infection with the human immunodeficiency virus. Since the main function of the immune system is to protect against infection, the main consequence of immune deficiencies is an increase in the frequency or severity of infections. The pattern and type of infections usually reflects the nature of the immunological defect. Failure to recognise and diagnose immunodeficiency at an early stage results in increased morbidity and mortality. However, a variety of therapeutic options are available that improve both quality of life and life expectancy for immunodeficient patients.

4.1 Introduction

Learning objectives

You should:
- be able to describe the major classifications of immunodeficiency
- know the most common causes of primary and secondary immunodeficiency
- know the clinical features of primary immuno-deficiency syndromes.

Immunodeficiency is a term generally applied to the state in which the immune system is unable to respond appropriately and effectively to infectious microorganisms. The main consequence of immunodeficiency is infection, although there may also be an increased incidence of autoimmune disease and malignancy in some patients. In contrast to typical infection that occurs in immunocompetent individuals, immunodeficient patients tend to have infections that are *serious, persistent, unusual* or *recurrent* (SPUR, Table 12). They may present with an acute infection or with features of organ damage as a result of repeated infection, for example bronchiectasis. Despite this guidance, it is often difficult to be sure when a patient should be investigated for immunodeficiency, especially in primary care; therefore, the '10 warning signs for primary immunodeficiency' have been developed as a more detailed guideline (Box 2). The type of infectious organisms encountered is related to the immunological components that are defective (Table 11). Antibody-deficiency syndromes tend to present with recurrent bacterial infection of the upper or lower respiratory tract, while T cell deficiency causes specific susceptibility to viral and fungal disease. Recurrent abscess formation may indicate a neutrophil disorder, while recurrent neisserial infection may suggest a complement defect. It is, however, important to realise that combined deficiencies occur, and a patient may present with multiple types of infections.

In addition to infection there may be other features in the immunodeficient patient.

Autoimmune diseases such as thyroid disease or autoimmune cytopenia may occur as a result of impaired immune regulation. The prevalence of malignancies is

Table 11 Typical clinical features of primary immunodeficiency states

Deficient immunological component	Bacteria	Viruses	Fungi	Graft versus host	Abscesses	Neisserial infection
Antibody	Common	Uncommon	Uncommon	No	Yes	May occur
T cells	No	Common	Common	Rarely	No	Rare
Combined B and T cell	Common	Common	Common	Common	Rare	Rare
Neutrophils	Common	Rare	Common	No	Common	Rare
Complement (classical pathway)	Common	Rare	Rare	No	Uncommon	Rare
Complement (terminal and alternate pathways)	Uncommon	No	No	No	No	Common

Box 2 Warning signs of immunodeficiency

The following 10 signs should alert to the possibility of immunodeficiency.
1. Eight or more new ear infections in a year
2. Two or more serious sinus infections in a year
3. Antibiotics for 2 months without effect
4. Two or more pneumonias in a year
5. Recurrent, deep skin or organ abscesses
6. Two or more deep-seated infections such as osteomyelitis, cellulitis or sepsis
7. Surgical intervention for chronic infection, e.g. lobectomy, recurrent incision of boils
8. Persistent thrush in mouth or elsewhere on the skin after age 1 year
9. Failure to thrive
10. Family history of primary immunodeficiency.

Table 12 Infections suggesting underlying immunodeficiency

SPUR	Example	Comment
Serious	Meningococcal septicaemia	Life-threatening infections
Persistent	Oral candidiasis resistant to local therapy	Infections that persist despite appropriate anti-microbial therapy
Unusual	*Pneumocystis carinii* pneumonia; *Mycobacteria avium intracellulare* infection	Infections may be unusual in terms of either site or organism involved
Recurrent	Recurrent upper or lower respiratory infection	Recurrent infection can be difficult to define (see text)

also increased in immunodeficiency and at least some of this increase is directly related to infection, for example lymphomas (Epstein–Barr virus) and Kaposi's sarcoma (human herpes virus 8). Additional features may be found with specific primary immunodeficiencies, for example eczema and thrombocytopenia in Wiskott–Aldrich syndrome; congenital heart disease, hypocalcaemia and dysmorphism in Di George syndrome. Failure to thrive is a common feature in children with immunodeficiency. Patients with immunodeficiency may present in many clinical environments, from primary care through to specialist clinics in tertiary referral centres. Unfortunately, there is often a long delay before a diagnosis of immunodeficiency is made, and this results in significantly increased morbidity and mortality. It is, therefore, important that awareness of these conditions is raised in order to prevent avoidable ill-health.

Classification of immunodeficiency

Underlying cause

Immunodeficiency states are classified as either **primary** or **secondary** depending on whether or not an 'external' cause can be identified as the underlying factor.

Primary immunodeficiencies are, by definition, not the result of such an 'external' insult. Many result from single genetic defects (Table 13); however, some are acquired problems, not apparently associated with a single gene defect, for example common variable immune deficiency (CVID).

Causes of secondary immunodeficiency include
- drugs (e.g. corticosteroids, etc.)
- infection (HIV, Epstein–Barr virus, malaria, etc.)
- malignancy (lymphoproliferative disease)
- malnutrition
- systemic disease (diabetes mellitus, liver/renal failure)
- splenectomy.

In numerical terms, secondary immunodeficiency is a much more common clinical problem than primary immunodeficiency. As such, it is necessary to have a high index of suspicion for infection in a very wide range of patients. The immunological mechanisms underlying secondary immune defects are often multiple and difficult to demonstrate by routine

Table 13 Antibody deficiency syndromes

Antibody deficiency syndrome	Immunoglobulin levels	Cellular abnormalities	Comments
IgA deficiency	IgA < 0.05 g/l; IgG and IgM normal	Normal	May be asymptomatic; 1:600 of population affected
Common variable immunodeficiency (CVID)	IgG < 5 g/l; IgA and IgM variable	Normal/may be reduced CD4 subset	Dual peak ages of onset in childhood and early adulthood
IgG subclass deficiency	Total immunoglobulins normal	Normal	May be asymptomatic
Antibody deficiency with normal immuno-globulins/specific antibody deficiency	Total immunoglobulins normal	Normal	Diagnosis rests on appropriate clinical history and demonstration of failed responses to test immunisation
X-linked agammaglo-bulinaemia	IgG < 2 g/l; IgA undetectable	Absent B cells (CD19⁺)	Usually present in early childhood
X-linked agammaglo-bulinaemia with hyper IgM (hyper-IgM syndrome)	IgG < 2 g/l; IgA undetectable; IgM normal/high	Absent CD40 ligand on activated T cells; neutropenia	May present with *Pneumocystis carinii* pneumonia; susceptible to cryptosporidiosis

immunological laboratory testing. HIV infection is, however, an exception to this rule and one in which laboratory testing provides a very valuable means of monitoring disease progression and identifying the need for specific therapies.

Deficient component in innate system

Deficiency of components of the innate immune system (Ch. 1) may occur in both primary and secondary immunodeficiency. Patients with breaches of the normal physical defences against infection (e.g. after severe burns and skin loss) are extremely vulnerable to infection and have secondary immunodeficiency. Primary immunodeficiency may also affect the innate system (e.g. with specific deficiencies of the complement or phagocytic systems).

Deficient component in adaptive system

The main components affected are antibody production or T cell function. The example of HIV infection leading to acquired immunodeficiency syndrome (AIDS) is an excellent example of a secondary immunodeficiency with a specific cellular defect. While some immunosuppressive drugs may target individual lymphocyte populations preferentially, the majority of secondary immunodeficiencies are associated with less well defined and sometimes generalised defects of the adaptive response. In contrast, understanding of primary immunodeficiency has increased rapidly over recent years with the identification of specific molecular lesions in a number of these previously poorly understood conditions.

4.2 Investigation for suspected immunodeficiency

Learning objectives

You should:
- understand the most appropriate hierarchy of investigations.

Investigation for immunodeficiency begins with a comprehensive history and examination. Particular attention should be paid to the infection history, family history (e.g. of unexplained deaths from infection) and risk factors for HIV infection. Other more common causes of recurrent infections (e.g. diabetes, cystic fibrosis) may need to be excluded first. Microbiological investigations play a vital role in the investigation for immunodeficiency but special samples may be required (e.g. induced sputum or bronchiolar lavage fluid for *Pneumocystis carinii* pneumonia (PCP)) and serological testing may be misleadingly negative in antibody-deficient patients. The pattern of infections present helps to identify the part of the immune system most likely to be dysfunctional in the patient and hence helps to prioritise the type of investigation required (Table 11). Immunological investigation for immunodeficiency addresses the following questions

- is the component present?
- is it at normal levels?
- does it work?
- if not, why not?

In the following discussion of immunodeficiency syndromes, conditions will be discussed according to the affected immunological components.

4.3 Antibody deficiencies

Learning objectives

You should:
- be aware of the susceptibilities of patients with antibody deficiencies
- know how to manage patients with the different defects
- know the clinical features that indicate the need to consider underlying immunodeficiency
- understand the genetic defects that may be involved.

There are a number of well-defined antibody-deficiency syndromes (Table 13) some with defined molecular defects (Table 14), others of unknown aetiology. Antibody-deficient patients share a susceptibility to recurrent bacterial infections (typically *Streptococcus pneumoniae* or *Haemophilus influenzae*), usually affecting the respiratory tract, which may lead to bronchiectasis. Each defined syndrome has particular characteristics, which are detailed below. The majority of patients require immunoglobulin-replacement therapy, either by the intravenous (ivIg) or subcutaneous (scIg) route. The clinical features of the different primary antibody deficiency syndromes are described below. The most common conditions are described first.

Antibody-deficiency syndromes

IgA deficiency

IgA deficiency is the most common primary immunodeficiency in the UK (prevalence approximately 1:600); however, many people with IgA deficiency are entirely asymptomatic and require no specific treatment. The challenge, therefore, is to identify those patients in whom there is a significant defect, which may require therapy. The history is crucial in this assessment. IgA deficiency is associated with an increased risk of pulmonary/sinus infections, allergy, coeliac disease, other autoimmune diseases and malignancy. Furthermore, IgA deficiency can be a presenting feature of some combined immunodeficiencies (e.g. ataxia telangectasia and Wiskott–Aldrich syndrome) and one should seek any associated clinical features suggestive of these diseases.

IgA deficiency is defined as serum IgA < 0.05 g/l. Many laboratories do not report IgA levels this low, and some patients will have intermediate levels of IgA, between 0.05 g/l and the normal range. For these reasons, not all reports of 'low' serum IgA necessarily indicate a diagnosis of IgA deficiency. Some patients have an associated IgG subclass deficiency and/or a failure of antibody responses to test immunisation. If a combined immunodeficiency syndrome is suspected, more extensive investigations are required.

It is only a minority of IgA-deficient patients who have a significant history of infection and there are usually other laboratory indicators of immunodeficiency in these patients (IgG subclass deficiency, failure of response to test immunisation, combined immunodeficiency syndromes). This supports the view that IgA IgG subclass and common variable immune deficiency forms a spectrum of related diseases. Therapeutic options include (a) prolonged high-dose antibiotics for infectious episodes, (b) prophylactic antibiotics, and (c) immunoglobulin-replacement therapy. Very few patients without IgG subclass deficiency or failure of immunisation responses require immunoglobulin replacement, which suggests that isolated IgA deficiency, in the absence of such defects, is a relatively benign condition.

IgA-deficient patients may form anti-IgA antibodies, which creates a high risk of transfusion reactions to IgA-containing blood products. If immunoglobulin-replacement therapy is required, a product containing the lowest possible concentration of IgA must be used in order to minimise the risk of infusion reactions.

Table 14 Genetic causes of immunodeficiency

Disease	Molecular lesion	Phenotype
X-linked severe combined immunodeficiency syndrome (SCID)	Interleukin-2 receptor γ chain	SCID with B cells
Autosomal recessive SCID	Adenosine deaminase deficiency	SCID with low T and B cells
Hyper IgM syndrome	CD40 ligand	Low serum IgG with normal/high serum IgM ± neutropenia
X-linked agammaglobulinaemia	Bruton's tyrosine kinase (BTK) gene	Absent B cells
Chronic granulomatous disease	Defects of cytochrome b_{588} or NADPH oxidase (see text)	Failure of neutrophil bacterial killing

Common variable immunodeficiency

Common variable immune deficiency is the most common form of antibody deficiency requiring treatment with replacement immunoglobulin. Unfortunately, diagnosis is typically delayed (on average for 7 years in the UK) because of a general lack of awareness of immunodeficiency disorders. Although CVID may present at any age, it typically develops in childhood or early adult life. Adults, typically present with established lung disease. Patients with CVID have an increased incidence of autoimmune phenomena including thrombocytopenia, haemolytic anaemia, malabsorption syndromes and organ-specific autoimmune disease. They also have a tendency to granuloma formation and may present with lymphadenopathy or hepatosplenomegaly, which is usually steroid responsive. Patients with CVID have an increased risk of developing malignancy, particularly lymphoma. The prevalence of CVID is estimated as 2–4:100 000 in the UK. Total serum IgG level is usually < 5 g/l; the levels of IgA and IgM are more variable. The diagnosis can, therefore, be difficult and before a diagnosis is made, careful evaluation of the clinical history and investigative results is required. There is no single diagnostic test but investigation should include assessment of antibody levels (including total immunoglobulins, IgG subclasses and vaccine-specific antibody levels) and lymphocyte subpopulations. In most cases, test immunisation with at least two vaccines (e.g. tetanus toxoid and pneumococcal vaccine (Pneumovax II)) with measurement of vaccine-specific antibody levels before and 4 weeks after immunisation is required. There is usually a failure to respond to immunisation and may be a low CD4+ T cell count. Unlike X-linked agammaglobulinaemia (XLA), a single genetic defect has not been described for CVID, but B cells from these patients do not develop normally into plasma cells. It is thought that there is an abnormality of T cell regulation in CVID. IgA, IgG subclass and specific antibody deficiencies are thought to be related conditions. Some patients who present with those conditions may progress to more typical CVID.

IgG subclass deficiency

The identification of a reduced level of an IgG subclass is not of itself sufficient to warrant a diagnosis of significant primary immunodeficiency. There are, therefore, similarities with IgA deficiency in that not all patients with a low level of the protein are clinically affected. There are four IgG subclasses (IgG_1–IgG_4). The most common clinical deficiency is of the IgG_2 subclass, which is particularly important in normal responses to bacterial polysaccharide antigens. Patients suspected of antibody deficiency in whom total serum immunoglobulins are normal should, therefore, have IgG subclass measurement usually in combination with test immunisation. Lymphocyte numbers and function are usually normal. In a patient with recurrent infection significantly low IgG subclass levels (usually < 50% of the lower limit of normal range) with abnormal responses to immunisation are suggestive of a significant defect. Occasionally, there may be a compensatory rise in the level of the non-deficient subclass (usually IgG_1).

Specific antibody deficiency (functional antibody deficiency/antibody deficiency with normal immunoglobulins)

The increasing use of test immunisation in the investigation of patients suspected of antibody deficiency has led to the identification of individuals with clinical histories suggestive of antibody deficiency in whom total serum IgG and IgG subclass levels are normal but immunisation responses are abnormal. Defining a 'normal' antibody response is difficult and expert assessment is required; however, such patients are deemed as suffering from *specific functional antibody deficiency*, also known as *antibody deficiency with normal immunoglobulins.*

X-linked agammaglobulinaemia (Bruton's type)

Boys affected with XLA (Bruton's type) usually present between 6 months and 2 years of age and there may be a history of affected male relatives. In addition to upper and lower respiratory infection, affected boys may present with joint infection or chronic diarrhoea (often caused by *Giardia lamblia*). Tonsils and other lymphoid tissue may be hypoplastic. Serum IgG levels tend to be < 2 g/l and IgA, IgM and IgE usually are undetectable. Characteristically, B cells (CD19+ lymphocytes) are undetectable in peripheral blood. This is a very helpful diagnostic test. Long-term complications include mycoplasma or ureaplasma arthritis, and enterovirus infection (polio, coxsackievirus or echoviruses). Oral polio vaccine (Sabin type) is contraindicated as it may cause paralysis but the killed (Salk) vaccine is safe.

The prevalence of XLA is thought to be approximately 1:100 000 in the UK, but with the advent of molecular testing, milder variants of the condition are being identified and, therefore, the prevalence may be higher. Carrier detection is also possible using molecular techniques. It has been shown that XLA is caused by a defect of the intracellular tyrosine kinase (Bruton's tyrosine kinase), which is encoded at X21.3-22. This enzyme is essential for normal B cell maturation; development is, therefore, arrested at the pre-B cell stage. This explains why B cells are usually undetectable.

X-linked immunodeficiency with associated hyper-IgM

Boys affected by X-linked immunodeficiency with associated hyper-IgM (hyper-IgM syndrome/CD40 ligand (CD40L) deficiency) may present with recurrent pyogenic infections or typically with PCP in infancy. PCP is seen in antibody-deficiency syndromes but occurs in hyper-IgM syndrome because of the underlying T cell defect. For the same reason, there is increased susceptibility to cryptosporidium infection, which can cause ascending cholangitis and chronic liver impairment. There is also an increased incidence of malignancy, particularly lymphoma and a range of autoimmune diseases. Serum levels of IgG are usually < 3 g/l but IgM levels may be as high as 10 g/l (normally< 3 g/l). Neutropenia is common, but T cell numbers and response to mitogens are normal. The underlying defect is a failure of CD40L expression on activated T cells (Fig. 25). This prevents T cells delivering essential signals to IgM-producing B cells (which express CD40) that would allow them to differentiate into IgG-producing plasma cells.

The gene is located at Xq26-27 and molecular confirmation of diagnosis and carrier status is possible.

Commencement of ivIg therapy usually results in normalisation of both serum IgM and neutrophil counts. The particular susceptibility of those patients to PCP is an indication for primary/secondary prophylaxis with oral co-trimoxazole. Allogeneic bone marrow transplantation is the definitive treatment in childhood. For those (usually older) patients with established chronic liver disease, combined liver and bone marrow transplantation is now considered.

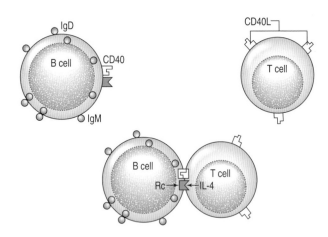

Fig. 25 CD40 ligand (CD40L) is expressed on T cells. Binding of CD40 to CD40L links IgM-producing B cells to T cells and enables class switching (i.e. a change from IgM to IgG production). In X-linked immunodeficiency with associated hyper-IgM, there is a failure of expression of CD40L on activated T cells. IL-2, interleukin-2.

Transient hypogammaglobulinaemia of infancy

There is a physiological phase of development in some infants where a gap occurs between the disappearance of passively acquired maternal immunoglobulin and the production of the infant's own immunoglobulin. This results in a low level of serum antibody level at 3–6 months of age, and in some infants this is associated with bacterial infections. There are no other specific features and this is a *diagnosis of exclusion*. The priority is to ensure that any child presenting with recurrent infection and low levels of serum immunoglobulin in the first year of life does not have primary immunodeficiency. Therefore detailed immunological investigation is often required to exclude the diagnoses of severe combined immunodeficiency (SCID), XLA or early-onset CVID.

Differentiation from primary antibody deficiency may be difficult at this stage and careful clinical and laboratory monitoring of such infants is required for evidence of emerging antibody production. A diagnosis of transient hypogammaglobulinaemia can only be made retrospectively when antibody levels have returned to normal and the baby is clinically well.

Management of patients with antibody deficiency

Replacement therapy with regular ivIg is now the standard treatment for clinically significant primary antibody deficiency (the majority of IgA-deficient patients *do not* require this treatment). This lifelong treatment is extremely effective in controlling infection, improving quality of life and preventing end-organ damage. The usual dose is 400 mg/kg, given every 3 weeks. Careful clinical review is required to ensure that infections have come under control and to monitor for the development of complications of the conditions/therapies. Regular preinfusion serum IgG levels are measured and should be maintained within the physiological range (usually > 8 g/l). Patients with established structural lung disease will often require higher doses of ivIg in order to maintain clinical well-being. Patients must be weighed regularly and appropriate increments in ivIg dose made because growth (in children) and weight (in adults) often increases significantly after the initial diagnosis and treatment. Various commercially available ivIg preparations differ in their content. These products are manufactured from pooled human immunoglobulin and are, therefore, potential sources of viral transmission to patients. This is an important factor in selection of ivIg products for treatment and indicates the need to hold preinfusion serum samples in long-term frozen storage to enable retrospective viral testing should infection be identified at a later date.

Selection of a replacement immunoglobulin product

The most common side effect of ivIg is reaction to the infusions. This may be related to infusion rate, intercurrent infection, or anti-IgA antibodies in IgA-deficient patients. Transmission of viral infection is now a very small risk because of careful viral screening and new antiviral steps in the production of ivIg from pooled donor sera. Some products are prepared as liquid formulations while others are lyophilised and require reconstitution prior to infusion. Recent advances in treatment include self-administration of ivIg at home and the development of subcutaneous immunoglobulin preparations (scIg), which is of particular value in the very young. More concentrated immunoglobulin products are required for subcutaneous use because smaller volumes (e.g. 20 ml) are administered more frequently (e.g. once per week). Once a patient is established on a particular product, it must not be changed without clear clinical indications.

Although immunoglobulin replacement is the mainstay of treatment for antibody deficiency, there are other aspects of therapy. When respiratory infection occurs, patients should be treated over an extended period (usually 10 days) with high-dose antibiotics, guided by antibiotic sensitivity. Patients should be encouraged to undertake regular breathing exercises to assist with expectoration of sputum, and, in those with established lung damage, postural drainage should be undertaken daily. Regular assessment of pulmonary function is advised; however, 'routine' use of radiograph and computed tomographic examination (e.g. at annual review) is not advised in patients with primary immunodeficiency. Many of these conditions predispose to malignant disease and 'non-essential' exposure to radiation should, therefore, be avoided.

4.4 Complement pathway deficiencies

Learning objectives

You should:
- be aware that defects can occur in both complement components and in pathway-controlling proteins
- be aware of the genetic defects that may be involved
- know the clinical features of the deficiencies
- know how to manage patients with the different defects.

Isolated complement component deficiencies are rare and in most cases are inherited as autosomal recessive conditions. The clinical features of deficiency depend on which part of the activation cascade is interrupted.

Defects in the pathway components

Classical pathway deficiency

Deficiencies of the early components of the classical pathway (C1, C2 and C4) may present with recurrent bacterial infection or with immune complex-mediated disorders (lupus-like syndromes). C2-deficient patients are especially prone to infection by *S. pneumoniae*. C3 deficiency is very rare; but it is associated with recurrent bacterial infection.

Alternate and terminal pathway deficiency

Deficiencies of the alternate pathway component **properdin** (X-linked) or the terminal pathway components C5, C6, C7, C8 and C9 are associated with recurrent neisserial (*Neisseria meningitidis* or *Neisseria gonococcus*) infections.

Investigation of the complement system is, therefore, indicated in any patient with symptoms of recurrent bacterial (especially neisserial) infection, 'lupus-like' disorders or angioedema. Total C3 and C4 levels are readily measured and low levels may be identified; however, the most useful screening tests for deficiency are assays that test the functional integrity of the classical and alternative pathways (the 50% haemolysing dose of complement (CH_{50}) and alternative pathway (AP_{50}, respectively). If an abnormality is detected, further characterisation is necessary to identify the individual component that is defective.

Management of complement deficiency

Management is dictated by the clinical presentation. For patients with recurrent bacterial infection, prophylactic antibiotics may be indicated. For those susceptible to infection, immunisation with pneumococcal capsular polysaccharide (Pneumovax II) and meningococcal vaccines is often advised. It is important to note that the tetravalent meningococcal vaccine protects against serotypes A, C, W135 and Y and is, therefore, preferred to the less-protective meningitis C vaccine in this group. In some cases, intramuscular penicillin is stored at home for emergency treatment of suspected meningococcal disease and patients are advised to wear a medical warning bracelet (Medic-Alert/SOS). For those patients with prominent joint symptoms possibly caused by a lupus-like syndrome, further rheumatological assessment is advised.

Defects in the proteins controlling the pathway

In addition to defects of the individual proteins in the complement cascade, there are a number of control proteins that regulate and control the activation of the pathways; these too may be defective, resulting in clinical disease. The most common is CI inhibitor deficiency.

C1 inhibitor deficiency

Defects of the control protein C1 inhibitor are inherited in an autosomal dominant manner and cause hereditary angioedema. In this condition there is a failure of the normal regulation of the classical pathway that results in uncontrolled activation of complement and kinin pathways in response to even minor trauma.

Clinical features

Patients present with recurrent deep-tissue swelling following apparently minor trauma (typically dental treatment). This may affect any part of the body but is of most concern when the airway is compromised. Symptoms usually begin in early adolescence, although late presentation is increasingly recognised. An interesting feature is that attacks may begin, or become more severe, in women after commencement of the oral contraceptive pill, hormone-replacement therapy or during pregnancy.

Although inherited as an autosomal dominant trait, many patients do not give a significant family history. It is therefore thought that approximately 20% of cases are caused by new mutations in the C1 inhibitor gene. As with other primary immunodeficiencies, there is often a period of diagnostic delay, during which patients will have suffered symptoms, often of a life-threatening nature. It is typical for children with this condition to suffer recurrent abdominal pain (caused by intestinal wall swelling), rather than swelling at other sites. In one series, 30% of patients had an undiagnosed relative who had died of laryngeal oedema, 34% had had an unnecessary laparotomy and 10% had had endotracheal intubation or tracheotomy prior to diagnosis.

Investigation

During an acute attack, there is a characteristic pattern of serum complement levels, which is caused by inefficient activation of the classical complement pathway. Serum C4 and C2 are low but C3 levels are usually normal. This is a very valuable pointer to the diagnosis of hereditary angioneurotic oedema. Measurement of C3 and C4 should be considered in any patient with angioedema to help differentiate allergic from hereditary angioneurotic oedema. In 85%, there is a low level of C1 inhibitor (usually < 50% of the lower limit of normal) but in 15% the enzyme level is normal. This latter group have 'functional C1 inhibitor deficiency', the enzyme being present but non-functional.

Management

Prophylactic treatment with androgenic steroids (danazol 200–400 mg daily; stanozolol 2.5–10 mg/day) or antifibrinolytic drugs (tranexamic acid up to 4 g/day) is usually effective. Antifibrinolytic drugs are the preferred option for female patients because of the virilising side effects of the androgens. If laryngeal oedema occurs (e.g. after dental extraction), it may obstruct the airway and become life threatening. This requires emergency intravenous administration of C1 inhibitor concentrate (1000–1500 U). It should be noted that this is a very different treatment approach to allergic angioedema, in which injectable epinephrine (adrenaline) is effective.

In long-term management, patients should be advised to wear a medical warning bracelet. C1 inhibitor concentrate should also be given prior to any surgical procedures. Otherwise 'routine dental work' should only be undertaken in hospital, where laryngeal oedema can be dealt with effectively.

4.5 Cellular immunodeficiency

Learning objectives

You should:
- understand the likely consequences of a defect in one of the cell types in the immune system
- be aware of the genetic defects that may be involved
- know the clinical features of the deficiencies
- know how to manage patients with the different defects.

Because of the central role of T cells in coordinating the immune response, isolated T cell deficiency is rare. In other words, if T cells are defective it is likely that there will also be evidence of associated B cell deficiency. In the following sections, those conditions in which the T cell defect is the major feature will be described first and then those in which a combined defect is more prominent.

T cell defects

Di George syndrome

This is a rare syndrome associated with a developmental abnormality of the third and fourth pharyngeal pouches. The clinical features of the fully expressed syndrome consist of:

- abnormal facies with low-set ears, 'fish-shaped' mouth, hypertelorism, notched ear pinnae, micrognathia and a downward slant of the eyes
- hypoparathyroidism (often presenting with neonatal hypocalcaemic tetany)
- congenital heart disease (particularly aortic arch defects: truncus arteriosus, interrupted arch or Fallot's tetralogy)
- cellular immunodeficiency.

However, not all of these clinical features are present in every case of Di George syndrome. Partial forms exist and most often these children will be diagnosed when they present with significant congenital heart disease. Significant immunodeficiency is estimated to occur in approximately 20% of cases and, interestingly, immune function in those children usually improves with time.

Di George syndrome is now recognised as one of a group of related disorders that share a common genetic lesion. This is usually a deletion at 22q11 and the group of conditions is referred to as the CATCH 22 syndrome:

- <u>c</u>ardiac anomalies
- <u>a</u>bnormal facies
- <u>t</u>hymic hypoplasia
- <u>c</u>left palate
- <u>h</u>ypocalcaemia.

Other clinical syndromes that are within the broader CATCH 22 group include velocardiofacial syndrome, Kallman's syndrome and Schprintzen's syndrome. Not all the CATCH 22-associated conditions are associated with immunodeficiency.

Investigation

Diagnosis is based on the typical morphological features associated with recurrent viral or fungal infections such as oral and perineal candidiasis or viral pneumonia. Chest radiograph may show an absent thymic shadow with abnormal cardiac outline. It is usual to find a reduced number of circulating T cells, but the degree of immunological deficiency is variable and is probably only significant in approximately 20% of patients identified by other criteria. Lymphocyte proliferation in response to mitogens (e.g. phytohaemagglutinin and phorbol myristate acetate) may be reduced. Antibody deficiency is rare. The chromosome 22q11 lesion is detectable by fluorescent in situ hybridisation. However, as the range of clinical associations of 22q11 lesions is wide and the degree of immunodeficiency variable, the simple demonstration of a 22q11 deletion does not necessarily imply that there is clinically important immunodeficiency.

Management

Awareness and early recognition of Di George syndrome is important, particularly as these infants may be subjected to neonatal cardiac surgery. Calcium levels must be monitored and supplemented as necessary. All blood transfusions must use X-irradiated (25 Gy/unit) blood only and live immunisations are contraindicated (MMR, BCG oral polio vaccine). Antibiotic prophylaxis to prevent PCP should be considered. Guidelines suggest that primary PCP prophylaxis should be instituted if the absolute CD4$^+$ cell count is $< 0.4 \times 10^9$/l or if there is reduced T cell proliferation in response to mitogens. In those with severe cellular immunodeficiency, bone marrow transplantation is suggested. The place of fetal thymus grafting is still experimental, although there have been some recent encouraging results showing reconstitution of T cells.

Chronic mucocutaneous candidiasis

Chronic mucocutaneous candidiasis is a rare condition that affects both males and females and presents with chronic candidal infection of skin and mucous membranes. There may be an associated autoimmune endocrine deficiency, most commonly hypoparathyroidism or Addison's disease (Ch. 6), which may precede the immunodeficiency. Investigation of such patients usually reveals normal T cell responses to nonspecific mitogens but a specific failure of proliferative response to *Candida* sp. Management can be challenging, with the need for regular antifungal chemotherapy often at high dose and for prolonged periods of time.

Natural killer cell deficiency

Natural killer cell deficiency is reported in the literature but is very rare in clinical practice. Patients have an increased susceptibility to herpes viruses. Absolute levels of natural killer cells are usually normal but their function is impaired. Functional studies of natural killer cells are only performed in specialist centres.

Combined immune deficiencies

Wiskott–Aldrich syndrome

The classical presentation of Wiskott–Aldrich syndrome, an X-linked disorder, is in young boys with a typical triad of eczema, thrombocytopenia and recurrent infection. However, the immunodeficiency may be mild and initially unrecognised, and eczema in childhood is common. The finding of thrombocytopenia is, therefore, usually the essential clue that there is a significant underlying diagnosis. The major differential at this stage is X-linked thrombocytopenia. Wiskott–Aldrich syndrome is associated with life-threatening complications occurring in the second and third decades of life. These include severe autoimmune vasculitis or glomerulonephritis and malignant lymphoma. If definitive treatment is not undertaken early in life, death from one of these causes is likely in the second or third decade.

Investigation

Platelets are small and have abnormal expression of surface glycoproteins (CD43 and gpIb). There are defects affecting the cytoskeletal proteins, including actin, and associated defects of T cell proliferation. The molecular defect is mutation of the *WASP* gene at Xp11.22. Characteristically there is a failure of response to polysaccharide antigens and progressive lymphopenia.

Management

These patients require careful clinical and laboratory assessment to establish optimum management. Increasingly, affected males are offered bone marrow transplantation in early childhood in order to reduce the risk of long-term complications and increase life expectancy.

Ataxia telangectasia

Ataxia telangectasia is a progressive neurological and immunological disorder that is inherited as an autosomal recessive condition and presents in early childhood with neurological manifestations, including cerebellar ataxia, nystagmus and oculomotor dyspraxia. Telangiectases are typically seen on the elbows, conjunctivae and ear lobes. There is a progressive, combined, immune defect that is variable in its immunological features. Patients ultimately develop lymphoid leukaemia/ lymphoma in the second and third decades and this, combined with progressive combined immunodeficiency, is the usual cause of death.

Investigation

The fundamental lesion is defective DNA repair, leading to increased radiosensitivity (similar to that seen in other disorders such as Bloom's syndrome, xeroderma pigmentosa, Nijmegen breakage syndrome). Chromosomal breaks, inversions and translocations are commonly seen at the gene for the T cell receptor and the gene complexes for immunoglobulins on chromosomes 7 and 14, respectively. The serum α-fetoprotein is often raised. Heterozygotes for the gene mutations in ataxia telangec-

tasia have an increased risk of developing a number of malignancies (including breast cancer), and family members need to be made aware of this. Patients with ataxia telangectasia gradually develop immunodeficiency and, after comprehensive immunological investigation at diagnosis, this is confirmed and monitored by regular review of the clinical and laboratory features.

Management

Careful, continuing, immunological assessment is essential in these patients and treatment is dependent on the degree of immunodeficiency. Patients commonly require ivIg by late childhood. There is no corrective treatment available for the underlying chromosomal instability. It is essential that the management of a child affected by ataxia telangectasia should be in the context of a multidisciplinary team in order to meet the needs of the family over time.

Severe combined immunodeficiency

SCID describes a group of conditions that have a number of causes but usually similar presenting features. By definition, both humoral and cellular responses are impaired or absent. SCID typically presents early (in the first weeks and months of life) with a history of failure to thrive, unexplained diarrhoea and recurrent bacterial, viral or fungal infection. Unexplained lymphopenia ($< 2.8 \times 10^9/l$) is often present and should always prompt investigation. Total lymphocyte counts may, however, be apparently normal in B cell-positive variants, T cell activation deficiencies and graft-versus-host disease (GVHD). GVHD is usually thought of in the context of bone marrow transplantation but in babies born with SCID, maternofetal transfusion of normally functioning maternal lymphocytes results in an almost identical syndrome of jaundice, typical skin rash and diarrhoea in the immunodeficient child. GVHD caused by maternofetal transfusion occurs in the first month of life but GVHD may also occur as a complication of blood transfusion in the baby with SCID. Therefore, all transfusions to potentially immunodeficient individuals should be irradiated (25 Gy/unit) to eradicate immunocompetent lymphocytes, the potential inducers of GVHD.

Investigation

When SCID is suspected, immunological advice should be urgently sought, with regard to both investigation and immediate management (Box 3). In general, serum immunoglobulins are low and there is a low lymphocyte count with diminished proliferative response to mitogens. Lymphocyte subset analysis is essential and a range of other investigations is needed to exclude SCID. The molecular basis of many variants of SCID is now recognised; each has a particular pattern of abnormali-

Box 3 Emergency management of severe combined immunodeficiency (SCID)

- Make the diagnosis (liaise with clinical immunologist, exclude HIV if appropriate)
- Treat current infections
- Look for other infections, e.g. *P. carinii* pneumonia, do not rely on serology
- Prophylactic co-trimoxazole/intravenous immunoglobulin/nystatin
- Avoid live vaccines
- Only use blood that is cytomegalovirus negative and irradiated
- Make an early referral to supraregional centre for bone marrow transplant.

ties and some of the more common are summarised in Table 14. Molecular characterisation allows greater precision in diagnosis and carrier detection.

Management

Early diagnosis, prevention of infection and rapid bone marrow transplantation are all crucial to ensure ultimate survival. Delay in making the diagnosis allows complications to occur (such as disseminated cytomegalovirus infection), which reduce the chance of survival. Bone marrow transplantation can be curative and, in the UK, is currently performed at two supraregional centres. Gene therapy has already been successful in small clinical trials and it is hoped this therapeutic approach will have a major impact on SCID management in the future.

Phagocytic disorders

Phagocytes may be defective in numbers or function. The more common disorders are described below.

Chronic granulomatous disease

Chronic granulomatous disease typically presents in childhood with recurrent, deep abscesses caused by catalase-positive organisms (*Staphylococcus aureus, Aspergillus, Serratia* and *Nocardia* spp.). Presentation may be with osteomyelitis, unexplained granulomatous lesions, malabsorption or recurrent pneumonia. New cases have been diagnosed in adulthood. Inheritance may be X-linked or autosomal recessive.

Investigation

The diagnosis rests on the demonstration of a failure of the neutrophil respiratory burst. The most common screening test of neutrophil function is the nitroblue-tetrazolium (NBT) test, in which normal neutrophils reduce the yellow dye formazan into blue intracellular crystals. This test may not be abnormal in all cases and

more sensitive flow cytometric screening techniques have been developed. The molecular defect can be in any of the following molecules:

- the 91 kDa chain of cytochrome b_{558} (X-linked chronic granulomatous disease/CGD X91)
- the 22 kDa chain of cytochrome b_{558} (autosomal recessive/CGD A22)
- the p47 component of the cytosolic NADPH oxidase (autosomal recessive/CGD A47)
- the p67 phox cytosolic component (autosomal recessive/CGD A67).

These proteins are all involved in the energy-dependent process of intracellular killing (Fig. 26). The definitive test is to demonstrate a failure of neutrophil mediated bacterial killing.

Management

Antimicrobial prophylaxis (usually with co-trimoxazole) is the mainstay of therapy. Interferon-γ may be a useful adjunct to conventional antibiotic and surgical management of abscesses but is not recommended for prophylactic use. Allogeneic bone marrow transplantation, in

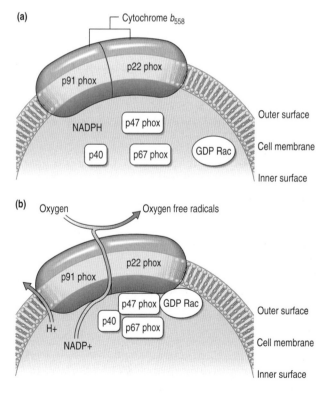

Fig. 26 The cytochrome b_{558} system and intracellular killing. (a) The individual components in a resting cell. (b) In an activated cell, the components interact to generate the respiratory burst. NADPH oxidase releases hydrogen and an electron, allowing the formation of superoxide. In chronic granulomatous disease, one of the membrane or cytosolic components of the complex is deficient (see text).

early childhood before the development of complications of infection, is now the treatment of choice for chronic granulomatous disease if a suitable donor can be found.

Cyclical neutropenia

Cyclical neutropenia may present in childhood or adult life and is characterised by recurrent abscesses, usually occurring at intervals of approximately 3 weeks although the periodicity can vary greatly. The neutrophil count is typically $< 1 \times 10^9/l$ at times of infection and the diagnosis should be suspected if there is clear periodicity to the history. Alternatively, the neutrophil count may be incidentally noted as low on a blood count during acute infection. The cause is unknown.

Investigation

Neutrophil counts should be measured on alternate days for a 4-week period and carefully analysed for any evidence of a cyclical pattern. A cyclical pattern may also be detected for other elements including platelets and other leukocytes.

Management

Management is dictated by the clinical severity of the condition. Prophylactic antibiotics may be adequate during times of low neutrophil numbers. In more severe cases, treatment with granulocyte colony-stimulating factor is considered.

Leukocyte adhesion deficiency type 1

Leukocyte adhesion deficiency type 1 is typically a disorder of infancy and childhood. Chronic/recurrent skin ulcers and periodontitis are common. There is characteristically little pus formation and an associated peripheral blood neutrophilia. There is likely to be a neonatal history of delayed separation of the umbilical cord stump (> 10 days).

Investigation

There is defective expression of the CD18 (β-chain) of the integrin family of adhesion molecules CD11a/CD18, CD11b/CD18 and CD11c/CD18. The lack of expression is demonstrated on both lymphocytes and phagocytes by flow cytometry. A second variant, type 2, is associated with defective expression of CD15.

Management

Antibiotics are the mainstay of therapy. Drug choice should be guided by antibiotic sensitivities. Prophylactic therapy may be necessary, depending on the frequency of infection. Bone marrow transplantation is necessary for severely affected individuals.

Type 1 cytokine pathway defects

The type 1 cytokine pathway defects form a group of recently described immunodeficiencies that includes defects both of cytokine secretion and expression of their cellular receptors. This affects secretion and expression of interferon-γ, interleukin-12, interferon-γ receptor (IFNγR) and interleukin-12 receptor (IL-12R). There is a spectrum of severity of these conditions, which affect both children and adults. Affected individuals typically develop infection with poorly pathogenic mycobacterial or salmonella species or with the live vaccine bacille Calmette–Guérin (BCG). The most severe forms are fatal in infancy; however, the more mild variants are treatable with combinations of antimicrobial chemotherapy and adjunctive cytokine therapy where appropriate.

Investigation

Investigation requires a specialist laboratory. Cell surface expression of IFNγR and IL-12R is detected by flow cytometry. Specialist functional assays of lymphocyte signalling are necessary to confirm and characterise the defects. Histologically, complete IFNγR deficiency is characterised by a failure to form granulomata while partial deficiency is associated with good granuloma formation.

Management

Once the diagnosis is established, appropriate antimicrobial chemotherapy must be commenced. Experience with adjunctive interferon-γ treatment in the partial forms is increasing, and discussion with specialist centres is advised.

4.6 Secondary immunodeficiency

Learning objectives

You should:
- be aware of the various causes of secondary immunodeficiency
- know the clinical features that would indicate such a deficiency
- know the clinical features of HIV infection
- know how to manage patients with secondary immunodeficiency.

Immunosuppressive drugs are widely used in the treatment of cancer and autoimmune diseases. They are an important cause of secondary immunodeficiency. When using these agents, it is essential to monitor treatment carefully and maintain the lowest level of immunosuppression compatible with effective treatment (Ch. 9).

Malnutrition, infection and other iatrogenic causes, including radiotherapy, are also important causes of secondary immunodeficiency. The mechanisms of secondary immunosuppression are usually multifactorial: specific intervention is not indicated but susceptibility to infection must be recognised in the patients who are at risk. Box 2 lists the warning signs of immunodeficiency.

Splenectomy

Splenectomy is an important cause of secondary immunodeficiency. These patients have a lifelong risk of sudden-onset overwhelming sepsis caused by encapsulated organisms. This is related to the important role of the spleen in the immune response to polysaccharide antigens. (See Ch. 3 for advice on long-term management of asplenic patients.)

Human immunodeficiency virus infection

The existence of AIDS has been recognised since the early 1980s when a number of young male homosexuals presented with severe opportunistic infections including PCP. From early in the epidemic, a sexually transmitted cause was suspected and the causative virus, HIV-1, was finally identified in 1983. HIV-2 was subsequently identified in AIDS patients from West Africa.

Unprotected sex between homosexual men was quickly identified as a high-risk factor for the condition. Subsequently, it was realised that semen, blood and cervical secretions were all highly infectious and HIV could readily be passed 'horizontally' by anal or vaginal intercourse and also 'vertically' in utero, at birth (intrapartum) and by breast-feeding. What originated as an unusual condition in a limited number of at-risk individuals rapidly developed into a pandemic. By the end of 1999, it was estimated that 32.4 million adults and 1.2 million children were infected with HIV (living with HIV) and that 16.3 million people had died since the start of the epidemic.

Human immunodeficiency virus

HIV-1 and HIV-2 are from the family of retroviruses; these are RNA viruses that possess an enzyme called reverse transcriptase, which is capable of synthesising a DNA copy of the viral RNA and integrating this into the host cell DNA. Therefore, infection of a cell with a retrovirus creates a potential source of new viruses: once the incorporated proviral DNA becomes activated, it synthesises new viral RNA, viral particles are assembled and shed from the cell. A schematic diagram of HIV and its life cycle is shown in Figure 27. HIV-1 and HIV-2 specifically infect cells expressing the CD4 surface antigen (T helper cells and macrophages/monocytes). This specificity is termed **viral tropism** and it occurs because the HIV protein gp120 specifically binds to the CD4 molecule, allowing entry to the cells. There are other cell-surface molecules (CCR5 and CXCR4) that act as cofactors for HIV entry. This selective infection of CD4$^+$ cells leads to their death by a variety of immunological mechanisms. The importance of CD4$^+$ cells as central coordinators of the immune response is nowhere more evident than in HIV-related disease. As CD4$^+$ cells are lost, a profound immunodeficiency

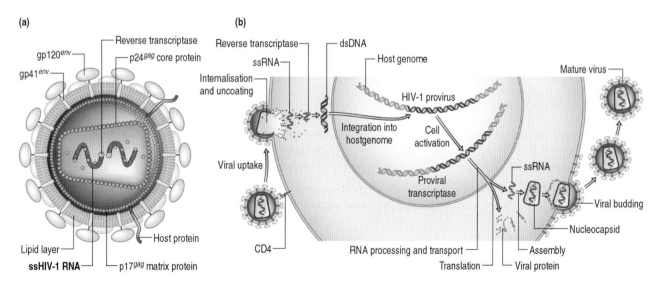

Fig. 27 The HIV particle and its life cycle. (a) The HIV particle. (b) The virus binds specifically to cell surface CD4 molecules and is internalised. The single-stranded (ss) RNA is released from the viral particles and reverse transcriptase synthesises double-stranded (ds) DNA, which is subsequently integrated into the host DNA. Upon activation of the cell, new viral ssRNA is synthesised, viral particles are assembled and shed from the cell.

results, with particular susceptibility to viral, fungal and other opportunistic pathogens.

Clinical presentation

Acute infection with HIV is usually unnoticed symptomatically; however, there may be an acute seroconversion illness characterised by fever and influenza-like symptoms. Patients who experience such a seroconversion illness may have a worse prognosis than those who do not.

About one-third of patients have persistent generalised lymphadenopathy, which is defined as enlarged lymph nodes in two or more non-contiguous sites for which no other cause can be found. The patient may be asymptomatic for a considerable period of time (up to many years); however, as the immune system is progressively damaged, the onset of AIDS becomes inevitable in the vast majority.

Early symptoms that may occur before the development of AIDS include:

- fatigue
- fever
- weight loss
- diarrhoea
- rashes
  —drug associated
  —eczematous
- bacterial infection
- fungal infection
- oral discomfort.

The clinical signs are:

- lymphadenopathy
- oral/pharyngeal candidiasis
- shingles
- herpes simplex
- leukoplakia of the tongue.

Acquired immunodeficiency syndrome

The definition of AIDS has developed over time but is generally accepted to have occurred if an HIV-positive patient develops one or more of a number of indicator infections or malignancies.

Pneumocystis carinii pneumonia
P. carinii is a common cause of pneumonia in AIDS. *P. carinii* is an airborne fungus and typical opportunistic pathogen (i.e. an organism that only infects those with significantly impaired immune systems). Clinical features include

- dry cough
- fever ± night sweats

- dyspnoea
- weight loss.

At least 90% of patients will have an abnormal chest radiograph with bilateral hazy infiltrates being common. Hypoxaemia is typical and diagnosis is best confirmed on bronchoalveolar lavage. Treatment with high-dose co-trimoxazole or intravenous pentamidine is necessary. Mortality associated with PCP is high, at approximately 20%. Survivors should be commenced on secondary prophylaxis (regular oral co-trimoxazole/pentamidine).

Oesophageal candidiasis
Oesophageal candidiasis may be asymptomatic or present with

- chest pain
- dysphagia
- nausea/vomiting.

Diagnosis is confirmed on barium swallow or endoscopy, and treatment with fluconazole is recommended.

Cytomegalovirus retinitis
Cytomegalovirus retinitis affects approximately 20% of patients and causes progressive visual loss. The retina develops segmental areas of necrosis and haemorrhage. Funduscopy findings are usually typical and there are no specific diagnostic tests. Treatment with antiviral agents including ganciclovir, foscarnet or cidofovir should be continued to delay the development of blindness. Cytomegalovirus retinitis is usually a poor prognostic indicator.

Mycobacterium avium intracellulare infection
Mycobacterium avium intracellulare is a ubiquitous non-pathogenic organism already alluded to in discussion of type 1 cytokine defects. It may present as an AIDS-defining illness with non-specific symptoms of

- fever ± night sweats
- cough
- diarrhoea
- weight loss
- anaemia.

Diagnosis is by positive culture either of abscess material, bone marrow or blood and treatment is by combination antituberculous medication.

Malignancy
The common cancers that occur in AIDS patients include Kaposi's sarcoma, central nervous system (CNS) and other lymphomas and squamous cell carcinomas. Kaposi's sarcoma presents as purplish nodules or plaques affecting the skin or mucous membranes.

Prior to the HIV pandemic, it occurred only rarely in Ashkenazi Jews. Caused by human herpes virus 8, the lesions respond to local radiotherapy, interferon-α or chemotherapy. The occurrence of lymphoma either within or outside the CNS is usually linked to Epstein–Barr virus proliferation and prognosis is poor. Squamous cell carcinoma of the rectum or cervix may partially respond to surgery or radiotherapy but the prognosis is also poor.

Neurological complications

There is a range of neurological features of HIV infection including dementia, peripheral neuropathies and depression. Dementia may be the presenting feature of AIDS development and, therefore, can be delayed by appropriate antiviral therapy. It is important to note that this is typically a slowly progressive condition and, in contrast, the acute development of a confusional state should raise the suspicion of intracerebral lymphoma or abscess. Computed tomography scanning is usually helpful as those with dementia should show cerebral atrophy. Peripheral neuropathy, when it occurs, tends to be progressive and unresponsive to therapy. Depression is common, as in other terminal illnesses, and management of all of these neurological complications is demanding of the multidisciplinary team.

Investigation of HIV infection

Investigation of patients with HIV infection should begin with a careful clinical history that identifies either risk factors for infection and/or symptoms consistent with HIV infection. Many infected individuals are diagnosed through their regular attendance at genitourinary medicine clinics; however, there are a significant number of people, particularly heterosexuals who might not consider themselves at particularly high risk, who are diagnosed in other settings. It is all too common for such individuals to be investigated extensively for a variety of other illnesses before HIV infection is recognised.

Diagnosis rests on the demonstration of positive antibody tests to HIV-1 and/or HIV-2. Before testing is undertaken, it is essential that the patient is fully informed as to the nature and purpose of the test and what the result will mean, both if it is positive and negative. Individuals must give fully informed consent for such testing.

It is crucial to explain the meaning of a negative HIV antibody test. The nature of antibody responses (Ch. 1) indicate that, after acute infection, an IgG antibody test may not become positive for 3 months. Therefore, patients need to know that a negative result does not necessarily exclude very recent infection and

the test will need to be repeated in 3 months to confirm negative antibody status. This is particularly relevant to individuals who may have experienced a single high-risk episode (needlestick injury, sexual assault, etc.). For those who regularly engage in high-risk practices, HIV antibody tests become a part of their regular clinical follow up.

Once HIV infection is diagnosed, a number of baseline tests are required to establish the degree of immune competence, coexisting infections and any evidence of organ impairment:

- confirm the HIV test
- full blood count
- lymphocyte subset analysis (CD4+ cell count)
- liver and renal function tests
- serology for
  —toxoplasma
  —syphilis
  —hepatitis B
- chest radiograph.

Thereafter the patient should be regularly reviewed to allow clinical, immunological and virological monitoring. Measurement of absolute numbers of CD4+ T cells in the blood is a very useful method of monitoring HIV-positive patients. The measurement of CD4+ cell counts should not, however, be used as a surrogate marker of HIV infection. There is no place for using this test as a means of avoiding the need for an HIV antibody test. Patients with HIV can have normal CD4+ cell counts while patients without HIV may often have low CD4+ cell counts for other reasons. Until relatively recently, the serial measurement of the CD4+ cell count was the most reliable test to monitor the progress of HIV infection. The introduction of a test to measure plasma HIV viral load adds a further dimension to monitoring. Figure 28 indicates the generally reciprocal relationship between viral load and CD4+ cell count during HIV infection.

During the acute phase, plasma viral load is high and there may be a transient dip in total CD4+ cell count. Thereafter, there is an initial recovery of CD4+ cells that can last for varying lengths of time but eventually there will be a progressive loss of CD4+ cells as viral proliferation continues and the disease progresses.

The experience of monitoring CD4+ cell counts in many patients since the 1980s has confirmed that once counts fall below certain levels, particular susceptibilities exist that warrant the introduction of prophylactic therapy. These are summarised in Figure 29.

Management of HIV infection

The management of HIV-infected patients has many aspects including drug and other treatments. It is

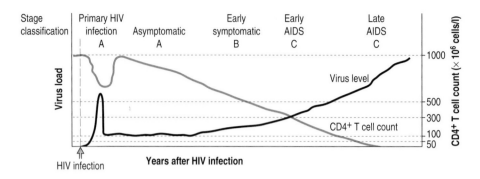

Fig. 28 Longitudinal patterns of immunological and virological parameters in HIV infection.

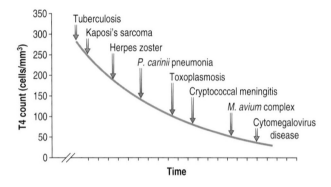

Fig. 29 Characteristic opportunistic infections and malignancies that occur in HIV infection as the CD4+ T cell count falls.

dependent on a dedicated multidisciplinary team that usually includes medical, nursing, psychology, social work and other disciplines, both hospital and community based. There are many issues around counselling and infection control that go beyond the scope of this chapter. It is also important to realise that AIDS is a terminal illness and the full range of issues associated with dying need to be addressed in an appropriate manner.

The development of specific anti-HIV therapy was a particular challenge, as once viral RNA had been copied and integrated into the host, these host cells effectively became viral production units. Treatment had, therefore, to be directed against the enzymes that allowed this integration to occur. Antiretroviral drugs specifically inhibit the proliferation of retroviruses and include the nucleoside reverse transcriptase inhibitors (NRTI: zidovudine, didanosine, lamivudine, etc.), the non-nucleoside reverse transcriptase inhibitors (NNRTI: nevirapine, efavirenz) and protease inhibitors (PI: sequinavir, ritonavir, etc.). These are used in combination (known as *highly active antiretroviral therapy* (HAART) to improve their effectiveness in preventing viral replication and avoiding the development of antiviral drug resistance. The availability of viral load monitoring has been a great asset in the management of HIV-infected people. Treatment is now guided by the measurement of the number of copies of viral RNA per millilitre of plasma. The aim of treatment is to maintain viral RNA at undetectable levels. This approach has led to greatly improved outcomes, with prolonged maintenance of higher CD4+ cell levels and, therefore, delays in the development of the complications of infection. The antiviral drugs are, however, both expensive and associated with significant side effects. Viral resistance to the drugs does occur. The current lack of availability of effective anti-HIV medication in the developing world is a source of major concern in these countries, where the prevalence of HIV infection is very high (8% of the population of sub-Saharan Africa were HIV positive in 1999).

Self-assessment: questions

Multiple choice questions

1. Specific susceptibility to infection by non-tuberculous mycobacteria is most likely to increase in the primary immunodeficiency:
   a. Common variable immunodeficiency
   b. Interferon-γ receptor deficiency
   c. Chronic granulomatous disease
   d. Classical pathway complement
   e. Factor B deficiency

2. A 70-year-old male with chronic lymphocytic leukaemia is admitted to hospital with bilateral pneumonia. He has had several courses of chemotherapy over the past 3 years and has been suffering from frequent upper respiratory infections over the previous 6 months. The component of the immune system that is most likely to be defective is:
   a. Macrophages
   b. Immunoglobulin G
   c. T lymphocytes
   d. Mast cells
   e. Complement pathway

3. A 17-year-old male with non-Hodgkin's lymphoma requires splenectomy for haemolytic anaemia; infection with following organism is likely to carry the greatest risk for him:
   a. *Mycobacterium tuberculosis*
   b. *Haemophilus influenzae*
   c. *Staphylococcus aureus*
   d. *Streptococcus pneumoniae*
   e. *Pseudomonas aeruginosa*

4. A 27-year-old female has been attending her dentist frequently because of recurrent dental abscesses. She is a smoker and her only regular medication is the oral contraceptive pill. The only other infective history is of admission to hospital with pneumonia at 23 years of age and osteomyelitis as a child. The following component of the immune system is most likely to be defective:
   a. Macrophages
   b. Immunoglobulin E
   c. Neutrophils
   d. B lymphocytes
   e. Complement pathway

5. Which of the following are features of the Wiskott–Aldrich syndrome?
   a. Low neutrophil numbers
   b. Thrombocytopenia
   c. Defective neutrophil function
   d. Hypocalcaemia
   e. Hypoadrenalism

6. A 42-year-old man presents with a 4-day history of progressive dyspnoea. He has a history of heavy alcohol and intravenous drug abuse. His chest X-ray showed diffuse shadowing and his oxygen saturation at rest is 78%. Which aspect of his immune function is most likely to be impaired?
   a. Basophils
   b. Immunoglobulin G
   c. T lymphocytes
   d. B lymphocytes
   e. Complement pathway

7. Deficiencies of which of the following complement components are most associated with an increased risk of recurrent neisserial infection?
   a. C1
   b. C2
   c. C4
   d. C3
   e. C5

8. Deficiency of which one of the following complement proteins is most associated with recurrent angioedema?
   a. C1
   b. C2
   c. Properdin
   d. C1 inhibitor
   e. Membrane attack complex

9. Deficiency of which one of the following complement components is most associated with an increased risk of disease mediated by immune complexes?
   a. C2
   b. C3
   c. Properdin
   d. C5
   e. C9

Case history questions

History 1

An 11-year-old boy was referred with a 1-year history of being unwell. He had presented with left lower lobe pneumonia 1 year previously, which had been treated in hospital with intravenous antibiotics. In the past he had had frequent ear infections and had bilateral vent insertion at 5 years of age. Since discharge, he had complained of occasional fevers and cough. His parents had noticed him to be easily tired and his school performance had deteriorated. On examination he appeared pale and was on the 50th percentile for height and 25th percentile for weight. Respiratory examination revealed some coarse crepitations at the left base. The referring paediatrician had undertaken a chest X-ray examination, which was reported as normal. The boy's serum immunoglobulins were measured (Table 15).

Table 15 Serum immunoglobulin measurements in case history 1

Immunoglobulin	Serum level (g/l)	Reference range (g/l)
IgG	4.6	5.4–16.1
IgA	< 0.07	0.5–1.8
IgM	0.28	0.5–2.8

1. What is your differential diagnosis?
2. What further investigations are indicated?

Results of further investigations are given in Tables 16 and 17. The total lymphocyte count included CD3, CD4, CD8, CD19, CD16/56.

Table 16 IgG subclasses and lymphocyte phenotypes

	Serum level	Reference range (g/l)
IgG subclasses (g/l)		
IgG$_1$	4.19	4.5–9.5
IgG$_2$	0.2	1.5–4.9
IgG$_3$	0.46	0.1–1.8
IgG$_4$	< 0.17	
Lymphocyte subsets (%)		%
CD3	68	62–69
CD4	40	30–40
CD8	28	25–32
CD19	21	21–28
CD16/56	10	8–15

Table 17 Immunisation studies

Parameter	T0 (ELISA units)	T0 + 4 weeks (ELISA units)
Tetanus toxoid IgG	3	9
Tetanus toxoid IgG$_1$	1	5
Pneumococcal capsular polysaccharide IgG	< 1	1
Pneumococcal capsular polysaccharide IgG$_2$	< 1	1

3. What diagnoses do these investigations exclude and why?
4. What is now the most likely diagnosis?
5. What other investigations might be helpful?
6. What treatment would you recommend?

History 2

A boy aged 3 years and 10 months was admitted to his local hospital with symptoms suggestive of chest infection. He was treated with intravenous antibiotics and made a good recovery. The past history indicated that he was born at full term (normal delivery) and had no significant problems in the neonatal period. From 4 months of age he had developed frequent loose foul-smelling motions. This was initially diagnosed as viral gastroenteritis and then thought to be temporary lactose intolerance. Milk protein exclusion was ineffective in controlling symptoms, which persisted until 2 years of age. He had also suffered repeated chest infections and was, on average, receiving antibiotics on a monthly basis. He had recurrent otitis media, conjunctivitis, and skin infections over his buttocks. Because of this history, he had been investigated for cystic fibrosis (CF) but that diagnosis was excluded by normal sweat test and negative genetic analysis for the common CF mutations. During his admission serum immunoglobulins were measured (Table 18).

Table 18 Serum immunoglobulin measurements in case history 2

Serum immunoglobulins	Value (g/l)	Reference range
IgG	0.19	4.9–16.1
IgA	1.0	0.4–2.0
IgM	2.67	0.5–2.0

1. What is your differential diagnosis at this stage?
2. What further investigations must be undertaken urgently?

3. Do you require further detailed antibody studies (IgG subclasses, functional/specific antibodies)?

Further tests gave the results shown in Table 19 and Figure 30.

Table 19 Lymphocyte phenotyping in case history 2

Class	Percentage	Normal range (%)
Lymphocyte subsets		
CD3	71	62–69
CD4	54	30–40
CD8	13	25–32
CD19	26	21–28
CD16/56	2	8–15

4. What conclusion can you draw from these investigations?
5. What is the diagnosis?
6. What treatment would you recommend and indicate your priorities?

Data interpretation

1. A 48-year-old man has a 20-year history of chest disease. He has a daily productive cough, and the sputum is often purulent. High-resolution computed tomographic scan of chest indicates some peribronchial thickening and moderate hilar lymphadenopathy. Moderate splenomegaly is also noted. Investigations gave the results shown in Tables 20 and 21. No compact band was detected in protein electrophoresis. The most likely diagnosis is:

a. Chronic granulomatous disease
b. X-linked agammaglobulinaemia

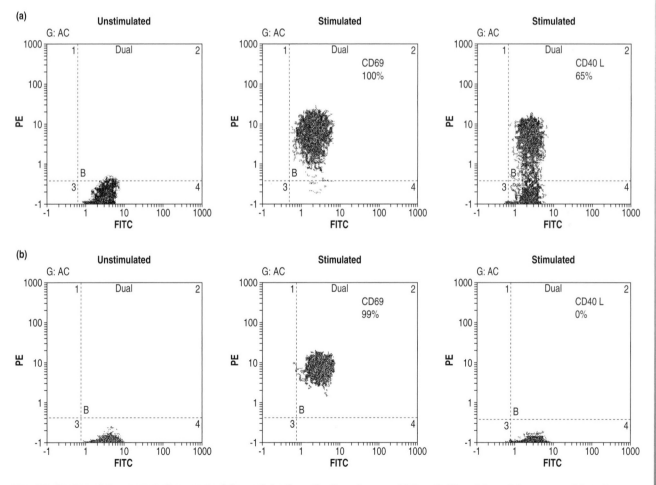

Fig. 30 Scatter plots generated as part of the cellular investigations in case history 2. The data points represent lymphocytes that have been stained with monoclonal antibodies with or without stimulation. Series (a) are from the mother and series (b) from her son. The monoclonal antibodies used in each scatterplot are as follows (X/Y). Left hand (CD3/CD40L), Middle (CD3/CD69), Right hand (CD3/CD40L). CD69 is a control activation marker.

Table 20 Data interpretation question 1

Parameter	Value	Normal range
Haemoglobin (g/l)	145	130–180
White cell count ($\times 10^9$/l)	15	4–10
Lymphocyte count ($\times 10^9$/l)	4.5	
Platelets ($\times 10^9$/l)	30	150–450

Table 21 Lymphocyte markers for data interpretation question 1

Parameter	Value	Normal range
Lymphocyte phenotype (%)		
CD3	73	62–69
CD4	38	37–64
CD8	43	11–36
CD19	18	3–13
Immunoglobulin subclass (g/l)		
IgG	3.2	7–16
IgA	< 0.07	0.8–4.7
IgM	0.5	0.5–3.0

c. Common variable immunodeficiency
d. Specific antibody deficiency
e. Acquired immunodeficiency syndrome (AIDS).

2. A 10-year-old boy with a long history of moderate eczema presents with a swollen knee joint. He has a history of recurrent upper respiratory infection and a maternal uncle died in his early teens. Investigations gave the results in Table 22. Aspiration of the joint reveals bloodstained fluid. The likely diagnosis is:

a. Di George syndrome
b. Common variable immunodeficiency
c. Wiskott–Aldrich syndrome
d. X-linked agammaglobulinaemia
e. Ataxia telangectasia.

Table 22 Data interpretation question 2

Parameter	Value	Normal range
Haemoglobin (g/l)	114	130–180
White cell count ($\times 10^9$/l)	8	4–10
Platelets ($\times 10^9$/l)	15	150–450

Self-assessment: answers

Multiple choice answers

1. a. **False.** Infection with capsulate bacteria is most common.
    b. **True.** Infection with non-tuberculous mycobacteria is characteristic of this condition.
    c. **False.** Chronic granulomatous disease typically presents with abscess formation or atypical pneumonia.
    d. **False.**
    e. **False.** Factor B deficiency predisposes to neisserial infection.

2. a. **False.** Macrophages are not affected in chronic lymphocytic leukaemia (CLL).
    b. **True.** This is a common complication of lymphoproliferative disease.
    c. **False.** Most CLL is of B cell origin.
    d. **False.** Mast cells are unaffected in CLL.
    e. **False.** Complement is unaffected in CLL.

3. a. **False.** No significantly increased risk of mycobacterial infection.
    b. **False.** While frequency of infection by a range of capsulate bacteria may be increased after splenectomy, it is overwhelming pneumococcal septicaemic illness that has the highest mortality.
    c. **False.** There is no significantly increased risk of staphylococcal infection.
    d. **True.** Overwhelming pneumococcal septicaemia is a significant risk after splenectomy and has a very high mortality.
    e. **False.** There is no increased risk of pseudomonas infection.

4. a. **False.** The history does not suggest a macrophage defect.
    b. **False.** IgE deficiency is not a significant immunodeficiency.
    c. **True.** The history of recurrent abscesses, pneumonia and osteomyelitis together make chronic granulomatous disease the most likely diagnosis.
    d. **False.** While antibody deficiency could explain the infections, the sites and pattern of infection would be unusual.
    e. **False.** While complement deficiency might be considered in the differential diagnosis, it is not the most likely condition to explain this history.

5. a. **False.** Neutrophil numbers are not affected by Wiskott–Aldrich syndrome.
    b. **True.** Thrombocytopenia, eczema and recurrent infection are the typical triad of features.
    c. **False.** Neutrophil function is not affected by Wiskott–Aldrich syndrome.
    d. **False.** Hypocalcaemia is associated with the Di George syndrome.
    e. **False.** Hypoadrenalism may be associated with chronic mucocutaneous candidiasis.

6. a. **False.**
    b. **False.**
    c. **True.** The clinical history suggests *Pneumocystis carinii* pneumonia, which is characteristically associated with T lymphocyte immunodeficiency.
    d. **False.**
    e. **False.**

7. a. **False.** Deficiency of classical pathway components C1, C4 and C2 is associated with increased incidence of disease mediated by immune complexes.
    b. **False.** See a.
    c. **False.** See a.
    d. **False.** Deficiency of C3 renders the individual susceptible to infection by a wide range of bacteria.
    e. **True.** C5 is part of the terminal complement pathway, deficiency of which causes failure to form the membrane attack complex and susceptibility to neisserial infection.

8. a. **False.** Deficiency of classical pathway component C1 is associated with increased incidence of immune complex-mediated disease.
    b. **False.** Deficiency of classical pathway component C2 is associated with increased incidence of immune complex-mediated disease.
    c. **False.** Deficiency of properdin is associated with recurrent neisserial infection.
    d. **True.** Causes hereditary angioedema.
    e. **False.** The membrane attack complex is crucial for bacterial killing.

9. a. **True.** Deficiencies of classical pathway components C1, C4 and C2 are associated with increased incidence of immune complex-mediated disease.

b. **False.** Deficiency of C3 is associated with recurrent infection.

c. **False.** Deficiency of properdin is associated with recurrent neisserial infection.

d. **False.** C5 deficiency causes failure of formation of the membrane attack complex and leads to susceptibility to neisserial infection.

e. **False.** C9 is also part of the terminal complement pathway.

Case history answers

History 1

1. The presentation with left lower lobe pneumonia at 11 years of age is unusual, but it was the persisting symptoms and clinical signs in the chest that triggered the paediatrician to undertake immunological investigation. The initial serum immunoglobulins indicated IgA deficiency; however, there were also slightly low levels of total serum IgG and IgM. The differential diagnosis, therefore, needs to include the causes of pan-hypogammaglobulinaemia: common variable immunodeficiency (CVID) and X-linked agammaglobulinaemia (XLA) as well as IgA deficiency. The absolute levels of immunoglobulins would be more consistent with CVID than XLA.

2. Further investigations include measurement of IgG subclasses, lymphocyte phenotype and test immunisation, the results of which were provided in Tables 16 and 17. The IgG subclasses are all below the normal range; however, IgG$_2$ is most notably low.

3. Lymphocyte phenotype indicates normal levels of CD19$^+$ cells (B lymphocytes), which effectively excludes XLA.

4. The failure of specific antibody titres to rise after immunisation confirms a functional defect of antibody production. Panhypogammaglobulinaemia with normal B cells and failure to response to immunisation makes the most likely diagnosis CVID.

5. Sputum culture to exclude persisting bacterial infection. Full respiratory assessment including pulmonary function tests to exclude reversible airway obstruction. High-resolution computed tomographic scan of the chest should be considered in order to document any baseline lung damage including bronchiectasis (unlikely in this case). Full blood count should be undertaken to exclude anaemia or thrombocytopenia, both of which can occur in CVID.

6. Immunoglobulin replacement therapy (either intravenous or subcutaneous) will be required to prevent further infection and the long-term development of chronic lung disease.

History 2

1. The presentation to hospital in this case is similar to case 1; however, there are important differences. This boy is presenting at a much younger age and his initial investigations indicated a very profound hypogammaglobulinaemia. These factors mean that XLA is much more likely than CVID. The possibility of severe combined immunodeficiency (SCID) must be considered urgently; however, the total IgM was above the age-related normal ranges and this suggested XLA with hyper-IgM (X-HIGM) as the most likely diagnosis.

2. With either of the last two differentials, urgent cellular investigations are required.

3. Hypogammaglobulinaemia of this degree means that further detailed antibody testing as suggested is unlikely to be helpful.

4. The cellular investigations undertaken indicate that major T and B lymphocyte populations are present, effectively excluding XLA and the more common forms of SCID. The scatter plots provided are the result of functional studies of the expression of CD40 ligand (CD40L). This is the cell-surface molecule that is deficient in X-HIGM syndrome. Scatter plots (a) from the mother indicate reduced CD40L expression compared with CD69 consistent with her carrier status. Scatter plots (b) from the boy indicate a complete lack of expression of the molecule and confirm the diagnosis.

5. X-linked hyper-IgM syndrome.

6. Immediately commence:

   • primary *Pneumocystis carinii* prophylaxis
   • intravenous immunoglobulin replacement
   • cryptosporidiosis avoidance precautions.

Discuss the case with the supraregional centre for paediatric bone marrow transplantation.

Data interpretation

1. a. **False.** Although chronic granulomatous disease can present with pneumonia, hypogammaglobulinaemia is not a feature and this is not a likely diagnosis.

   b. **False.** The presence of CD19$^+$ B cells makes X-linked agammaglobulinaemia very unlikely.

c. **True.** The age at presentation, IgG levels, associated thrombocytopenia and splenomegaly are typical of common variable immunodeficiency.
d. **False.** The low serum IgG excludes this diagnosis.
e. **False.** There are no features to suggest AIDS.
2. a. **False.** There are no features to suggest Di George syndrome.

b. **False.** Although there is recurrent infection, the family history and joint swelling do not suggest common variable immunodeficiency.
c. **True.** The history of eczema, thrombocytopenia and suggestion of a haemarthrosis are typical of Wiskott–Aldrich syndrome.
d. **False.** The history does not suggest X-linked agammaglobulinaemia.
e. **False.** There are no features of ataxia telangectasia.

5 Allergy

Chapter overview

The prevalence of allergic disorders is increasing rapidly in developed societies. Allergic sensitisation occurs when the immune system recognises agents such as pollens, foods or drugs and generates allergen-specific IgE molecules. These molecules then bind via specialised Fc receptors to the surface of mast cells, which are distributed throughout the body. When allergen subsequently enters the body, it binds to the mast cell-surface IgE molecules and this causes the mast cell to release chemical mediators into the local microenvironment. It is this local release of histamine and other mediators into the tissues (e.g. nasal epithelium, conjunctivae, bronchi) that is responsible for organ-based allergic symptoms (rhinitis, conjunctivitis, asthma). If there is systemic release of mast cell mediators into the bloodstream, the most severe form of allergic reaction occurs—an anaphylactic reaction.

This chapter will describe the immunological mechanisms that underlie allergic disorders, how to approach the diagnosis of allergy, the common clinical syndromes and strategies for their management.

5.1 Introduction

Learning objectives

You should:
- understand the possible reasons for the increase in allergic disorders
- understand how the molecules and cells of the immune system interact to produce an allergic reaction.

It is recognised that the prevalence of allergic disorders is increasing rapidly in the 'developed' world. Data from many such countries indicate that conditions including allergic rhinitis, asthma and eczema are now extremely common. In the UK, it is estimated that up to 30% of teenagers suffer from asthma. The prevalence of true food allergy is probably 1–2% of the population. What are the reasons for this increased burden of allergic disease? There is no single cause, rather a number of factors are implicated in this phenomenon, which are associated with 'developed' or westernised societies. Although there are genetic associations for atopy, no single genetic factor can account for the rapid increases in allergic disease seen recently. A reduction in family size is associated with a higher risk of allergy, as is a lower position in birth order within a family. Environmental pollution (particularly diesel exhaust fumes) is often suggested as a potential factor in the development of airway allergy, and experimental models to explain the role of pollution have been developed. A major area of current interest is the interrelationship of the declining incidence of infectious and the rising incidence of allergic disease. Children in developed societies live in cleaner environments and are relatively protected from early nosocomial infection being brought into the home because they have fewer siblings than previous generations. They are also protected from infection by mass immunisation programmes. These and other factors have led to the development of the 'hygiene hypothesis' of allergy. This hypothesis suggests that, because of the reduced exposure of the immune system to pathogens, especially at mucosal sites (gut, lungs, etc.), there is a preferential switch of the immune response from a

T helper (Th) type 1 profile to a type 2 profile (see below), which favours the development of allergic responses. While this is probably an oversimple model, as our knowledge of T cell regulation increases, it is likely to be developed further to help us to understand the current 'allergic epidemic'.

Immunological mechanisms

Allergic reactions are caused by the immune system reacting to antigens that are mainly harmless and are referred to in this context as **allergens**. The immune system forms IgE antibody on first exposure to the allergen. These IgE molecules bind (via Fc receptors) to mast cells and basophils, which are widely distributed throughout the body. Subsequent exposure to allergen allows cross-linking of mast cell-bound IgE molecules; these, in turn, initiate an intracellular signal for the mast cell to degranulate and release **preformed**

mediators (histamine, heparin, lysosomal enzymes and proteases, neutrophil chemotactic factor and eosinophil chemotactic factor). Furthermore, intracellular metabolism of arachidonic acid via the lipooxygenase and cyclooxygenase pathways is activated to generate a second set of chemical mediators (leukotrienes, prostaglandin, thromboxanes and chemotactic and activating factors) that are released into the local tissues approximately 4–8 hours later (**late phase mediators**). These two sets of mediators cause the local vasodilatation, swelling and itch that characterise allergic reactions (Table 23).

5.2 Diagnosis

Learning objectives

You should:
- be able to differentiate typical allergic from non-allergic conditions
- recognise the clinical features of history and examination that are typical of allergic disorders
- know the value of specialist investigation in the diagnosis of complex allergic disorders.

History

Although the diagnosis of allergy is often thought to be difficult and to require complex investigations, in the majority of cases a carefully taken clinical history will provide all the information necessary for including or excluding allergy from the differential diagnosis. The typical features of an allergic reaction are

- rhinitis, conjunctivitis, wheezing, urticaria, angioedema and anaphylaxis
- rapid onset of symptoms after exposure to the allergen
- recurrence of symptoms after each exposure to the allergen
- seasonality of symptoms (for pollen allergy)
- resolution of symptoms during periods of complete allergen avoidance.

The particular allergen and route of exposure will influence the detail of the history and the severity of any reaction. For example, in allergic rhinitis, seasonality is a crucial indicator of pollen as the likely allergen, whereas allergic rhinitis symptoms that occur throughout the year are more likely to be caused by house dust mite. In a patient with penicillin allergy, administration by the intravenous route is likely to be associated with a more severe reaction than oral administration.

Table 23 Causes of urticaria and angioedema

Type	Causes
Idiopathic	
Allergic	Foods, drugs, hymenoptera venom, contact
Physical	Pressure, heat, solar, aquagenic, vibratory
Cold induced	Autosomal dominant, cryoprotein
Cholinergic	Exercise or heat induced
Adrenergic	Stress induced
Vasculitis	Hypocomplementaemic urticarial vasculitis
Autoimmune	Systemic lupus erythematosus, antibodies to IgE/FcER1/C1q
Infection	Hepatitis B, *Helicobacter pylori*, Epstein–Barr virus, Lyme disease, cutaneous larva migrans, larva currens
Insect bites	Papular urticaria
Drug induced	Aspirin, angiotenisin-converting enzyme inhibitors, opiates, muscle relaxants, radiocontrast allergen-specific IgE media
Hypothyroidism	
Urticaria pigmentosa (reddish brown macules that urticate on rubbing; Darier's sign)	
Systemic mastocytosis	Systemic form of urticaria pigmentosa
Angioedema with deafness, urticaria (Muckle–Wells syndrome)	
Malignancy	

The causes of rhinitis symptoms include:

- allergic (aeroallergens)
- drug induced (decongestant sprays, cocaine, anti-hypertensive)
- vasomotor
- infectious
- irritant
- vasculitis
- hormonal (pregnancy)
- cerebrospinal fluid rhinorrhoea.

Skin prick tests

Skin prick testing (SPT) is a very useful technique to confirm allergic sensitisation. It involves the application of small drops of liquid allergen extracts, usually to the flexor aspect of the forearm, through which a lancet or needle is inserted to create a superficial epidermal scratch. The introduction of minute quantities of allergen into the epidermis is sufficient, in allergic sensitised individuals, to cause a **weal and flare** reaction. The weal diameter is measured 15 minutes after application. The diameter is compared with the positive (1% histamine) and negative (saline) controls, which should always be included. The positive control should produce a weal of > 3 mm diameter and the negative control should cause

no weal. In these circumstances, an allergen producing a weal diameter of > 3 mm would be regarded as positive (Fig. 31). In the uncommon cases where the negative control is associated with a small weal, an allergen weal diameter > 3 mm greater than that elicited by the negative control indicates a positive response. There are limitations to the use of SPT as it is not suitable for the following patient groups:

- those with severe atopic eczema (as it may cause a flare of the condition)
- patients dependent on antihistamines (as these will suppress skin reactivity)
- very young children who are unable to sit still
- patients with dermographism (because they will have false-positive results).

Nevertheless, SPT provides a rapid, cheap and painless form of in vivo challenge in the majority of patients. When it not possible to use SPT, blood tests (see below) are an alternative. Although SPT became less popular in the 1980s, it is now returning to practice. Although the use of SPT for inhaled allergens is largely confined to hospital clinics, it is beginning to develop within the primary care setting. The use of SPT for the investigation of food allergy is probably best reserved for specialist hospital practice because of the difficulties of interpretation and the possibility of anaphylactic reactions.

Blood tests

Measurement of total serum IgE is of very limited value in the diagnosis of allergy. Total IgE levels vary widely in the healthy, non-allergic population, as they do in allergic individuals. There is, therefore, no clear cut-off level of serum IgE above which all patients are allergic and below which they are not. There is, however, diagnostic value in identifying allergen-specific IgE in the serum. Laboratory techniques for the identification of allergen-specific IgE in serum are semi-quantitative and are commonly reported as scores (e.g. 1–6). Detection of allergen-specific IgE does not require specialist clinical skill other than venepuncture and is widely available for over 100 different allergens. It is, therefore, equally suitable for use in primary and hospital-based care. There are limitations, however, and although allergen-specific IgE results correlate well with skin testing for most allergens, the results are not always directly comparable for every allergen. The interpretation of any conflicting results obtained by the two methods must be guided by the clinical history. Furthermore, individuals with high total serum IgE have high false-positive rates. Therefore, measurement of allergen-specific IgE should not be used as a screening test for allergy, the diagnosis of which should always be based on careful clinical history taking.

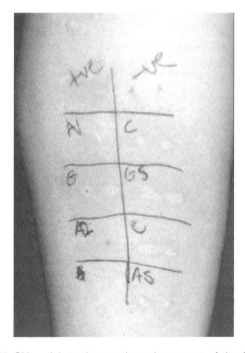

Fig. 31 Skin prick testing on the volar aspect of the forearm. Note the positive weal reaction with the histamine control (+ve) and absence of weal with the negative control (−ve). Multiple positive weals are identified in this patient after skin testing with A1, A2 and AS (apple), C (celery), G and GS (grapes). She suffered from oral allergy syndrome.

Challenge tests

Challenge tests are used when there is uncertainty regarding diagnosis despite careful history taking and the use of SPT and allergen-specific IgE measurement. Challenge tests are most frequently used by immunologists in the diagnosis of food and drug allergy; however, bronchial challenge testing is used in the diagnosis of occupational asthma. Bronchial challenge testing is only available in specialist respiratory units.

Oral challenge

Oral challenge testing is normally employed to *exclude allergy* to certain substances and *is contraindicated* if there is a recent history of anaphylactic collapse after exposure to the specific allergen. It has a very useful role in confirming the development of tolerance to foods in children. Such challenge testing should only be undertaken by specialists with appropriate expertise, in an appropriate hospital environment.

Open challenge

As the name suggests, in an open challenge, both the patient and the clinical team know what food or drug is being used in the challenge. The patient usually attends as a day case and is exposed to the allergen in a progressively graded fashion. For example, in food challenge, there will usually be a progressive exposure to skin, lip and sublingual mucosa over several hours followed by swallowing of the food. There is close monitoring of vital signs and the procedure is stopped if the patient develops any signs of allergic reaction. It is essential that full resuscitative facilities are available. Open challenge is a valuable diagnostic technique but is, however, susceptible to false-positive interpretation (e.g. an anxious patient may develop tachycardia because of anxiety rather than an allergic reaction).

Double-blind placebo-controlled food challenge

The definitive test for food allergy, the double-blind placebo-controlled food challenge is only available in specialist centres. A multidisciplinary team including allergy specialists, dieticians and nurses is required as well as inpatient facilities. Detailed description of the protocols is beyond the scope of this book; however, the principles are as follows. The patient is required to eat only a restricted ('low allergen') diet for a period of time prior to admission to hospital. During admission, the patient will be fed either placebo or challenge food, but neither they nor the clinical team will know which is being used (double blind). Following a period of care-

ful inpatient observation, the patient is allowed home and subsequently the procedure is repeated using the alternative challenge food or placebo, again in a double-blind fashion. By comparing clinical observations on the two occasions, a decision regarding the presence or absence of allergic sensitisation is made. The double-blind placebo-controlled food challenge is, therefore, a resource-intensive technique but is needed in a small number of complex cases of suspected food allergy.

5.3 Clinical allergic disorders

Learning objectives

You should:
- understand the common clinical presentations of allergic disorders
- be aware of the principles of allergen avoidance
- be familiar with the range of drugs that may benefit patients with allergic disorders.

The common clinical presentations of allergic disorders are detailed in this section. For each of the conditions there is a brief account of clinical features, investigation and management.

- atopy
- allergic rhinitis
- allergic asthma
- urticaria
- angioedema
- food allergy
- oral allergy syndrome
- venom allergy
- drug allergy
- anaphylactic reactions.

Atopy

Atopy is a term used to describe the triad of eczema, allergic rhinitis and asthma occurring in a single patient and the term is often used to imply a genetic susceptibility to allergy. The term **atopic eczema** is often used to describe the flexural distribution of eczema that typically occurs in such children (Fig. 32).

Allergic rhinitis

Clinical features

Allergic rhinitis usually presents little diagnostic difficulty or need for specific investigation. The symptoms

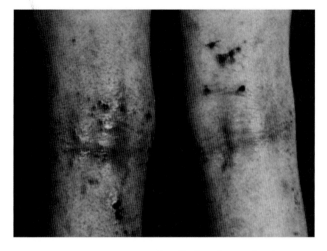

Fig. 32 Atopic eczema typically affecting the popliteal fossae.

of a red, itchy, runny nose with associated swelling and itchy watery eyes are easily recognised. A history of seasonal exacerbation may indicate allergy to specific airborne pollens/moulds (Fig. 33) while year round (perennial) symptoms are more likely to be associated with allergens such as house dust mite or domestic pet (dog/cat) allergy. It is also important to remember non-allergic causes of rhinitis (see the differential diagnosis, above).

Investigation

The history usually indicates which of the airborne allergens is likely to be causative. Particular enquiry should be made regarding exposure to animals, and any seasonal variation in symptoms. Patients may present with symptoms of secondary bacterial sinusitis. SPT or allergen-specific IgE may be used to confirm the suspected sensitivity or to exclude allergy when another cause is suspected.

Management

The most important aspect in management of any allergic disorder is *allergen avoidance*. Little can be done to reduce exposure to airborne pollens, although avoiding exposure to animals can be achieved if the patient is willing to modify their lifestyle. House dust mite allergy is an important cause of both allergic rhinitis and allergic asthma.

House dust mite avoidance measures are focused on the bedroom environment:

- reduction of clutter (especially furry toys)
- bed linen laundering > 55°C
- damp dusting
- mite-proof bed, duvet and pillow covers
- HEPA-filtered vacuum cleaners
- floor covering replacement
- possibly with chemical acaricides measures.

This list summarises the advice given to patients in order to reduce house dust mite exposure. Attention is mainly focused on the bedroom environment, where house dust mite thrive on the shed human skin in a warm humid environment. Floor coverings, bedding, cleaning and laundering procedures all need to be reviewed to ensure maximum killing of house dust mite. It is believed that reducing exposure to house dust mite results in symptomatic improvement in both rhinitis and asthma, and that effective control of nasal allergy in asthmatic patients can improve their overall airway disease. It is likely, however, that rigorous allergen control is required for significant clinical effect; therefore, partial eradication measures contribute little to clinical management. Conclusive research studies are required in this area of practice.

The pharmacological treatment of allergic rhinitis usually begins with the use of daily non-sedating antihistamines. If this is inadequate, nasal corticosteroid sprays are added to the regimen; however, young

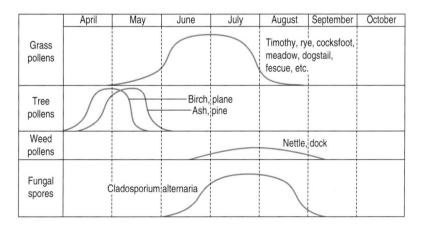

Fig. 33 Seasonal patterns of airborne allergens.

children may find the use of these difficult. Desensitisation is returning to clinical practice for grass pollen and house dust mite allergy but should only be undertaken in specialist allergy units.

Allergic asthma

The allergens implicated in allergic asthma are the same as those associated with rhinitis. In the history, therefore, it is important to determine if asthmatic control deteriorates in certain seasons or if exposure to specific allergens (animals, pollens, etc.) results in an acute asthmatic attack. Investigation and allergen avoidance is as discussed for rhinitis; however, the detailed drug management of asthma goes beyond the scope of this book. It is true to say that there are similarities in the pathogenesis of asthma and rhinitis and the management of the two conditions in an individual patient should be considered in an integrated way, particularly to ensure that there is not overuse of inhaled steroids.

Urticaria and angioedema

Clinical features

Urticaria and angioedema are considered together in this section because, while the clinical features are distinct, the two conditions commonly coexist in the same patient and share the same aetiology. Urticarial lesions are raised red itchy weals (often described as like 'nettle stings' or 'hives') that are caused by mast cell activation and

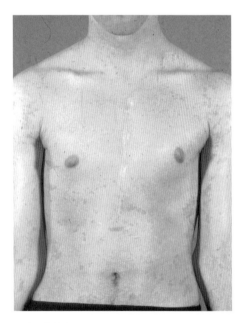

Fig. 34 Urticarial lesions over the trunk of a young man. In this case infection with scabies had caused the urticarial rash, which resolved after successful antiscabetic treatment.

degranulation within the epidermis (Fig. 34). In contrast, angioedema is non-itchy, non-dependent swelling that occurs as a result of mast cell activation in the deep dermis. Activation of the kinin system is important in causing angioedema. Angioedema commonly affects the lips, eyes, tongue (angioedema: Fig. 35) and peripheries, including arms and legs. Bilateral angioedema of the tongue, or more particularly of the larynx, can cause life-threatening respiratory obstruction, necessitating emergency medical treatment (see below). A number of specific triggers for both urticaria and angioedema may be identified (Table 23) but in the majority (approximately 90%) of individuals referred to clinics, no specific allergic cause is identified. Physical factors are commonly implicated. Individual patients often report that 'stress' factors aggravate their condition.

Therefore, the vast majority of cases are **idiopathic urticaria/angioedema**. If symptoms persist for more than 6 weeks **chronic idiopathic urticaria/angioedema** is diagnosed. This can be a very distressing condition and the natural history is quite variable. Many patients experience prolonged relapses interspersed with remissions that may last many years.

It is important to note that the *individual urticarial lesions* in idiopathic urticaria should resolve within 24 hours and leave no mark on the skin. If *individual lesions* last longer than 24 hours, the rare conditions of urticarial vasculitis or urticaria pigmentosa should be considered. In the latter, there are often pigmented lesions that if rubbed will become raised and itchy (urticate); this is known as Darier's sign. Urticaria pigmentosa may be associated with the more severe condition of systemic mastocytosis.

Rarely, angioedema occurs in the *absence* of urticaria; in this situation, hereditary or acquired deficiencies of C1 esterase inhibitor should be considered (see below).

Investigation

A thorough clinical history is essential to determine the pattern of symptoms and any associated trigger factors. Most patients with urticaria believe they are 'allergic to something' and it is essential to address this issue but not to overinvestigate. Screening tests for allergy are not recommended; however, the wide variety of disorders associated with combined urticaria/angioedema (Table 23) may justify further investigation in individual patients including full blood count, thyroid function tests, C-reactive protein and complement levels. Skin biopsy is helpful in confirming urticaria pigmentosa and urticarial vasculitis. Serum complement levels are especially useful in confirming a diagnosis of hereditary or acquired deficiencies of C1 esterase inhibitor. In this deficiency, serum levels of C2 and C4 should be low, while C3 levels remain rela-

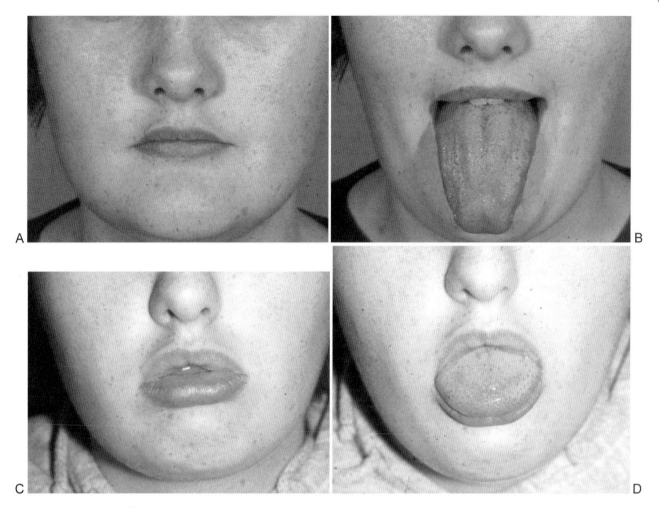

Fig. 35 Angioedema affecting the lips and tongue. The four images indicate the changes that occurred after an oral milk challenge in a 19-year-old female. A and B indicate the normal shape of the patient's lips and tongue when protruded. 1 ml of milk was absorbed sublingually and almost immediately the patient reported a 'tingling' sensation in the lips. C and D, taken 45 minutes after the milk challenge, demonstrate significant swelling of the lips and an inability to protrude the swollen tongue.

tively normal. If this pattern of complement components is identified in the context of angioedema, testing for C1 esterase inhibitor is indicated. In contrast, a patient with urticaria and normal complement levels should not have such testing performed.

Management

If an associated medical condition is identified (e.g. hypothyroidism, infection), the urticaria should respond to management of that disorder. In patients with episodic acute urticaria/angioedema, short-acting oral antihistamines (e.g. acrivastine) will be adequate. In most cases of chronic idiopathic urticaria/angioedema, however, daily long-acting, non-sedating antihistamines are necessary (e.g. fexofenadine, loratidine and cetirizine). If necessary, older sedating antihistamines can be added at night (e.g. hydroxizine hydrochloride).

The H_2 antagonists (cimetidine and ranitidine) are often tried for refractory conditions, as is doxepin (an antidepressant with potent antihistamine effects). Experience with oral disodium chromoglycate in chronic idiopathic urticaria has been disappointing. However, this drug does appear to have a useful role in the management of urticaria pigmentosa. Urticarial vasculitis often responds to therapy with non-steroidal anti-inflammatory drugs, and delayed pressure urticaria may respond to dapsone.

The relapsing, remitting nature of chronic idiopathic urticaria/angioedema makes it difficult to be certain of the efficacy of some of the therapeutic interventions and it is essential that, once regular therapy is commenced, the dose is periodically reduced or the drug withdrawn to determine whether continued treatment is necessary. The management of C1 inhibitor deficiency is discussed in Chapter 4.

Food allergy

IgE-mediated allergy to food has been described since the 1920s but remains a source of controversy. There are several reasons for this, one of which is that exaggerated claims are made both for the prevalence and for the effects of food allergy.

Prevalence

In one large population study, 20% of a randomly selected adult population reported food intolerance; however, the actual prevalence of food allergy was only 1–2% when confirmed by double-blind placebo-controlled food challenge. This figure is accepted as a reasonable estimate of the prevalence of food allergy in adults. In children, the figure is higher at approximately 2–8%. One potential explanation for the great overreporting of food allergic symptoms is that foods may produce clinical symptoms by non-allergic mechanisms: most correctly termed **food intolerance**. For example, the triggering of migraine headaches by ingestion of cheese or chocolate is well recognised clinically; however, the mechanism is probably mediated by vasoactive amines contained in the foods and does not involve the immune system. A second reason for overreporting is that the routinely available diagnostic blood tests (allergen-specific IgE) are not useful when used as screening tests and are prone to give false-positive results, particularly in atopic individuals, who often have very raised total serum IgE.

Effects of food allergy

Food allergy is often invoked as a potential cause for complex multisystem disorders or obscure symptoms such as chronic fatigue or non-specific arthralgia or myalgia. Food allergy rarely, if ever, causes such symptoms and expert opinion is that the symptoms typically caused by IgE-mediated food allergies are restricted to:

- urticaria
- angioedema
- rhinitis
- asthma
- gastrointestinal symptoms (chiefly acute vomiting and/or diarrhoea)
- oral allergy syndrome
- anaphylactic reactions.

Clinical features

The most common foods that elicit allergic reactions are milk, eggs and seafood but since the late 1980s nut allergy has been increasingly recognised (nut allergy is discussed in detail below). Food-allergic children develop typical allergic symptoms during the course of normal weaning. They may have an atopic background, but this is not an essential requirement. Typically, the first recognised exposure to egg, cow's milk or fish will cause either a cutaneous weal and flare reaction or acute vomiting. Such reactions can be florid and very frightening for the parents; they are, however, rarely life threatening. Diagnosis of food allergy is not always easy, and a particular problem occurs because of the complex nature of commercially prepared foods and the often confusing and misleading nature of food labelling. The expert advice of a dietician is invaluable in the assessment of the food-allergic patient.

Eczema and food allergy

A specific challenge in paediatric allergy practice is the contribution of food allergies to poorly controlled atopic eczema. This is a question frequently put to the allergy specialist and can be very difficult to answer. In the first place, atopic eczema has a naturally relapsing and remitting course and, therefore, relapses or remissions may erroneously be ascribed to a recent dietary modification. Second, the diagnostic tests available are more than usually confounded. If the eczema is severe, SPT may not be possible because of the extent of skin involvement and the child's dependence on antihistamines. Furthermore, most such children have high serum levels of IgE, which are often associated with a high false-positive rate for allergen-specific IgE tests. Nevertheless, some affected children do have associated food allergies, but the relative contribution to eczema control can be very difficult to assess. In such cases, diagnosis is often based on a careful food and symptom diary, which includes periods of single food withdrawal and reintroduction (usually for periods of 2 weeks at a time).

Investigation

If the history is clear-cut, there is no need for extensive investigation; however, confirmatory SPT or allergen-specific IgE is helpful in the baseline assessment. It is important to note that the weal size in SPT or the 'score' on blood testing *does not* correlate with the clinical severity of the food allergy.

Management

The mainstays of management are:

- avoidance of allergenic foods
- adequate nutritional assessment and supplementation

- availability of medication at home to treat incidental allergic reactions
- regular review to assess the development of food tolerance.

Most children will become tolerant to common foods by mid-late childhood. Rigorous avoidance of the allergenic food probably contributes to the development of tolerance although the immunological mechanisms underlying this process are incompletely understood. Regular review is important to assess normal growth and development and adequacy of any dietary supplementation. A key aspect of the management of anyone, especially a child, who has a restricted diet is regular nutritional assessment. *All children in whom food allergy is suspected, and whose diet is restricted, must be regularly assessed by a suitably experienced dietician.* A reduction in SPT or allergen-specific IgE reactivity may herald the development of tolerance. However, subtle changes in either investigation should not be overinterpreted, and one would expect both tests to be negative before considering repeating challenge tests. In any case, challenge testing should not be repeated more frequently than annually in most cases.

Children with egg allergy are often advised that they are at increased risk of severe allergic reactions to routine immunisations. The currently used influenza vaccine in the UK is contraindicated in egg-allergic subjects; however, most concern centres on the administration of the combined measles, mumps and rubella (MMR) vaccine in children. Despite previously published advice, it is now clear that *egg allergy is not a contraindication to the administration of MMR.* Large clinical studies have confirmed that egg-allergic children are no more likely to suffer allergic reactions to this vaccine than non-egg-allergic children.

Nut allergy

Peanut allergy was a relatively unknown condition until the late 1980s; however, the prevalence of peanut allergy has increased considerably. Amongst the UK preschool population, it is now estimated to be as high as 1:50–100. While peanuts are most commonly implicated, approximately 50% of affected individuals also report symptoms when exposed to tree nuts. This phenomenon is difficult to explain biologically as peanuts are members of the legume family. Peanut allergy sufferers are sometimes allergic to other members of the legume family, including peas, lentils and beans. Nut allergy is different in many important respects from other food allergies:

- it develops in very young children
- reactions to nuts typically cause angioedema of the mouth, tongue and larynx
- anaphylactic reactions may result from exposure to even trace amounts of nut
- indirect exposure (smell or touch) may cause life-threatening reactions in highly sensitive individuals
- nut allergy appears to be a lifelong problem in the majority of those affected.

Management of nut allergy is a major challenge facing those who look after children. Successful management requires the complete avoidance of all nut-containing foods, and the education of family, friends and school staff regarding the symptoms and signs of allergic reactions. Children and young adults account for the majority of cases at present although this profile will change with time. Those with associated asthma appear to be at the greatest risk of the most severe reactions and it is essential that their asthma is well controlled on regular medication (including inhaled corticosteroids if necessary). Overdependence on β_2-adrenoceptor agonists to control asthma may limit the effectiveness of injected epinephrine (adrenaline) in an emergency.

An emergency medication kit should be available at all times and include both oral antihistamines and injectable epinephrine (adrenaline) (for life-threatening reactions). Patients are encouraged to wear a medical warning bracelet. Nut allergy has now overtaken bee/wasp sting allergy as the most common cause of anaphylactic reactions occurring outside hospital.

Oral allergy syndrome

A small number of individuals present with oral allergy syndrome. Presenting symptom is usually swelling of the lips or tongue after eating fresh fruit (not jams or other cooked fruits). Patients usually have coexistent allergy to tree pollens (most frequently birch pollen) and the underlying mechanism is thought to be a cross-reactivity of highly conserved structural proteins called profilins that are present in both pollens and fresh fruit. The profilins are structurally altered during cooking and this explains why most affected people can tolerate cooked fruit.

Venom allergy

Allergy to bee and/or wasp stings is important and may manifest as either minor/limited or major/systemic reactions. As stated above, allergy to stinging insects was, until recently, the most frequent cause of anaphylactic reactions outside hospital. As with other allergies, most individuals demonstrate stereotypical reactions; however, interestingly, many patients who have suffered a severe life-threatening reaction may have a less-severe reaction on subsequent stinging. This reduction in severity of attacks may be influenced by the time interval between stings. It has been estimated that the average interval between stings is 15 years in the UK. There are, however, occupational groups who are at higher risk including bee keepers and others such as forestry workers (who may occasionally disturb wasps' nests).

Management

Treatment decisions are based both on the severity of previous reactions and the risk of future stings. Treatment options include prescription of an emergency medication kit including oral antihistamines and injectable epinephrine (adrenaline) as in nut allergy. Desensitisation is also considered for those at high risk of systemic/generalised attacks. Desensitisation is based on the principle that repeated injection of tiny quantities of allergen into an allergic person can induce tolerance to that allergen and thus prevent allergic reactions. Desensitisation was commonplace in the UK in the 1980s; however, a series of patients' deaths led to its withdrawal. The appropriate use of desensitisation in specialist hospital clinics for defined patient groups is now re-emerging and is proving therapeutically useful. Currently treatment is limited to venom, grass pollen and house dust mite allergies. Best results are achieved in patients with single allergen sensitisation.

Drug allergy

Drug allergy is a very difficult area of clinical practice because drugs have many complex effects and side effects that may mimic, mask or aggravate allergic reactions. There are few reliable investigations to confirm or exclude drug allergy; diagnosis, therefore, requires considerable expertise. Not all adverse reactions to drugs are caused by allergy and it is important to distinguish between IgE- and non-IgE-mediated reactions (Table 24). A careful history is again essential in differentiating allergy and pseudo-allergy from the other causes of adverse drug reaction. In contrast to the community setting, administration of drugs is the most common cause of anaphylactic reactions occurring in hospital. Two of the most common groups of drug to be implicated in allergic reactions are antibiotics and anaesthetic agents.

Antibiotic allergy

Allergic reactions to antibiotics have been recognised since the early days of their clinical use. IgE antibodies

Table 24 Classification of adverse reactions to drugs

Type of reaction	Features
Reactions that may occur in anyone	
Overdose	Toxic effects caused by excess intake or reduced excretion
Side effects	Undesired effects occurring at recommended dose
Interactions	Effect of one drug on the effectiveness or toxicity of another
Reactions that only occur in susceptible individuals	
Intolerance	Unusual susceptibility to normal pharmacological effect
Idiosyncrasy	Genetically determined abnormal reaction to a drug
Allergy	Drug-specific, IgE-mediated reaction
Pseudo-allergy	Drug-specific, non-IgE-mediated reaction that mimics allergy

are directed either against the β-lactam ring (major determinant allergy) or one of its components, metabolites or side chains (minor determinant allergy). Major anaphylactic reactions can occur in penicillin-allergic patients, particularly if the drug is administered parenterally (intramuscular or intravenous). Because of concern regarding this potential risk, it has become common for anyone developing a rash while taking penicillin to be labelled as 'penicillin allergic'. While this precautionary approach is understandable, it unnecessarily limits the range of antibiotics available to many people. It is, therefore, important that, when a patient indicates they suffer from 'penicillin allergy', this should as far as possible be critically evaluated by the doctor. To confirm a diagnosis of penicillin allergy, typical allergic features occurring rapidly after ingestion of the drug (certainly within 24 hours) should be sought. Specific IgE testing for penicillin allergy is only about 85% sensitive for major determinant allergy and most tests do not detect minor determinant allergy. A negative test does not, therefore, exclude the diagnosis. SPT is complex in both its practice and interpretation and carries a risk of sensitisation and/or clinical reaction. However, it is only a history of systemic reaction to penicillin that is an absolute contraindication to its use, not simply the occurrence of a rash. The many other causes of rash while taking antibiotics (infection, fever, coprescribed medication) must be considered in the differential. The increased risk of systemic reaction following parenteral rather than oral administration must also be considered before determining whether a patient may safely be prescribed penicillin.

Anaesthetic reactions

Reactions occurring during anaesthesia were once thought to be extremely rare; however, research indicates they may occur in up to 1:3500 anaesthetic administrations. The process of modern anaesthesia involves the administration of both intravenous and inhaled drugs. Usually several drugs are administered in close succession and so it is very difficult from the history to identify the cause of any allergic symptoms. In addition to anaesthetic drugs, the patient may also be exposed to antibiotics, latex, antiseptics such as chlorhexidine, or radiocontrast media, all of which may provoke allergic or pseudo-allergic reactions. Most major teaching hospitals should have agreed protocols for the investigations of such events. These should include taking blood samples at the time of reaction for measurement of mast cell tryptase and follow-up SPT to identify causative agents and drugs to which the patient is not sensitised.

5.4 Anaphylactic reactions

Learning objectives

You should:
- be aware of the principles of allergen avoidance
- be familiar with the protocol for emergency treatment of anaphylactic reactions in adults and children.

As should be clear from the preceding sections, anaphylactic reactions are the most severe forms of allergic reactions and can have many causes. Because of the precautionary approach to medical practice, it is not uncommon for an individual presenting with urticaria and perhaps some angioedema to be initially suspected of suffering an anaphylactic reaction. It is often only in hindsight, once the response to therapy and subsequent clinical pattern of symptoms are clear, that it is possible to classify the clinical presentation correctly. It is important to classify allergic symptoms correctly to ensure that the patient is given the most appropriate advice and therapy. The following section attempts to define the characteristics of the most severe reactions; however, it must be recognised that in clinical practice it is often difficult to be absolute regarding classification and often we ask patients or their carers to make difficult but essential therapeutic decisions on their own behalf. It is, consequently, essential that patients and parents are educated regarding the clinical features and appropriate management of both minor and major types of reaction.

Clinical classification

Allergic reactions may be divided into the *minor/limited* or *major/systemic* types.

Minor/limited reactions. Minor/limited reactions include urticarial rashes, oral allergy syndrome and non-life-threatening angioedema. Non-life-threatening angioedema usually implies swelling of lips, face or peripheries that does not impair airway patency. It is also possible, however, to have angioedema affecting the tongue that does not impair breathing. Such reactions will almost always respond to oral antihistamine treatment.

Major/systemic reactions. Major/systemic reactions include those that are associated with narrowing of the upper airway (typically the larynx), acute severe asthmatic symptoms and anaphylactic collapse. It is these types of reaction that may require intramuscular epinephrine (adrenaline) and patients who are recognised to be at risk of major/systemic reactions are usually prescribed an emergency self-administration pack containing both antihistamines and epinephrine (adrenaline) in a spring-loaded syringe.

This classification represents the two ends of a spectrum of possible allergic reactions. Patients' reactions will often fall somewhere between these two extremes and in such circumstances they may wait to see the effect of oral antihistamine before deciding whether to progress to the use of epinephrine (adrenaline). A more formal classification system (the Ring classification of anaphylactic reactions) is indicated in Table 25; this is often used in classifying acute anaphylactic reactions occurring in hospital, particularly those occurring during induction of anaesthesia (see Ch. 12).

It is a common misconception that individuals who suffer repeated allergic reactions will inevitably progress to the most severe type. This is not the case. It is most typical for an individual patient to suffer stereotypical reactions. In other words, the best predictor of the severity of future attacks is the severity of previous attacks. Decisions regarding the requirement for an individual to carry epinephrine (adrenaline) are, therefore, best based on the history of previous attacks rather than other assumptions. Protocols for emergency treatment of anaphylactic reactions in children and adults are given in Figures 36 and 37.

Table 25 Ring classification of anaphylactic reactions

Grade	Reactions
I	Rash only, no cardiovascular symptoms
II	Cardiovascular reaction: tachycardia, hypotension
III	Shock, life-threatening spasm of smooth muscles
IV	Cardiac and/or respiratory arrest

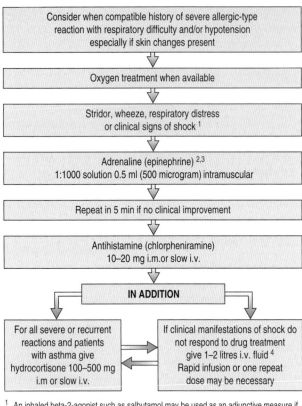

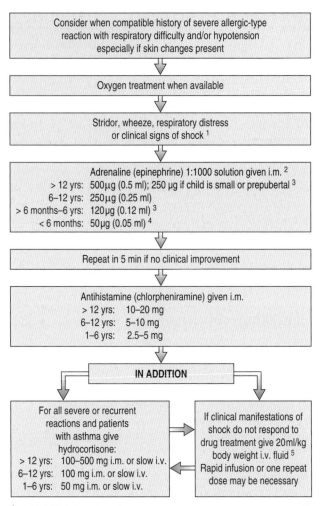

¹ An inhaled beta-2-agonist such as salbutamol may be used as an adjunctive measure if bronchospasm is severe and does not respond rapidly to other treatment.

² If profound shock is judged **immediately** life threatening give CPR/ALS if necessary. Consider **slow** i.v. adrenaline (epinephrine) 1:10000 solution. This is hazardous and is recommended only for an experienced practitioner who can also obtain i.v. access without delay. Note the different strength of adrenaline (epinephrine) that may be required for i.v. use.

³ If adults are treated with Epipen, 300μg will usually be sufficient. A second dose may be required. Half doses of adrenaline (epinephrine) may be safer for patients on amitriptyline, imipramine, or beta blocker.

⁴ A crystalloid may be safer than a colloid.

Fig. 36 Resuscitation protocol for first medical responders to anaphylactic reactions in adults. i.m., intramuscular; i.v., intravenous; CPR/ALS, cardiopulmonary resuscitation/advanced life support. (Reproduced with permission from the Resuscitation Council UK.)

¹ An inhaled beta-2-agonist such as salbutamol may be used as an adjunctive measure if bronchospasm is severe and does not respond rapidly to other treatment.

² If profound shock is judged **immediately** life threatening give CPR/ALS if necessary. Consider **slow** i.v. adrenaline (epinephrine) 1:10000 solution. This is hazardous and is recommended only for an experienced practitioner who can also obtain i.v. access without delay.

³ For children who have been prescribed Epipen, 150μg can be given instead of 120μg, and 300μg can be given instead of 250μg or 500μg.

⁴ Absolute accuracy of the small dose is not essential.
Note the different strength of adrenaline (epinephrine) that may be required for i.v. use.

⁵ A crystalloid may be safer than a colloid.

Fig. 37 Resuscitation protocol for first medical responders to anaphylactic reactions in children. i.m., intramuscular; i.v., intravenous; CPR/ALS, cardiopulmonary resuscitation/advanced life support. (Reproduced with permission from the Resuscitation Council UK.)

Self-assessment: questions

Multiple choice questions

1. The following immunoglobulin isotype is bound specifically to the surface of mast cells:
   a. IgA
   b. IgD
   c. IgE
   d. IgG
   e. IgM

2. Which of the following allergens is the most frequent cause of anaphylaxis outside hospital?
   a. Bee venom
   b. Eggs
   c. Peanuts
   d. Penicillin
   e. Wasp venom

3. Angioedema is the result of mast cell degranulation at which location?
   a. Dermis
   b. Dermis–epidermal junction
   c. Epidermis
   d. Intramuscular
   e. Subcutaneous

4. Open food challenge is:
   a. The definitive diagnostic test for food allergy
   b. Indicated to confirm the cause of suspected food-related anaphylaxis
   c. Contraindicated if there is a history of angioedema
   d. Associated with a lower reaction risk than skin prick testing
   e. Susceptible to false-negative reactions

5. Idiopathic angioedema is:
   a. A very common condition
   b. Associated with significant mortality
   c. Requires treatment with intramuscular epinephrine (adrenaline) for the majority of attacks
   d. Rarely associated with urticaria
   e. Typically responds to oral antihistamines

6. Skin prick testing:
   a. Is a controlled, objective diagnostic test
   b. For food allergy, is safe in a general practice setting
   c. Is not associated with a risk of anaphylactic reactions

   d. Should not be performed in those under 10 years of age
   e. Detects type I hypersensitivity reactions

7. Patch testing:
   a. Detects type III hypersensitivity reactions
   b. If positive, causes a wheal and flare reaction
   c. Is performed, using multiple antigens simultaneously
   d. Is useful in the investigation of reactions to latex
   e. Is a suitable alternative to skin prick testing

8. The oral allergy syndrome is most associated with pollen allergy to:
   a. *Alternaria* sp.
   b. Birch
   c. Grass
   d. Nettles
   e. Weed

9. Which of the following is the most common cause of chronic urticaria in European adults?
   a. Cosmetic allergy
   b. Drug allergy
   c. Food allergy
   d. Idiopathic
   e. Parasitic infestation

10. The most appropriate first-line therapy for seasonal allergic rhinitis is:
    a. Oral antihistamine
    b. Oral steroids
    c. Depot steroids
    d. Desensitisation
    e. Inhaled steroids

11. The natural history of oral allergy syndrome usually includes:
    a. Spontaneous resolution within 5 years of onset
    b. Progression to involve increasing number of allergens
    c. Progressive increase in severity of attacks
    d. Progressive reduction in intervals between attacks
    e. Unpredictable development of spontaneous anaphylaxis

12. Severe allergic reactions to latex is most associated with:
    a. Mucosal route of exposure
    b. Associated asthma
    c. Skin contact
    d. Severe eczema
    e. Perennial rhinitis

13. A 30-year-old nurse is allergic to latex. She develops an anaphylactic reaction after eating lunch. The fruit most likely to have triggered the attack is:
    a. Orange
    b. Grape
    c. Banana
    d. Kumquat
    e. Pear

Case history questions

History 1

> A 34-year-old man attends you complaining of repeated allergic attacks. He describes repeated episodes of a generalised itchy raised rash. Several of these have occurred while playing soccer. He has been to a health food store where he underwent some tests and was advised to avoid all wheat and dairy products in his diet. He was additionally prescribed a herbal remedy to take on a daily basis. On questioning, he does not think that his symptoms have improved since commencing the diet 6 months previously, although he has lost some weight.

1. What is the differential diagnosis?
2. What further information would you require?
3. What tests would you undertake and why?
4. What treatment would you prescribe?
5. What is the prognosis?

History 2

> A mother brings her 2-year-old son to the clinic concerned that he may have allergies. He was exclusively breast-fed until the age of 6 months when he was changed to formula milk. This transition was difficult because the baby became very agitated and screamed whenever she tried to give him the bottle. A friend suggested that he might be allergic to milk and, therefore, she tried him on goat's milk. This he began to take and has remained on goat's milk ever since. More recently at a Halloween party, her son had developed a florid urticarial rash and became wheezy and unwell. She thought he may have inadvertently drunk some milk and initially gave some oral antihistamine syrup. However, he became progressively wheezier and had to be taken to hospital. There he has given nebulised medication and an injection. He was kept overnight prior to discharge.

1. Do you think the child is allergic to milk?
2. What investigations would you perform?
3. What is the most likely cause of the recent severe reaction and how would you investigate this?
4. What advice would you give?

Data interpretation

A mother attends her GP because she is concerned about her child's atopic eczema. Despite using topical emollients and hydrocortisone 1% cream sparingly, the child continues to have flares of the condition. On examination, there are chronic eczematous changes in the popliteal and antecubital fossae and also around the eyes. The mother reports that the child is constantly scratching at night and she has read that unrecognised food allergy can be an important cause of poorly controlled eczema. She has a list of foods and other allergens that she thinks may be causing a problem and asks her doctor to test for these. A blood sample is, therefore, sent to the immunology laboratory; results for IgE testing to the specified foods are given in Table 26. Total IgE was 4690 kU/l.

1. How would you interpret these results?
2. What dietary advice would you give?
3. Are further tests required?

Table 26 Immunology laboratory results for specific IgE testing for the specified foods in the data interpretation question

RAST scores (range 0–6)	Allergen
6	House dust mite, grass pollen, peanut
5	—
4	Cat, cow
3	Dog, orange, potato, milk, egg white
2	Wheat, oats, maize, sesame seed, soybean, strawberry, feathers
1	Chicken, seafood
0	Pork, beef

Self-assessment: answers

Multiple choice answers

1. a. **False.** IgA is secreted at mucosal sites.
   b. **False.** IgD is found mainly on B cell membranes.
   c. **True.** IgE molecules bind via Fc receptors to mast cells.
   d. **False.** IgG is found in the bloodstream and can attach to phagocytic cells.
   e. **False.** IgM is found in the bloodstream and activates complement and agglutinates antigens.

2. a. **False.** Nut allergy has now overtaken bee/wasp sting allergy as the most common cause of anaphylactic reactions occurring outside hospital. Some occupational groups will still be at high risk from allergy to stinging insects.
   b. **False.** However, allergy to egg or milk tends to be identified when a child is very young.
   c. **True.** Peanut allergy was a relatively unknown condition until the late 1980s; however, the prevalence has increased considerably and is estimated to be as high as 1:50–100 in the UK preschool population.
   d. **False.** Major anaphylactic reactions can occur in penicillin-allergic patients and this potential risk has resulted in anyone developing a rash while taking penicillin to be labelled as penicillin allergic.
   e. **False.** See (a) above.

3. a. **True.** It results from mast cell activation in the deep dermis.
   b. **False.** It occurs in the deep dermis.
   c. **False.**
   d. **False.**
   e. **False.**

4. a. **False.** The definitive diagnostic test for food allergy is the double-blind placebo-controlled challenge.
   b. **False.** Should only be undertaken to exclude a cause of suspected food-related anaphylaxis.
   c. **False.** Non-life-threatening angioedema is not a contraindication.
   d. **False.** There is a higher reaction risk than for skin prick testing.
   e. **False.** It is susceptible to false-positive reactions.

5. a. **True.** Although prevalence figures are not well established.
   b. **False.** Truly idiopathic angioedema is rarely, if ever, associated with life-threatening episodes.
   c. **False.** The majority of attacks are controlled by oral antihistamines.
   d. **False.** Urticaria commonly occurs in association with idiopathic angioedema.
   e. **True.** Oral antihistamines are first line treatment of choice.

6. a. **True.** Positive and negative controls should always be used.
   b. **False.** This should only be undertaken in specialist units for reasons both of safety and interpretation of results.
   c. **False.** There are a few reports of anaphylactic reactions occurring during a skin prick test.
   d. **False.** Skin prick testing is very suitable for most children.
   e. **True.** Skin prick testing identifies type I sensitisation.

7. a. **False.** Patch testing detects type IV hypersensitivity reactions.
   b. **False.** A positive patch test causes an eczematous type appearance.
   c. **True.** Multiple antigens are tested simultaneously.
   d. **True.** Latex can induce both types I and IV reactions.
   e. **False.** Skin prick testing and patch testing are complementary but not interchangeable.

8. a. **False.**
   b. **True.** A coexistent allergy to tree pollens (most frequently birch pollen) results in a reaction to eating fresh fruit. This is believed to be caused by cross-reactivity of profilins, which are present in both pollens and fresh fruit.
   c. **False.** It is a tree pollen allergy.
   d. **False.** It is a tree pollen allergy.
   e. **False.** It is a tree pollen allergy.

9. a. **False.**
   b. **False.** It can cause urticaria but not commonly.
   c. **False.** It can cause urticaria but not commonly.
   d. **True.** Approximately 90% of patients referred to clinics have idiopathic urticaria and so no specific allergic cause is identified.
   e. **False.**

10. a. **True.** Daily non-sedating antihistamines are the first line.
    b. **False.** Oral steroids should rarely if ever be required.
    c. **False.** Depot injection of steroids has been associated with serious side effects.
    d. **False.** Desensitisation is indicated in those who fail to respond adequately to conventional treatment.
    e. **False.** Nasally inhaled steroids are used in combination with antihistamines as a second-line approach.

11. a. **False.** Spontaneous resolution is unusual.
    b. **True.** This is characteristic.
    c. **False.** Severity of reactions tends to remain relatively constant.
    d. **False.** If offending fruits are avoided, this should not be the case.
    e. **False.** Spontaneous anaphylaxis does not occur in this condition.

12. a. **True.** The mucosal route has been associated with a significant number of fatal reactions.
    b. **False.** Although asthma may be exacerbated.
    c. **False.** A severe reaction does not occur although local skin reactions do.
    d. **False.** Severe eczema is not associated with latex allergy.
    e. **False.** Perennial rhinitis is not associated with latex allergy.

13. a. **False.**
    b. **False.**
    c. **True.** Bananas cross-react with latex and are a significant cause of food reactions in patients with latex allergy.
    d. **False.**
    e. **False.**

Case history answers

History 1

1. The rash sounds reasonably typical of urticaria, although you might want to confirm this by asking the patient if they have any photographs (many often will). From the initial history, the patient is highlighting an association with exercise rather than food consumption and this should be clarified.
2. Further clinical details on the frequency of attacks, severity of symptoms and triggering factors. Were any episodes associated with angioedema or ana-

phylactic collapse? Were there any episodes that came on rapidly after the consumption of either wheat or dairy products? If not, the likelihood of allergy to those foods is low. Were any other foods implicated from the history?

3. If having reviewed the history, the diagnosis appears to be physical urticaria associated with exercise, testing should be kept to a minimum. It may be reasonable to undertake skin prick testing to exclude wheat and milk allergy, but undertaking a 'screening approach' with multiple allergens is not recommended.
4. The mainstay of treatment should be the use of non-sedating oral antihistamines. Depending on the frequency and predictability of attacks, it may be possible in this case to achieve a satisfactory outcome by prescribing antihistamine to be taken 1 hour before exercise. Alternatively, if attacks are frequent and unpredictable, a daily non-sedating antihistamine may be required.
5. The natural history of chronic idiopathic urticaria is very variable. Some patients experience infrequent symptoms over a period of months; others have a daily rash for a prolonged period of time, possibly for years. There is a tendency for relapse and remission of symptoms. Patients should, however, be reassured that in the majority symptoms can be well controlled and a diagnosis of chronic idiopathic urticaria does not imply that the patients will become allergic to foods, drugs or insect stings; nor does this condition progress to anaphylaxis.

History 2

1. There is little in the history that would suggest milk allergy. Difficulties transferring babies from breast to bottle feeding are common but are not usually caused by milk allergy. The fact that he subsequently tolerated goat's milk without adverse effect virtually excludes cow's milk protein allergy as the proteins in the two types of milk are immunologically very similar.
2. It may be helpful to undertake skin testing with milk protein to reassure the parents that their baby is not sensitised to milk protein.
3. The clinical features of the recent event suggested an acute severe allergic reaction. The occurrence at a Halloween party raises the possibility of nut exposure as nuts are commonly eaten on these occasions and are a very important cause of acute severe allergic reactions. It would be important to enquire from the parents whether nuts had been served and if so what types. A nut-allergic child may react to apparently minor exposure to nuts

and so a history of consumption of nuts is not necessarily required. Testing for nut sensitisation would be important

4. If skin tests are positive for nut, one would make a presumptive diagnosis of nut allergy and advise avoidance of all nut-containing foods. The home should become a 'nut-free zone' and the parents would need an emergency medication pack to include oral antihistamine syrup and in this case an adrenaline autoinjector. The parents, and any other carers, would need advice on how and when to use both types of medication.

Data interpretation

1. In the absence of further clinical details, it is impossible to interpret these results adequately. It would be overly simplistic to say that all results greater than an arbitrary level (e.g. 3/6) are significant. The most important point is that the child has a very high level of total serum IgE and, therefore, there is a significant risk of false-positive results.
2. Dietary advice should be aimed at complete avoidance of foods to which a child is known to be allergic but should not be overly restrictive and should ensure a nutritionally complete diet. Excessive or inappropriate dietary restriction in children is potentially very harmful to normal growth and development and, therefore, dietary advice should be cautious and should be reviewed by a qualified dietician. In this case, there is not enough information to justify dietary restriction because we do not yet know whether the blood results confirm true sensitisation or whether these are false-positives associated with a very high level of serum IgE.
3. Further laboratory tests are not required but what is required is a critical analysis of the history looking for any clear association between specific food consumption and immediate flare of eczema symptoms. Ideally this should happen before requesting the blood tests! In this case, review of the history confirmed that many of the foods were eaten without adverse effect on the eczema. There was uncertainty as to whether milk or wheat might be causing symptoms and, consequently a 2-week exclusion diet was tried but produced no significant improvement in eczema control. The child was returned to a normal diet and referred to a dermatologist for expert advice on eczema management.

6 Autoimmune diseases

Chapter overview

The immune system has developed to protect the individual from infectious microorganisms and achieves this by molecular recognition of specific 'foreign' antigenic structures. The success of this protection depends on the ability of the immune system to distinguish 'self' antigens from 'non-self' and to prevent immunological responses against self-antigens.

Autoimmunity is the term used to describe specific immunological reactions against components of the individual's own body. These may occur in a wide range of clinical situations and are not always associated with harmful effects or disease. There are, however, a distinct group of **autoimmune diseases**, which may be organ specific or non-organ specific. The nature of autoimmune responses and the spectrum of autoimmune disease will be discussed in the chapter. The major focus will be on organ-specific disease as the non-organ-specific conditions are discussed in separate chapters on vasculitis and connective tissue diseases.

6.1 Introduction

Learning objectives

You should:
- be familiar with the concept of self/non-self discrimination
- understand the concept of autoimmune disease
- know the theoretical mechanisms by which autoimmune reactions may occur
- be familiar with the spectrum of clinical autoimmune disorders
- understand the diagnostic value of auto-antibody measurements.

The immune system has evolved to protect the host against invading pathogens. As described in Chapter 1, this involves a complex set of interactions between different types of immune cell, including antigen-presenting cells and T cells. These interactions require specific molecular recognition of foreign amino acid sequences or proteins and it is clear that the immune system must be able to distinguish between self- and non-self-sequences/proteins.

Self-reactivity is prevented by a number of processes that occur early during lymphocyte development and result in **immunological tolerance** of self-antigens. Under certain circumstances, these mechanisms break down and the body reacts against itself.

Immunological tolerance

During T cell maturation in the thymus, self-reactive T cells are identified and undergo **apoptosis** or programmed cell death. A small percentage of self-reactive T cells do escape into the peripheral circulation but these are generally incapable of stimulating an effective immune response and so remain harmless. Autoimmune B cells also occur during development, but these are generally deleted or rendered unresponsive during development in the bone marrow. The full detail of how autoreactive cells are controlled at a molecular level is outside the scope of this book; however, the principle that there are immunological mechanisms to control potentially autoreactive cells is important. These mechanisms are important clinically as the majority of people who develop autoimmune reactions (e.g. after infection, surgery, etc.) do not develop autoimmune disease.

Mechanisms of autoimmunity

The occurrence of autoimmune reactions and diseases implies that, in certain circumstances, the normal immunological control mechanisms have been bypassed in some way. Several mechanisms are thought to be important in allowing the occurrence of these reactions (Fig. 38).

Cross-reactivity and molecular mimicry

The classical association between group A streptococcal infection and rheumatic heart disease is explained on the basis of cross-reactivity: the streptococci express antigens that are structurally similar to self-antigens (cardiac muscle) and, consequently, the immune response to the microorganism also causes damage to the self-proteins.

At a molecular level, the concept of molecular mimicry has also been postulated. This states that short molecular sequences (e.g. of five amino acid residues) are commonly shared between microorganisms and self-proteins. However, modelling studies have indicated that such molecular mimicry is extremely common and its contribution to the generation of autoimmune responses is uncertain.

Provision of T cell epitopes

The potential linkage of foreign proteins (e.g. drugs or chemicals) to self-proteins provides another mechanism whereby normal immunological control may be by-passed. B cells binding to the self–non-self complex have the potential to process and present the non-self component to T cells reactive to the foreign epitopes. Thus, it is possible for T cells to deliver helper signals to B cells binding the self-component, stimulating an autoimmune reaction.

Release of sequestered/cryptic antigens

Some self-antigens are not normally exposed to cells of the immune system and are said to be sequestered (e.g. lens proteins from the eye). Tissue damage can release such antigens and allow an immune response to occur. In the example of traumatic damage to one eye, the release of proteins can cause autoimmune damage to the other: **sympathetic ophthalmia**.

Cryptic antigens are those that are only released during the normal turnover of body proteins by anti-

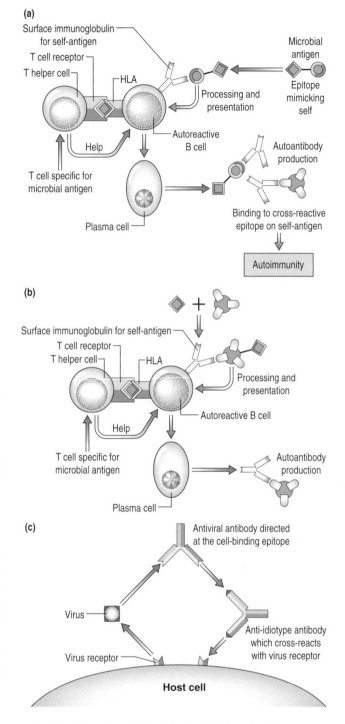

Fig. 38 Cellular mechanisms that underlie autoimmune reactions. (a) Cross-reactivity and molecular mimicry; (b) linkage of foreign proteins to self-proteins; (c) anti-idiotypic responses.

gen-presenting cells. Because they are not normally expressed, tolerance does not develop and their release can allow the generation of autoimmune responses. It is likely that cryptic epitopes are normally only released in low concentrations; however, coincidental factors such as infection or inflammation may be necessary to initiate the autoimmune response.

Failure of suppressive mechanisms

The concept of a 'suppressor T cell' is not well defined; however, it is recognised that the balance of cytokines secreted in the microenvironment is important in influencing the nature of an immune response to a microorganism (Ch. 2). It is known that altering the T cell constitution of experimental animal systems can result in autoimmune disease and it is, therefore, thought that the balance of T cell cytokine secretion in humans may be important in influencing autoimmune responses.

Anti-idiotypic responses

The antigen-binding sites of antibody molecules are known as **idiotypes**. It is possible that, during a normal response to infection, a 'second wave' of anti-idiotype antibodies is generated, directed against these idiotypic sites. In the case of viral infection, because such anti-idiotype antibodies may have significant similarity to the original virus, it is possible that the antibody could bind to the viral cell-surface receptor, so becoming an autoantibody.

Autoimmune reactions

Autoimmune reactions may occur as a consequence of infection, surgical procedures, drug treatment or be associated with increasing age. Such reactions are often only identified incidentally by the detection of auto-

antibodies in blood. Such phenomena may only be temporary, indicating that the immune system can regain control of autoreactive lymphocyte clones after the 'external insult' has been withdrawn. Autoimmune *reactions* are much more common than autoimmune *disease*. The detection of autoantibodies in blood, even in an unwell patient, does not, therefore, necessarily mean that the patient is suffering from an autoimmune disease. Serum autoantibodies may be an incidental finding. In the elderly, it is thought that 10% of the population over 70 years of age have detectable antinuclear antibodies in serum.

Autoimmune disease is said to be present only when tissue damage and symptoms occur and autoreactive antibodies or T cells are detected. Autoantibodies may be primary or secondary. **Primary autoantibodies** are rare in clinical practice and are antibodies that are known to directly cause disease. Examples include the antibody against the thyroid-stimulating hormone receptor antibody in Graves' disease, that against the acetylcholine receptor in myasthenia gravis or that blocking the voltage-gated calcium channel in Lambert–Eaton myasthenic syndrome (LEMS). **Secondary autoantibodies** are those that occur as part of an autoimmune process, may be associated with specific disease (and be diagnostically helpful) but do not directly cause disease. Examples of secondary autoantibodies would include antinuclear antibodies in systemic lupus erythematosus (SLE) and other connective tissue diseases, antimitochondrial antibodies in primary biliary cirrhosis and anti-gastric parietal cell antibodies in pernicious anaemia.

Table 27 The more common autoimmune diseases and their target antigens

Diseases	Autoantigen	HLA type
Organ specific		
Hashimoto's thyroiditis	Thyroid peroxidase and thyroglobulin	DR3, B8
Graves' disease	Thyroid-stimulating hormone receptor	DR3, B8
Pernicious anaemia	Intrinsic factor	DR4, DR2, DR3
Addison's disease	Secretory cells of adrenal cortex	DR3, B8
Type 1 (insulin-dependent) diabetes mellitus (IDDM)	Pancreatic islet cells	DR3, DR4, B8, B15
Goodpasture's syndrome	Glomerular and alveolar basement membrane	DR2, B7
Myasthenia gravis	Acetylcholine receptor	DR3, A1, B8
Pemphigus vulgaris	Intercellular component of epidermis	DR4, DR6
Bullous pemphigoid	Epidermal basement membrane	No known associations
Primary biliary cirrhosis	Bile ducts of liver	DR3, B8
Systemic		
Autoimmune haemolytic anaemia	Red blood cells, rhesus antigen	B8
Sjögren's syndrome	Extractable nuclear antigens	DR3, DR4, DR1, A1, B8
Rheumatoid arthritis	IgG rheumatoid factor	B44, B15
Dermatomyositis	Soluble nuclear proteins	DR3, B8, B14
Scleroderma	Nucleoli	DR5, B8
Mixed connective tissue disease	Ribonucleoprotein	DR4
Systemic lupus erythematosus	Double-stranded DNA	DR3, DR2, B5, B8

The spectrum of autoimmune disease

Autoimmune diseases may be classified as either *organ specific* where the autoantigen is localised in one organ only (e.g. thyroid peroxidase and thyroglobulin in Hashimoto's thyroiditis) or *systemic* where the autoantigen is widespread (e.g. components of the cell nucleus in SLE). The more common autoimmune diseases together with their target antigens are shown in Table 27. As with any clinical classification system, some of the disorders considered as organ specific have some systemic features (e.g. arthropathy is a common feature of primary biliary cirrhosis) and there is also some overlap between conditions. Patients with autoimmune thyroid disease often have detectable gastric parietal cell autoantibodies and/or pernicious anaemia. Some patients with SLE may have some of the clinical features more typically associated with scleroderma or rheumatoid arthritis. In some cases of systemic autoimmune disease, it may be virtually impossible to classify the patients at presentation and such patients are often diagnosed with 'undifferentiated connective tissue' disease at presentation; however, their clinical features may evolve over time to fit one of the more classical autoimmune diseases. The following is a brief description of the major organ-specific autoimmune diseases. The common clinical presentation, diagnostic features and principles of therapy are discussed, where appropriate, for each condition.

6.2 Endocrine disease

Learning objectives

You should:
- know the theoretical mechanisms by which autoimmunity can give rise to endocrine diseases
- know the common endocrine diseases that have an autoimmunity facet.

Autoimmunity is a common cause of endocrine diseases and both antibody- and cell-mediated immune responses are involved in pathogenesis. Some endocrine diseases involve classical hypersensitivity mechanisms and these will be described; others involve several immunological mechanisms occurring in the one disease process. There are some clear examples of primary autoantibody-mediated disease, whereas in others, autoantibodies are thought to be a secondary phenomenon. Endocrine disease results from autoimmune processes because there may be one or several of the following effects on the gland:

- destruction
- cellular infiltration
- uncontrolled stimulation
- blockade of stimulation.

Addison's disease

Addison's disease is the common name for adrenal insufficiency. The clinical symptoms of Addison's disease result from the deficient production of adrenocortical hormones, both glucocorticoid and mineralocorticoid. Globally, the most common cause is tuberculosis affecting the adrenal glands; other causes include adrenal haemorrhage, secondary malignancy, drugs, sarcoidosis and other viral or fungal infections. In the UK, however, the most common cause is autoimmune adrenal insufficiency. In this condition, secondary autoantibodies directed against adrenal tissue are detected in serum.

The clinical presentation is generally insidious, with fatigue, somnolence and depression, but may be acute as an Addisonian crisis, which is characterised by collapse, abdominal pain, hypotension and signs of salt and water depletion. There may be increased pigmentation, particularly of skin folds, buccal mucosa and scars, and occasionally signs of associated autoimmune disorders including thyroid disease or vitiligo.

The diagnosis primarily depends on having a high index of suspicion and identifying biochemical disturbances (hyponatraemia, hyperkalaemia, hypercalcaemia and occasionally hypoglycaemia) along with typical hormonal changes (low serum cortisol with high adrenocorticotrophic hormone). Acute management of an Addisonian crisis consists of fluid and electrolyte replacement along with intravenous hydrocortisone. Confirmation of the autoimmune nature of Addison's disease is by demonstration of anti-adrenal autoantibodies. In women, there is a strong association with autoimmune ovarian failure, and the possibility of autoimmune polyglandular syndrome should be considered in all patients with autoimmune Addison's disease.

Gonadal disease

Autoimmune gonadal dysfunction occurs in some patients with Addison's disease as the autoantibodies directed against steroid-producing cells in the adrenal cortex also bind to steroid-producing cells in the ovary and testis. Typically, this occurs as part of an autoimmune polyglandular syndrome (see below).

It is also thought that up to 20% of women with premature ovarian failure (menopause before the age of 40) may have an autoimmune basis and for this reason it is worth screening such women for anti-ovarian and anti-adrenal antibodies.

Diabetes mellitus

Type 1 diabetes mellitus (insulin-dependent diabetes mellitus (IDDM)) is an autoimmune disorder caused by the immunological destruction of the pancreatic islets of Langerhans. This results in deficient insulin production and the development of hyperglycaemia. A detailed discussion of diabetes presentation and acute and chronic management is outside the scope of this book; however, the immunological nature of type 1 diabetes does have potential clinical importance. Anti-islet cell autoantibodies are detectable in approximately 70% of type 1 diabetics at presentation and have been shown to precede the development of clinical diabetes. The autoantibodies do not, however, persist in the long term. Studies have indicated that prescription of immunosuppressive therapy at presentation can delay the requirement for insulin therapy; however, as yet, it has not been possible to prevent or reverse the autoimmune destruction of the insulin-producing cells. It is also recognised that the previously rigid differentiation between type 1 and type 2 diabetes may no longer be appropriate as adults presenting with diabetes may have a latent autoimmune form of the condition.

Thyroid disease

The thyroid is the endocrine gland most commonly affected by autoimmune disease, causing Graves' disease, Hashimoto's thyroiditis or autoimmune hypothyroidism. These conditions are related and occasionally an individual patient may present with one autoimmune thyroid disorder but progress to develop another. These disorders are significantly more common in women than men.

Graves' disease

This is the most common cause of hyperthyroidism, a condition that is characterised by the clinical effects of excessive thyroxine production. There is an approximately 10:1 female to male ratio. Common symptoms include weight loss, increased appetite, heat intolerance, irritability, tremor, anxiety, diarrhoea and, in women, oligomenorrhoea. On examination, there may be typical signs of Graves' disease, which include exophthalmos, ocular palsies or rarely pretibial myxoedema. General signs of thyrotoxicosis include goitre, tachycardia (possibly atrial fibrillation or other tachyarrhythmia), proximal myopathy, heart failure and eyelid retraction.

Graves' disease is caused by antibodies against the thyroid-stimulating hormone (TSH) receptor that overstimulate the thyroid gland, and the presence of these autoantibodies is measured in some diagnostic laboratories. Other autoantibodies are also detected, including anti-thyroid peroxidase in 50–80% and anti-thyroglobulin in 20–40% of those with Graves' disease. Detection of these serum autoantibodies in a patient with an appropriate clinical history and biochemical disturbance is usually considered adequate confirmation of diagnosis.

Management of Graves' disease is usually by the administration of anti-thyroid drugs including carbimazole or propylthiouracil. Thyroidectomy or iodine-131 treatment may be considered if the patient relapses.

Autoimmune hypothyroidism

Hypothyroidism in adults is almost always caused by either autoimmunity or previous treatment of thyrotoxicosis. The most common cause is **primary atrophic hypothyroidism** in which there is typically no goitre but circulating anti-thyroid peroxidase autoantibodies are detected in approximately 80% of patients. It is possible that this may represent the end stage of a subacute thyroiditis as histology reveals a marked lymphocytic infiltrate with fibrosis in many cases.

In **Hashimoto's thyroiditis** there is an autoimmune lymphocytic infiltration of the thyroid gland that causes a firm rubbery goitre, and affected patients have high-titre anti-thyroid autoantibodies (typically higher titres than in Graves' disease). A small percentage of patients with Hashimoto's disease initially present with a short phase of hyperthyroidism: so-called Hashitoxicosis.

Previous ablative therapy for Graves' disease is also an important cause for hypothyroidism and the development of this late complication underscores the need for careful longitudinal review of such patients.

Hypothyroidism affects 1–2% of women and < 0.5% of men. Common symptoms include gradual onset of fatigue, weight gain, mental slowness, cold intolerance, dry skin, hair loss and constipation. In severe cases, patients may be hypothermic and develop coma. On examination, there may be slowness in response to questioning, puffiness below the eyes and thinning of the hair. The voice may be hoarse and there is often a bradycardia.

Investigations reveal a raised serum TSH with low total and free thyroxine; detection of anti-thyroid peroxidase antibodies indicates an autoimmune cause. Hypothyroidism in a child may have several non-autoimmune causes that require expert investigation. In any patient presenting with hypothyroidism, it is essential to ensure that there is not associated pituitary or adrenal insufficiency, which also requires treatment. In treatment of primary hypothyroidism, a starting replacement thyroxine dose of 50–100 µg/day is usually adequate and treatment is monitored by clinical response and the serum TSH levels returning to normal. In patients with ischaemic heart disease, the initial dose of thyroxine should be reduced to avoid precipitation of cardiac failure.

Subacute (de Quervain's) thyroiditis

The term thyroiditis implies inflammation of the thyroid gland and in de Quervain's syndrome, the gland is enlarged, painful and the patient may be febrile. There is often an initial phase of hyperthyroidism followed by hypothyroidism, and the underlying aetiology is thought to relate to viral infection of the thyroid. Thyroid-specific autoantibodies are detected (usually at low titre) in < 50% of patients. Treatment is initially with aspirin or a short course of oral prednisolone.

Postpartum thyroiditis

Postpartum thyroiditis typically occurs around 3 months after giving birth and is characterised by a painless goitre. Affected women will be hyperthyroid initially, followed by a period of hypothyroidism and finally a return to the euthyroid state. Often there will be high titres of anti-thyroid peroxidase autoantibodies detected in serum. Recurrence in subsequent pregnancies is common and there is an increased risk of autoimmune thyroid disease later in life.

Polyglandular syndromes

Some patients with autoimmune endocrine disease have features that suggest more than one gland is affected. Two main patterns of such polyglandular autoimmunity exist: type 1 and type 2.

Type 1: autoimmune polyendocrinopathy candidiasis ectodermal dysplasia

Type 1 is a rare, autosomal recessive condition related to chronic mucocutaneous candidiasis (Ch. 4). Patients affected by autoimmune polyendocrinopathy candidiasis ectodermal dysplasia have at least two of the following features: Addison's disease, hypoparathyroidism and mucocutaneous candidiasis; they may also have alopecia, vitiligo, ovarian failure, hypothyroidism, enamel hypoplasia or nail dystrophy. Onset is usually in childhood.

Type 2: autoimmune polyglandular syndrome

Type 2 is inherited as an autosomal dominant with incomplete penetrance and is, therefore, a much more common condition that type 1. The main features are at least two of hypothyroidism, Graves' disease, type 1 diabetes and Addison's disease, with additional features of alopecia/vitiligo, coeliac disease, myasthenia gravis, chronic active hepatitis, Sjögren's syndrome, dermatitis herpetiformis or autoimmune pituitary failure.

6.3 Non-endocrine organ-specific autoimmune disease

Learning objectives

You should:
- know the common organ-specific diseases that have an autoimmunity facet
- understand the interaction of genetic and environmental factors in the development of organ-specific autoimmune disease
- understand the diagnostic value of autoantibody detection.

Coeliac disease

Coeliac disease is also known as **gluten-sensitive enteropathy**, reflecting the pathogenesis of the condition. Coeliac disease is a condition with strong genetic influences, but it is exposure to dietary gluten that activates a series of immunological mechanisms leading to small intestinal damage. It is the gliadin fraction of gluten that is the toxic component of wheat, barley and rye. Exposure to these components in the diet activates CD4+ T cells in the lamina propria layer of the small bowel mucosa. This leads to damage that manifests as gross changes in the small bowel mucosal architecture (Fig. 39):

- loss of villi
- crypt hyperplasia
- chronic inflammatory infiltrate.

There is, therefore, immunologically mediated damage, triggered by a dietary factor. The detection of autoantibodies directed against the endomysial sheath is an important aspect of diagnosis (see below) and taken together, these justify its inclusion here with other autoimmune conditions. It is important to note, however, that, in coeliac disease, avoidance of the triggering agent allows at least partial resolution of the conditions and this leads many to classify coeliac disease as a discrete inflammatory disorder.

Clinical features

The classical features of coeliac disease when first described were of cachexia, oedema, gross vitamin deficiency and anaemia, but these are now fortunately very rare. The most common age of presentation is in those under 5 years of age, but there is also a peak in

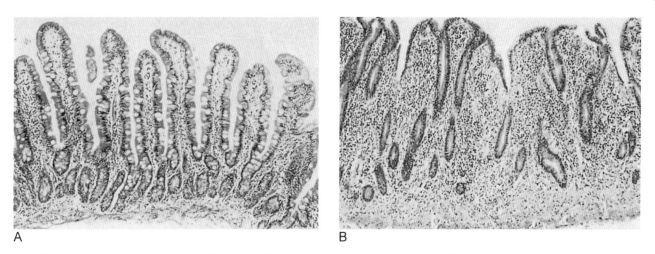

Fig. 39 The histological changes seen in the small bowel mucosa in coeliac disease. Note the partial or complete loss of the normal villous structure, with marked inflammatory cell infiltrate. (From Souhami RL, Moxham J 2002, Textbook of Medicine, 4th edn, Churchill Livingstone, Edinburgh.)

the third and fourth decades of life. There is an increased incidence of coeliac disease in patients with IgA deficiency (Ch. 4).

The most common features in childhood are

- poor energy
- failure to thrive
- diarrhoea
- anaemia.

The presentation, therefore, tends to be with non-specific symptoms and the diagnosis is usually suspected when investigation reveals anaemia with either iron or folate deficiency. Diarrhoea is more common in adults than children, but constipation may be a feature and many patients present with aphthous ulcers. Patients may have an itchy rash called **dermatitis herpetiformis** (see below).

A major long-term concern is the increased risk of lymphoma. This is usually a T cell, non-Hodgkin's type localised within the small bowel. There is also a higher incidence of other gastrointestinal malignancies, including squamous cell carcinoma of the oesophagus. These increased risks should be borne in mind in patients with coeliac disease who develop any unusual change in gastrointestinal symptoms. It is thought, however, that earlier diagnosis and better adherence to a gluten-free diet has reduced the incidence of malignancy.

Investigation

Diagnosis is still dependent on demonstrating abnormal villous architecture on small bowel biopsy. Previously it was considered necessary to perform three biopsies: the first at presentation, the second after a period on a gluten-free diet and the third after reintroduction of gluten into the diet. The aim was to confirm that the changes initially resolve on gluten withdrawal, but deteriorate upon rechallenge. However, this is now considered excessive and the improved diagnostic performance of coeliac-associated autoantibodies (Ch. 12) means that most adults undergo only a single biopsy to confirm typical histological findings at presentation. Most centres would, however, recommend a second biopsy in children to confirm response to gluten exclusion.

A combination of coeliac antibodies is used. Formerly, **anti-gliadin** antibodies were used as screening tests with **anti-endomysial** antibody detection as a more specific confirmatory test. Anti-endomysial antibody tests commonly become negative when patients are adhering to a gluten-free diet. The more recent introduction of **anti-tissue transglutaminase** antibody detection has superseded anti-gliadin antibody detection in many centres. It is important to note that IgA class antibodies are detected in most laboratories and there is a risk that these may be *falsely negative* in patients with coeliac disease with IgA deficiency or in young children with poorly developed IgA responses. For that reason, it is occasionally necessary to request IgG class coeliac serology (which should be positive in such patients).

If biopsy shows subtotal villous atrophy, but serology is negative and there is no response to gluten exclusion, the possibilities of giardiasis and tropical sprue should be considered. Other laboratory findings in coeliac disease include anaemia, hypocalcaemia and vitamin deficiencies. The potential clinical consequences of these are indicated in Table 28.

Management

Management of coeliac disease is by strict gluten-free diet and, therefore, flour from barley, wheat and rye must be avoided. In practice, this means avoidance of

Table 28 Clinical and laboratory features of coeliac disease

Pathological feature	Related symptoms and signs
Iron, folate deficiency	Anaemia, malaise
Malabsorption	Diarrhoea, steatorrhoea, weight loss; in children: failure to thrive, delayed development
Hypoproteinaemia	Oedema
Vitamin D and calcium deficiency	Bone pains and muscle weakness
Vitamin K deficiency	Bleeding tendency/bruising
Vitamin A deficiency	Night blindness
Bowel distension	Abdominal pain and bloating

most breads, cakes and biscuits. Rice and maize can be used as substitutes. Gluten-free foods are available on prescription in the UK. Depending on the duration and severity of the condition before diagnosis, a range of element and vitamin supplements may be necessary, including iron, folic acid, calcium and vitamins B_{12}, A, D, E and K. Osteoporosis is a significant risk for all patients with coeliac disease and, therefore, regular DEXA (dual-energy X-ray absorptiometry) scanning is recommended.

Haematological disease

Autoimmune haemolytic anaemia

Autoimmune haemolytic anaemia (AIHA) is classified according to whether the anti-erythrocyte antibodies bind at 37°C (warm AIHA) or at room temperatures (cold AIHA).

Warm anti-erythrocyte antibodies. These are usually of the IgG class and they bind directly to red cells. They do not fix complement and cause red cell lysis nor do they directly cause agglutination, but by opsonising red cells these are cleared through the reticulo-endothelial system. Warm AIHA is most commonly idiopathic but may occur secondary to a number of conditions including SLE, common variable immunodeficiency and lymphoproliferative disorders (e.g. chronic lymphocytic leukaemia). The autoantibodies are polyclonal.

Cold anti-erythrocyte antibodies. These are usually of the IgM class and are described as *complete* because they do cause direct red cell agglutination. Cold antibodies are more common than warm and often cause few clinical problems. When cold antibodies are associated with:

- lymphoproliferative disease, they are monoclonal and cause cold haemagglutinin disease
- infectious mononucleosis, they have anti-i blood group specificity

- mycoplasma pneumonia, they have anti-I blood group specificity.

Clinical features

Warm AIHA may cause acute severe or a mild chronic anaemia. It may be associated with immune thrombocytopenia. Cold AIHA may also be asymptomatic or give rise to cold haemagglutinin disease. The idiopathic form occurs most commonly in the elderly. There may be episodic haemolysis on exposure to cold, with cyanosis and Raynaud-like symptoms. In between acute episodes, the haemoglobin may be normal.

Investigation

There is usually a mildly macrocytic anaemia (caused by reticulocytosis) and raised erythrocyte sedimentation rate. The blood film may show spherocytes and red cell aggregates (in cold antibody disease). The diagnostic test is the direct and indirect antiglobulin test (Fig. 40).

Management

In idiopathic warm AIHA, high-dose oral steroids (1 mg/kg daily) are often effective. Blood transfusion may be necessary during acute anaemia, and splenectomy may be required for those with recurrent attacks or those who are not responsive to steroids. In cold AIHA, avoidance of cold is essential and if transfusion is required during acute episodes, a blood warmer must be used. Steroids and splenectomy are usually not helpful in cold AIHA and cytotoxic therapy with chlorambucil or cyclophosphamide is often required.

Autoimmune neutropenia

Autoimmune neutropenia may occur in patients with autoimmune or malignant disorders or as an isolated phenomenon. The diagnosis is often suspected in patients with autoimmune disease and a low

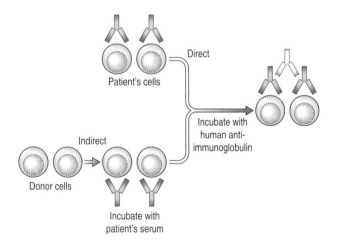

Fig. 40 The direct and indirect antiglobulin test.

neutrophil count; however, positive identification of anti-neutrophil antibodies is not routinely possible. This is because neutrophils have many Fc receptors on their cell surface and such non-specific immunoglobulin binding impairs the ability to distinguish specific Fab-mediated binding. Patients with significant neutropenia should, however, have a bone marrow examination to exclude alternative haematological diagnoses. Treatment with antibacterial and antifungal prophylaxis is usually recommended if the neutrophil count is < 0.5 $\times 10^9$/l. Injection of granulocyte colony-stimulating factor (G-CSF) may produce transitory rises in neutrophil count and prove helpful during periods of infection.

Immune thrombocytopenic purpura

Immune thrombocytopenic purpura is the most common cause of thrombocytopenia. Specific anti-platelet IgG binds to platelets and allows them to be phagocytosed and disposed of by the reticuloendothelial system. Most commonly, immune thrombocytopenia is idiopathic but it may be triggered by a preceding viral infection or occur as a complication of autoimmune or lymphoproliferative disorders.

Clinical features
The presenting feature is acute onset of purpura, bruising and often nose bleeds. The peak age of onset is between 2 and 5 years, when children suffer frequent viral infections. Because of the purpura, the child may initially be suspected of suffering from meningococcal septicaemia. Platelet count is usually $< 50 \times 10^9$/l at presentation.

Investigation
In idiopathic cases, it is often possible to demonstrate platelet-associated antibodies and some platelets may appear abnormally large. Other features would reflect underlying autoimmune/malignant conditions if present.

Management
In childhood, immune thrombocytopenic purpura is usually self-limiting and treatment is only necessary if bleeding is a significant problem. When required, treatment of both children and adults is initially with high-dose oral prednisolone (1 mg/kg daily). Intravenous methylprednisolone may be more rapidly effective. Splenectomy is rarely required or desirable in children; however, it is beneficial in 50–75% of adults who require long-term maintenance steroids. High-dose intravenous immunoglobulin (ivIg) can help to maintain an acceptable platelet count. The mechanism of action is thought to be by blockade of Fc receptors on macrophages. A similar clinical effect is seen in

Rhesus-positive individuals with immune thrombocytopenia after injection of anti-D immunoglobulin.

Pernicious anaemia

Pernicious anaemia causes deficiency of vitamin B_{12} and, therefore, a megaloblastic anaemia. It can occur at any age but is more common in the elderly. Affected people are not necessarily anaemic, but a macrocytosis is expected. Serum B_{12} levels are low and a number of autoantibodies are detected. Anti-gastric parietal cell antibodies are found in 90% of patients. These autoantibodies are directed against the gastric H^+/K^+-ATPase. Other autoantibodies present, but not normally requested in clinical practice, include anti-intrinsic factor antibodies. These are of two types: one that binds to intrinsic factor preventing its binding to vitamin B_{12} and a second that blocks the absorption of the intrinsic factor–vitamin B_{12} complex in the terminal ileum. The **Schilling test** is the definitive diagnostic test for pernicious anaemia, although it is seldom performed in clinical practice. It involves the administration of a loading dose of parenteral vitamin B_{12} to saturate plasma and liver binding sites followed by the oral administration of radioactively labelled vitamin B_{12} with or without intrinsic factor. The pattern of excretion of the radiolabelled vitamin B_{12} identifies whether there is malabsorption of the vitamin, correctable by the administration of intrinsic factor, consistent with pernicious anaemia. Treatment of pernicious anaemia is by monthly intramuscular injections of vitamin B_{12} either as hydroxocobalamin or cyanocobalamin.

Pernicious anaemia and autoimmune thyroid disease commonly coexist and, therefore, it is important to consider the possibility of incipient thyroid disease in patients with pernicious anaemia, especially those in whom fatigue is a prominent symptom. The most serious complication of the condition is *subacute combined degeneration* of the spinal cord in which the lateral and posterior columns of the cord degenerate along with the development of a peripheral neuropathy. Typical symptoms of this degeneration include numbness or painful hands and feet, which may progress to the development of a paraparesis. Neurological complications may not respond to B_{12}-replacement therapy.

Kidney disease: glomerulonephritis

Inflammation of the glomerulus is an important cause of acute renal disease and has many causes. Patients often present with rapidly progressive glomerulonephritis (RPGN) and in such circumstances it is essential to consider the potential immunological causes including the non-organ-specific immune diseases such as Wegener's granulomatosis, microscopic polyarteritis, SLE and also

Goodpasture's syndrome. Goodpasture's syndrome (anti-glomerular basement membrane (anti-GBM) disease) typically presents with pulmonary haemorrhage and/or RPGN. Unlike the relapsing and remitting course of many of the vasculitides, this is typically a monophasic illness that is caused by primary autoantibodies directed against the α_3-chain of type IV collagen (in the glomerular basement membrane). These autoantibodies bind to both glomerular and alveolar basement membrane and cause damage by a type II hypersensitivity mechanism (Ch. 2). As discussed in Chapter 12, it is, therefore, essential that any patient presenting with RPGN should have serological assessment at presentation and, as the level of anti-GBM appears to correlate with disease activity, also during treatment. Therapy in Goodpasture's syndrome usually includes plasmapheresis to remove the primary autoantibodies, cytotoxic therapy and renal-replacement therapy (usually dialysis) if required.

Liver disease

Autoimmune hepatitis

Autoimmune hepatitis is a disorder that mainly affects young women and there is a strong genetic association with HLA-B8, HLA-DR3 and HLA-DR4. Approximately 60% of patients present with an acute hepatitic illness that is very similar to acute viral hepatitis and the remainder manifest a more insidious onset of malaise, fatigue and jaundice, indicating underlying cirrhosis. Systemic symptoms are also common, with arthralgia, autoimmune thyroid disease, haemolytic anaemia and vitiligo.

Diagnosis rests on the exclusion of other causes of hepatitis (viral, drug, toxic, metabolic, etc.) and liver biopsy, findings of piecemeal necrosis with a lymphocytic infiltrate of T and B cells. Later in the disease, a cirrhotic pattern emerges. There is a marked elevation of hepatic transaminases, a marked polyclonal elevation of serum immunoglobulins and the detection of serum autoantibodies. Typically, antibodies are detected against nuclear material, double-stranded (ds) DNA, smooth muscle, liver-kidney microsomes (LKM) and mitochondria, and the pattern of autoantibodies is helpful in clinical classification of the subtypes. There are two main subtypes of autoimmune hepatitis, types 1 and 2.

Type 1. This presents in the fourth or fifth decade of life and 90% of those affected are female. It is common to have extrahepatic symptoms and a range of autoantibodies are detected including anti-nuclear, anti-dsDNA and anti-smooth muscle antibodies. There is also hypergammaglobulinaemia. This was formerly known as **lupoid hepatitis**. The condition responds well to oral corticosteroids, often used in combination with azathioprine as a steroid-sparing agent. Longitudinal monitoring of liver function is important and repeat liver biopsy can be helpful in determining whether treatment can be withdrawn. Relapse is, however, common and requires reintroduction of therapy. The 10-year survival is approximately 60%.

Type 2a. This occurs in childhood in approximately 50% of those affected and is typically associated with high-titre anti-LKM antibodies. The sex ratio is approximately equal and type 2a autoimmune hepatitis is frequently associated with extrahepatic symptoms.

Type 2b. This is associated with hepatitis C infection, affects the sexes equally and typically occurs in middle-aged and older age groups. There are no associated extrahepatic autoimmune features but anti-LKM1 antibodies are detected, probably on the basis that certain hepatitis C viral antigens cross-react with the P450 cytochromes. Treatment of this subtype is targeted antiviral therapy with interferon-α and/or other antiviral agents.

Primary biliary cirrhosis

Primary biliary cirrhosis is a condition that chiefly affects middle-aged and older women; less than 10% of affected individuals are male. The condition causes a slow progressive destruction of the intrahepatic bile ducts and, therefore, cirrhosis is not typically a feature at presentation. This may develop later in the disease or in a subset of patients with overlapping features of chronic active hepatitis. There is a strong genetic link to HLA-DR8 and the presence of serum autoantibodies directed against components of mitochondria is very helpful in diagnosis.

With the widespread availability of autoantibody detection and biochemical analysis, many patients are diagnosed early, before developing symptoms. Early symptoms, when they occur, include generalised itch and arthralgia and there is a progressive development of jaundice and skin pigmentation. On examination, periorbital xanthelasma are common and there may be features of other autoimmune disorders. Primary biliary cirrhosis is strongly associated with Sjögren's syndrome, thyroid disease, cryptogenic fibrosing alveolitis, CREST syndrome (calcinosis, Raynaud's phenomenon, oesophageal dysfunction, sclerodactyly and telangectasia) and renal tubular acidosis.

Diagnosis rests on a typical clinical picture, supported by the detection of anti-M2 mitochondrial autoantibodies and the development of an *obstructive pattern* of liver function tests (raised alkaline phosphatase and gamma-glutaryltransferase). There is commonly a polyclonal increase in total serum IgM and other autoantibody patterns may be detected, depending on the spectrum of autoimmune disease in the individual patient. Liver biopsy provides the definitive diagnostic test. The detection of anti-mitochondrial antibodies (anti-M2) in an otherwise healthy individual with normal liver function tests should indicate to the clinician that the patient is at increased risk of developing primary biliary cirrhosis in later life, and that annual monitoring of liver function is indicated, but it does not of itself indicate a diagnosis of primary biliary cirrhosis at that time.

Management is largely supportive. Oral ursodeoxycholic acid may reduce itch as it chelates retained bile acids. Similarly, cholestyramine may be helpful. Supplementation of fat-soluble vitamins is important where malabsorption has developed. Immunosuppressive therapy has no role to play, corticosteroids being associated with an increased risk of osteoporosis. Once symptomatic, the average lifespan is approximately 6 years and hence liver transplantation is considered when life expectancy is estimated at between 12 and 18 months.

Nervous system

Guillain–Barré syndrome

Guillain–Barré syndrome is an acute demyelinating, mainly motor, neuropathy that usually occurs 1–3 weeks after infection, either of the upper respiratory or gastrointestinal tracts. *Campylobacter jejuni* has been specifically implicated. Initial symptoms are typically distal paraesthesia and weakness. However, the demyelination quickly ascends and may involve the cranial nerves; bulbar weakness and diaphragmatic involvement are common and patients often require ventilation support in the most severe phase of the illness. Circulating autoantibodies against membrane gangliosides (anti-GM1) are detectable in serum but are not thought to be primarily pathogenic. Indirect evidence that this is an autoimmune disorder comes from the fact that early plasma exchange or treatments with high-dose ivIg are both effective therapies. The majority of patients (80–90%) make a full recovery over a period of months.

Chronic inflammatory demyelinating polyneuropathy

Chronic inflammatory demyelinating polyneuropathy is a related condition that has a more chronic course and may require repeated course of therapy with high-dose ivIg.

Myasthenia gravis

Myasthenia gravis is a condition characterised by fatiguable weakness of skeletal muscle. Women are affected twice as often as men and the clinical presentation is usually in early adult life. There is an association with HLA-A1, HLA-B8 and HLA-DR3 in younger patients

Symptoms may be limited in distribution (e.g. weakness of external ocular muscles) or more generalised, involving bulbar, neck, respiratory and shoulder and pelvic girdle muscles. In approximately 10% of those affected, the condition remains limited to ocular muscles. Patients may, therefore, complain of blurred vision—sometimes only at the extremes of gaze—difficulties with speech or swallowing, progressive 'breathlessness' or difficulty lifting or standing. The characteristic fatiguability on repetitive or sustained movement underpins the diagnostic techniques of asking the patient to maintain an upward gaze and observing for increasing ptosis. Similarly, testing the full range of ocular movements may reveal diplopia. It is common for intercurrent illnesses such as respiratory infection to trigger a relapse in symptoms.

There is a strong association of myasthenia gravis with thymic abnormalities: thymoma is common in the older patients and thymic hyperplasia in the younger patients.

The underlying aetiology is interruption of the normal neuromuscular signalling by **anti-acetylcholine receptor antibodies** (Fig. 41). These autoantibodies are detectable in the serum of approximately 90% of patients with systemic myasthenia gravis and approximately 55% of patients with ocular myasthenia gravis. Detection of serum autoantibodies to striated muscle is strongly associated with the presence of thymoma.

Autoantibody detection is, therefore, diagnostically helpful; however, the definitive test in patient suspected of myasthenia gravis is the **Tensilon test**. This involves intravenous injection of edrophonium, a short-acting anticholinesterase drug. A dose of 5–10 mg (after a test dose of 1–2 mg) should result in an improvement of muscle weakness. The test should only be undertaken by an expert as there are risks to the patient and the interpretation of the result can be difficult.

All patients with myasthenia gravis should be investigated for the presence of thymoma, as this may be malignant and require removal. Thymectomy often results in a symptomatic improvement, particularly if undertaken early in the course of the disease.

The principles of management include oral administration of long-acting anticholinesterase drugs (e.g. pyridostigmine). Immunosuppressive agents including

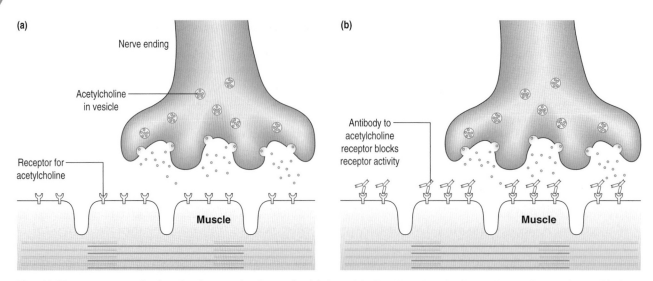

(a)

Nerve ending

Acetylcholine
in vesicle

Receptor for
acetylcholine

Muscle

(b)

Antibody to
acetylcholine
receptor blocks
receptor activity

Muscle

Fig. 41 The neuromuscular junction in myasthenia gravis. (a) Acetylcholine receptors in the postsynaptic membrane bind acetylcholine during neurotransmission. (b) In myasthenia gravis, anti-acetylcholine receptor antibodies bind to the endplate and cause receptor blockade and secondary damage and recycling of the receptor, impairing neuromuscular signalling.

prednisolone, azathioprine and methotrexate may be useful in long-term management, while plasma exchange and high-dose ivIg have been demonstrated to be helpful in acute myasthenic crisis.

Lambert–Eaton myasthenic syndrome

LEMS results from a rare defect of neuromuscular signalling and is clinically characterised by fatiguable muscle weakness. Typically, there is proximal limb weakness and occasionally ptosis, but bulbar muscles are spared. There may be signs of autonomic dysfunction of the parasympathetic system, causing dry mouth and impotence. A clinical sign useful in differentiating myasthenia gravis from LEMS is that in the former tendon reflexes are present/brisk whereas in LEMS they are usually absent. However, in LEMS, a brief maintained isometric contraction can restore reflexes: so-called post-tetanic potentiation.

In LEMS, the neuromuscular junction is defective in that there is a reduced number of voltage-gated calcium channels, which causes a reduction in acetylcholine release and impaired signalling. The reduction in these channels is mediated by the presence of anti-voltage-gated calcium channel autoantibodies (Fig. 42). As in myasthenia gravis, these are primary or disease-causing autoantibodies and they provide for very specific diagnostic tests.

Approximately 50% of those with LEMS are affected by a paraneoplastic phenomenon associated with small cell carcinoma of the lung; in the remaining 50%, LEMS appears to be a primary autoimmune condition. The latter form occurs in both adults and children and is associated with HLA-B8.

In treatment of the paraneoplastic form of LEMS, chemotherapy for the tumour is the first priority and this may relieve symptoms. Prednisolone and azathioprine are useful in both forms as is the use of guanidine and 3,4-aminopyridine, both of which increase the release of acetylcholine from the presynaptic terminal.

Paraneoplastic syndromes

Carcinoma of the breast or ovaries is in rare cases associated with a degenerative cerebellar syndrome. Symptoms and signs are those typical of cerebellar

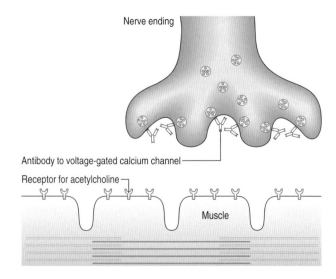

Nerve ending

Antibody to voltage-gated calcium channel

Receptor for acetylcholine

Muscle

Fig. 42 The neuromuscular junction in Lambert–Eaton myasthenic syndrome (LEMS). Antibodies block the voltage-gated calcium channels in the presynaptic membrane, preventing the release of acetylcholine. This results in impaired neuromuscular signalling.

disease and in some cases the cerebellar syndrome may be the presenting feature, requiring the doctor to seek out underlying malignancy. Two main types of autoantibody are associated with carcinoma of the breast: anti-Yo antibodies are directed against cerebellar Purkinje cells and a specific anti-neuronal nuclear antibody (anti-Ri) binds to more widely distributed autoantigens and is associated with ataxia and myoclonus.

Patients with small cell carcinoma of the lung and a paraneoplastic sensory neuropathy have a different type of anti-neuronal cell antibody: anti-Hu.

All these autoantibodies are detectable in serum and should form part of the investigation of otherwise unexplained neurological syndromes.

Skin conditions

There are a number of skin conditions in which immune depositions can be detected in the skin (Fig. 43).

Bullous pemphigoid

Bullous pemphigoid is a relatively common disease of the elderly and is characterised by the development of subepidermal blisters. The skin may initially appear urticarial or eczematous with itchy papules. Once blisters appear, these are tense and heal after rupture. The mucous membranes are spared in the majority of patients. Direct immunofluorescence indicates a linear deposition of IgG and C3 along the lamina lucida of the basement membrane. Treatment is with oral prednisolone and azathioprine.

Dermatitis herpetiformis

Dermatitis herpetiformis also causes chronic, intensely itchy subepidermal blistering. Lesions typically occur in crops over extensor surfaces, including the elbows, knees and buttocks. There is a close association with gluten-sensitive enteropathy (coeliac disease) and dermatitis herpetiformis may be the presenting feature of this condition. Skin biopsy indicates granular deposition of IgA in the dermal papillae of unaffected skin. Once a diagnosis of dermatitis herpetiformis is made, it is essential to investigate further for coeliac disease, both by serology (Ch. 12) and jejunal biopsy. A gluten-free diet is helpful in most patients, but some will require additional treatment with dapsone.

Pemphigus vulgaris

Pemphigus vulgaris is a rare blistering disorder that typically affects middle-aged men and Ashkenazi Jews. It is associated with HLA-A10 and also HLA-DR4/DQw3 or HLA-DR6/DQw1. It usually presents with non-healing erosions of the mucous membranes and, subsequently, flaccid blisters appear on the skin. The characteristic clinical sign (Nikolsky's sign) is that lateral pressure causes sloughing of existing blisters and will generate new blisters when applied to apparently unaffected skin. The underlying pathology is **acantholysis** or separation of keratinocytes in the epidermis. Direct immunofluorescence of snap-frozen skin biopsy indicates deposition of IgG and C3 in a chicken-wire pattern within the epidermis (Fig. 43). Pemphigus vulgaris is an almost invariably fatal condition, with fluid loss and super infection of erosions developing similar to those seen in a patient with severe burns. Treatment is with high-dose corticosteroids, usually with azathioprine or another steroid-sparing agent. Plasmapheresis appears to be ineffective; however, high-dose ivIg has been used with some success.

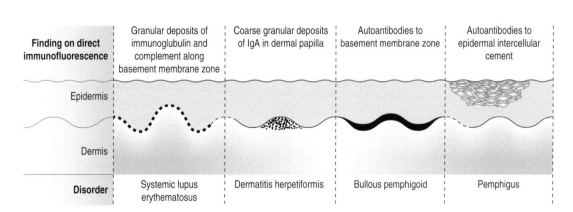

Finding on direct immunofluorescence	Granular deposits of immunoglubulin and complement along basement membrane zone	Coarse granular deposits of IgA in dermal papilla	Autoantibodies to basement membrane zone	Autoantibodies to epidermal intercellular cement
Epidermis				
Dermis				
Disorder	Systemic lupus erythematosus	Dermatitis herpetiformis	Bullous pemphigoid	Pemphigus

Fig. 43 Immune deposition in skin diseases.

Self-assessment: questions

Multiple choice questions

1. The following antibody is a *primary* auto-antibody:
   a. Anti-nuclear antibody
   b. Anti-double-stranded DNA antibody
   c. Anti-acetylcholine receptor antibody
   d. Anti-mitochondrial antibody
   e. Anti-voltage-gated calcium channel antibody

2. Primary biliary cirrhosis is associated with HLA type:
   a. DR2
   b. DR4
   c. DR5
   d. DR6
   e. DR8

3. Myasthenia gravis is associated with HLA:
   a. A1, B8, DR3
   b. DR2, B7
   c. B44, B15
   d. DR4
   e. B27

4. Pemphigus vulgaris is associated with which of the following features?
   a. Separation of the dermal–epidermal junction
   b. Complement deposition at the dermal–epidermal junction
   c. Autoantibodies to intracellular cement
   d. Mucosal ulceration
   e. Tense skin blisters

5. The following biochemical abnormalities would be expected in Addison's disease:
   a. Hypernatraemia
   b. Hyperkalaemia
   c. Hypercalcaemia
   d. Hyperglycaemia
   e. Hyperuricaemia

6. Type 1 polyglandular syndrome is characterised by:
   a. Autosomal dominant inheritance
   b. Mucosal candidiasis
   c. Vitiligo
   d. Hyperparathyroidism
   e. Hyperthyroidism

7. The lamina propria of the small bowel in coeliac disease is infiltrated by:
   a. Neutrophils
   b. CD4+ T cells
   c. CD8+ T cells
   d. B cells
   e. Eosinophils

Case history questions

History 1

A 24-year-old woman is referred with symptoms of weight loss and recurrent chest infections. She reports occasional diarrhoea only. On examination she is mildly anaemic but there are no other remarkable findings. You undertake a number of investigations the results of which are given in Table 29.

Table 29 Investigation results in case history 1

Parameter	Value	Normal range
Haemoglobin (g/l)	91	130–180
Mean cell volume (fl)	70	76–100
Platelets (× 10⁹/l)	239	150–450
Erythrocyte sedimentation rate (mm/h)	5	—
C-reactive protein (mg/l)	14	0–10
Total IgE (kU/l)	26	0–130
Food allergy screen	Negative	—
IgG (g/l)	10.3	7–16
IgA (g/l)	< 0.05	0.8–4.7
IgM (g/l)	1.28	0.5–3.0
Anti-nuclear antibody (IgG)	Negative	
Anti-mitochondrial antibody (IgG)	Negative	
Anti-endomysial antibody (IgA)	Negative	
Anti-tissue transglutaminase antibody (IgA)	Negative	

1. What is the significance of these results?
2. What further investigations would you advise?
3. What would be the appropriate treatment?

History 2

A 34-year-old doctor attends the immunology clinic because of recurrent oral candidiasis. This has on occasions responded to oral antifungal agents but is now persistent. She has a history of diabetes that is well controlled by insulin and has also had hypoparathyroidism since childhood. On examination, she has marked candidal growth in the mouth and appears to have fungal infection of the great toe nails. A number of investigations are undertaken to look for evidence of primary immunodeficiency (Table 30).

Table 30 Investigation results in case history 2

Parameter	Value	Normal range
Haemoglobin (g/l)	145	130–180
Platelets ($\times 10^9$/l)	285	150–450
Erythrocyte sedimentation rate (mm/h)	18	
C-reactive protein (mg/l)	8	0–10
IgG (g/l)	15.4	7–16
IgA (g/l)	2.3	0.8–4.7
IgM (g/l)	1.2	0.5–3.0
Anti-nuclear antibody (IgG)	Negative	
Lymphocyte subset analysis	Normal	

1. How would you interpret these results?
2. Are you able to reassure the patient regarding her immune function?
3. Could there be a link between her endocrine disorder and her recurrent infection?

Data interpretation

1. In a patient with Graves' disease, which of the following patterns of thyroid function test would you expect? (thyroid-stimulating hormone (TSH) normal range is 0.5–5.0 mU/l; free thyroxine normal range is 7–20 pmol/l).

   a. TSH > 50 mU/l; free thyroxine 2 pmol/l
   b. TSH < 0.1 mU/l; free thyroxine 40 pmol/l
   c. TSH 1.0 mU/l; free thyroxine 6 pmol/l
   d. TSH 10 mU/l; free thyroxine 7 pmol/l
   e. TSH 3.5 mU/l; free thyroxine 10 pmol/l

Self-assessment: answers

Multiple choice answers

1. a. **False.** Anti-nuclear antibodies are secondary autoantibodies; these do not directly cause disease but occur as part of an autoimmune process; may be associated with a specific disease, in this case systemic lupus erythematosus and other connective tissue diseases.
   b. **False.** Anti-double-stranded DNA is associated with autoimmune hepatitis.
   c. **True.** Anti-acetylcholine receptor antibodies are primary autoantibodies in that they directly interfere with neuromuscular signal transmission to cause the symptoms of myasthenia gravis.
   d. **False.** Anti-mitochondrial antibodies are secondary autoantibodies associated with primary biliary cirrhosis.
   e. **True.** The anti-voltage-gated calcium channel antibody is a primary antibody causing Lambert–Eaton myasthenic syndrome.

2. a. **False.**
   b. **False.**
   c. **False.**
   d. **False.**
   e. **True.** There is a strong genetic link to HLA-DR8.

3. a. **True**. There is an association with HLA-A1, HLA-B8 and HLA-DR3 in younger patients.
   b. **False.**
   c. **False.**
   d. **False.**
   e. **False.**

4. a. **False.** This is a feature of bullous pemphigoid.
   b. **False.** This occurs in a number of other skin conditions.
   c. **True.** These give a characteristic appearance on direct immunofluorescent examination of biopsy tissue.
   d. **True.** Mucosal ulceration is common.
   e. **False.** Blisters are not typically tense.

5. a. **False.** Hyponatraemia is a feature of Addison's disease.
   b. **True.** Hyperkalaemia is a feature of Addison's disease.
   c. **True.** Hypercalcaemia is a feature of Addison's disease.

d. **False.** Hypoglycaemia related to a lack of glucocorticoid is typical.
   e. **False.**

6. a. **False.** It is inherited in an autosomal recessive pattern.
   b. **True.** Mucosal candidiasis is a feature.
   c. **True.** Vitiligo may occur.
   d. **True.** Hypoparathyroidism may occur.
   e. **False.** This syndrome is characterised by multiple endocrine gland failure.

7. a. **False.** However, neutrophils will be part of the chronic inflammatory infiltrate that occurs as a result of damage to the small bowel mucosal architecture.
   b. **True.** Gliadin fraction of gluten is thought to activate CD4$^+$ T cells in the lamina propria layer of the small bowel mucosa.
   c. **False.**
   d. **False.**
   e. **False.** Eosinophils are involved in host defences against helminth infection in the gut.

Case history answers

History 1

1. The results indicate that this patient has a microcytic anaemia and is IgA deficient. Food allergy screening is negative, as is coeliac-associated serology. The history of recurrent infections suggests that the IgA deficiency might be significant. The cause of the anaemia is not clear; however, there is an association between coeliac disease and IgA deficiency and, in such patients, IgA autoantibodies may be falsely negative. These results, therefore, do not exclude coeliac disease as the cause of her symptoms.
2. Testing should be undertaken for IgG anti-endomysial antibodies and if these are positive, referral should be made to a gastroenterologist for jejunal biopsy. She needs a full nutritional assessment to look for evidence of malabsorption of other essential elements and vitamins. In view of the IgA deficiency identified in her investigations, measurement of IgG subclasses and vaccine-specific antibody levels should be considered along with test immunisation. Computed tomography of the chest may be appropriate if the further history suggests

recurrent chest infection and structural lung damage.

3. If coeliac disease is confirmed, commencement of a gluten-free diet is the mainstay of treatment. Element and vitamin supplementation may be needed depending on the outcome of further investigation. If she has significant IgG subclass deficiency and failure to respond to immunisation, intravenous immunoglobulin therapy may be indicated to prevent recurrent chest infection (Ch. 4).

History 2

1. These results show no significant abnormality. Total immunoglobulins and lymphocyte subsets are all normal.

2. No, the history is suggestive of chronic mucocutaneous candidiasis and, therefore, T cell proliferative responses to *Candida* spp. must be assessed. In this case, these were demonstrated to be abnormally low, consistent with a diagnosis of chronic mucocutaneous candidiasis.

3. Given the history of insulin-dependent diabetes and hypoparathyroidism, the possibility of type 1 polyglandular syndrome (autoimmune polyendocrinopathy candidiasis ectodermal dysplasia: APCED) should be considered. The patient should be assessed for the presence of autoantibodies against adrenal, ovarian and thyroid antigens as well as having functional biochemical studies to assess these organs.

Data interpretation

1. a. This pattern is typical of primary hypothyroidism not Graves' disease.
   b. This pattern would be consistent with hyperthyroidism; Graves' disease being the classical cause.
   c. This pattern is suggestive of secondary hypothyroidism not Graves' disease, as TSH has not risen as expected with a low thyroxine level. The possibility of pituitary failure should be considered.
   d. This pattern suggests compensated hypothyroidism not Graves' disease; the TSH has risen to compensate for falling thyroxine production.
   e. These results are normal.

Inflammatory arthritis and connective tissue disorders

Chapter overview

Inflammatory arthritis and connective tissue disorders encompass a wide range of conditions that are characterised by inflammation affecting the joints, synovial tissue, cartilage, bone as well as muscle, pleura, cardiac and many other tissues. These disorders have many features in common, but each has its own characteristic presentations, and long-term complications. The prognosis in each of the conditions can be quite different and, therefore, it is important to differentiate them early in their presentation so that accurate diagnostic and prognostic advice can be given and appropriate treatment commenced where necessary. Use of specialist investigations, including autoimmune serology, can be very helpful in distinguishing each condition; however, it is important to emphasise at the outset that diagnosis of inflammatory arthritis or connective tissue disorders must be based on careful overall clinical assessment.

7.1 Introduction

Learning objectives

You should:
- be familiar with the range of clinical conditions known as inflammatory arthritis or connective tissue disorders
- know the factors that can give rise to joint pains
- be aware of significant other features to look for in a history
- know the typical laboratory and radiological features of each condition.

The musculoskeletal system comprises all the bones and associated voluntary muscles while the 'connective tissues' comprise tendons, ligaments, joints and their associated soft tissues. The conditions described in this chapter are truly multisystem disorders because, while their main impact is on the joints and soft tissues, they may have very significant effects on other organs. The extent of 'extra-articular disease' can be very important prognostically.

The patient with joint pains

There is a very wide range of potential factors in the history that may contribute to a patient presenting with pain or stiffness of the musculoskeletal system. These include age, gender, ethnicity and family history. Social factors, including occupation, hobbies and recent activity, are important not only in identifying potential causes for symptoms but also in assessing the impact of symptoms on functional capacity. A careful drug history may identify symptom-triggering factors (some antibiotics, steroid withdrawal, etc.) as well as indicate the current level of analgesic requirement. Past medical history is very important, particularly to identify any previous similar episodes or other conditions known to be associated with musculoskeletal complications (e.g. inflammatory bowel disease, psoriasis, etc.). Recent infection can be an important historical feature, for example

- streptococcal sore throat preceding episodes of rheumatic fever
- a triad of urethritis, arthritis and iritis indicating Reiter's syndrome
- gastrointestinal or sexually transmitted infection preceding a reactive arthritis.

The key historical features will be highlighted under each condition (below).

Physical examination

The physical examination is a vital and informative aspect of the patient's assessment and begins as soon as the patient enters the consulting room. The **GALS screen**, the visual inspection of *g*ait, *a*rms, *l*egs and *s*pine, is a useful strategy for identifying locomotor abnormality. The patient is observed walking, asked to demonstrate a full range of movements of arms and legs and finally the spine is observed and the full range of movement established. General assessment of the limbs for their position and muscle bulk is important. Prior to examining specific joints, it is essential to establish which are painful and to ensure that examination is appropriately gentle.

Patients complain of joint pain (**arthralgia**) but examination must establish whether there is also joint swelling and evidence of inflammatory joint disease (**arthritis**). Joint swelling may be caused by

- synovitis (usually a soft, warm, tender swelling)
- effusion (fluctuant swelling)
- bony overgrowth (hard swelling).

It is essential to establish the pattern of joints affected by any apparent abnormality. Are the small joints of the hands and feet affected symmetrically or asymmetrically? Alternatively, are the central joints (spine, sacroiliac, knees and ankles affected)? The distribution of clinical signs can give important clues to the underlying aetiology and will also be important in determining the nature and extent of disability caused by the condition.

In addition to evidence of acute swelling, examination of the joints should include an assessment of range of movement, tenderness, evidence of deformity or palpable capsular thickening. General examination is also essential, for example to look for signs of anaemia, iritis, dry eyes/mouth, oral ulceration or skin rash, as well as a careful examination of the other major systems to establish any evidence of coexistent pathology or extra-articular disease.

Diagnosis

Diagnosis of connective tissues diseases is based on an overall clinical assessment of the history, examination, including the results of imaging and laboratory investigations. Laboratory investigations can help to classify subtypes of connective tissue diseases, but the results should only be interpreted in the light of the individual patient's clinical features. The American College of Rheumatology has produced diagnostic criteria for some of the connective tissue disorders (Tables 31 and 32, see below). While originally produced for the definition and categorisation of research studies, these criteria are useful aids to diagnosis, particularly where individual patients have features of more than one of the classical conditions. It is, however, important to remember that, in general, patients may not fit classification systems exactly and these diagnostic criteria should not be rigidly applied in clinical practice.

7.2 Inflammatory arthritis: rheumatoid arthritis

Learning objectives

You should:
- know the common presenting features of rheumatoid arthritis
- know the typical laboratory and radiological features
- be aware of the potential long-term complications
- be familiar with commonly used treatments.

Rheumatoid arthritis (RA) is a condition of unknown aetiology that causes a symmetrical, peripheral inflammatory arthritis (Table 31).

Table 31 The American College of Rheumatology criteria for the classification of rheumatoid arthritis[a]

Signs	Symptoms
1. Morning stiffness	Duration > 1 hour
2. Arthritis of three or more joint areas[b]	Soft tissue swelling or effusion
3. Arthritis of hand joints	Wrist, metacarpophalangeal joints, or proximal interphalangeal joints
4. Symmetric arthritis[b]	At least one area
5. Rheumatoid nodules	As observed by a physician
6. Serum rheumatoid factor	As assessed by a method positive in < 5% of control people
7. Radiographic changes	As seen on anteroposterior films of wrists and hands

[a]Diagnosis requires four out of seven of the criteria. The joint symptoms or signs must be continuous for at least 6 weeks for criteria 1 to 4.
[b]Possible areas: proximal interphalangeal joints, metacarpophalangeal joints, wrist, elbow, knee, ankle, metatarsophalangeal joints (observed by a physician).

Table 32 American College of Rheumatology criteria for the diagnosis of systemic lupus erythematosus[a]

Criterion	Definition
1. Malar rash	Fixed erythema, flat or raised, over the malar eminences, tending to spare the nasolabial folds
2. Discoid rash	Erythematous raised patches with adherent keratotic scaling and follicular plugging; atrophic scarring may occur in older lesions
3. Photosensitivity	Skin rash as a result of unusual reaction to sunlight, by patient history or physician observation
4. Oral ulcers	Oral or nasopharyngeal ulceration, usually painless, observed by physician
5. Arthritis	Non-erosive arthritis involving two or more peripheral joints, characterised by tenderness, swelling or effusion
6. Serositis	(a) Pleuritis (convincing history of pleuritic pain or rubbing heard by a physician or evidence of pleural effusion) or (b) pericarditis (documented by electrocardiograph, rub or evidence of pericardial effusion)
7. Renal disorder	(a) Persistent proteinuria > 0.5 g/day (or > 3+ if quantification not performed) or (b) cellular casts (may be red cell, haemoglobin, granular, tubular or mixed)
8. Neurological disorder	(a) Seizures in the absence of offending drugs or known metabolic derangements (e.g. uraemia, ketoacidosis or electrolyte imbalance) or (b) psychosis in the absence of offending drugs or known metabolic derangements (e.g. uraemia, ketoacidosis or electrolyte imbalance)
9. Haematological disorder	(a) Haemolytic anaemia, with reticulocytosis or (b) leukopenia ($< 4 \times 10^9$ cells/l total on two or more occasions) or (c) lyphopenia ($< 1.5 \times 10^9$ cells/l on two or more occasions) or (d) thrombocytopenia ($< 100 \times 10^9$ cells/l in the absence of offending drugs)
10. Immunological disorder	(a) Positive LE cell preparation or (b) anti-DNA (antibody to native DNA in abnormal titre) or (c) anti-Sm (presence of antibody to Sm nuclear antigen) or (d) false-positive serological test for syphilis known to be positive for at least 6 months and confirmed by *Treponema pallidum* immobilisation or fluorescent treponemal antibody absorption test
11. Anti-nuclear antibody	An abnormal titre of anti-nuclear antibody by immunofluorescence or an equivalent assay at any point in time and in the absence of drugs known to be associated with 'drug-induced lupus' syndrome

[a]A person shall be said to have systemic lupus erythematosus if any four or more of the 11 criteria are present, serially or simultaneously, during any interval of observation.

Clinical features

The small joints of the hand and feet (proximal interphalangeal, metacarpophalangeal, metatarsophalangeal) are most commonly affected (Fig. 44) followed by wrists, knees and ankles. RA is more common in women (female to male ratio 3:1) and tends to present in the third or fourth decade of life. Early morning stiffness (rather than pain) is a common presenting symptom and there may also be systemic symptoms of fever, weight loss and fatigue early in the presentation.

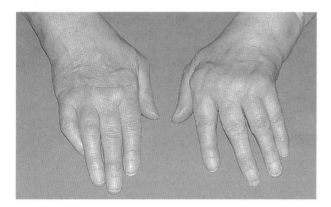

Fig. 44 Characteristic deformities of the hands in advanced rheumatoid arthritis. (From Forbes CD, Jackson WF 2003 Color Atlas and Text of Clinical Medicine, 3rd edn, Mosby, Edinburgh.)

On examination, in addition to the comments above, it is important to examine the extensor aspects of the forearm for **rheumatoid nodules**, which are subcutaneous, non-tender masses up to several centimetres in diameter. These occur in approximately 25% of patients and are associated with an increased incidence of extra-articular disease. It is also essential to note that RA is a systemic disease and that the majority of patients will experience extra-articular features at some stage during their illness. Clinical signs of extra-articular disease should also, therefore, be sought on examination.

Investigation

Mild anaemia is common and may be normochromic normocytic, reflecting disease activity, or hypochromic microcytic if iron deficiency has developed. Drug therapy and Felty's syndrome (see below) may also cause anaemia. Autoimmune haemolytic anaemia occurs rarely and folate deficiency can also occur (causing macrocytosis). The erythrocyte sedimentation rate (ESR) is typically elevated and is a good indicator of disease activity. The C-reactive protein (CRP) is also typically raised but falls much more quickly in response to therapy than the ESR and is, therefore, a very good test of response to therapy. The white cell count may be raised if the patient is taking oral steroids, but an important feature to look for in patients with RA is neutropenia, which may herald the onset of **Felty's syndrome** (see below). Immunological tests reveal a positive rheumatoid factor (RF) in approximately 75% (seropositive RA). This is a useful test in classification of patients, those who are seropositive for RA having a higher frequency of extra-articular complications than those with seronegative RA. There is, however, no benefit in serial RF measurements as the serum level of this autoantibody does not correlate with disease activity. Approximately 30% of patients with RA will have detectable anti-nuclear antibodies and those who develop secondary Sjögren's syndrome will have antibodies to the extractable nuclear antigens (ENA) Ro and La. There is often polyclonal hypergammaglobulinaemia (with a relative increase in total IgA levels compared with IgG and IgM) in RA, reflecting the chronic inflammatory process. Serum complement (C3 and C4) levels are usually elevated; however, if cryoglobulinaemia has developed, there will be the expected reduction in C4 levels with preservation of relatively normal C3 levels. RA is associated with HLA-DR4 and seven specific alleles are identified as having prognostic significance. It may, therefore, be helpful to identify their presence in patients with early RA.

Radiological findings in RA are very unhelpful in early disease and ultrasound scanning or magnetic resonance imaging of joints are much more sensitive indicators of disease at this stage. In established disease, plain radiographs of hands and feet may reveal increased soft tissue shadowing caused by joint effusion, periarticular osteopenia, narrowing of the joint space and erosion of bone at the joint margins (Fig. 45). As the disease progresses, chronic joint deformity will be demonstrable on radiographs.

Management

In assessing the need for therapy of any type, it is essential to differentiate between active inflammatory disease (synovitis, etc.) and damage that is the consequence of prior inflammatory activity. In general terms, inflammation should respond to drug therapy whereas established tissue damage will not.

Drug therapy

The aim of drug therapy is to reduce inflammation and, therefore, relieve pain and prevent joint damage. Historically, the management of RA was based on the minimum number of drugs at the lowest possible dose necessary to achieve effective control. The commonly used drugs include simple analgesics, salicylates and other non-steroidal anti-inflammatory drugs (NSAIDs). However, current evidence suggests that early intervention with disease-modifying drugs can improve long-term prognosis in RA. Disease-modifying antirheumatic drugs (DMARDS) include sulfasalazine, methotrexate,

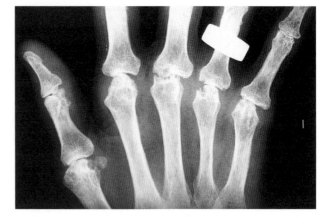

Fig. 45 Radiograph of the hands in rheumatoid arthritis indicating destruction of the metacarpophalangeal joints (MCP) with periarticular erosion and joint space narrowing. (From Forbes CD, Jackson WF 2003 Color Atlas and Text of Clinical Medicine, 3rd edn, Mosby, Edinburgh.)

penicillamine, gold and hydroxychloroquine and the new antitumour necrosis factor agents infliximab and etanercept. Examples of effective combination drug regimens include (a) methotrexate, hydroxychloroquine and salazopyrine or (b) methotrexate and infliximab. These drugs have a wide range of potential adverse effects and require careful clinical monitoring. These are discussed in Chapter 9.

Non-drug therapy

Drug therapy of RA is only one aspect of the management of the disease. It is essential that patients are well educated regarding the chronic nature of the condition both to ensure good compliance with therapy and enable realistic expectations. Physiotherapy and occupational therapy both have much to offer the patient with RA. Efforts focus on achieving an appropriate balance between rest and exercise, maximising joint mobility and maintaining functional ability. Local therapies, including application of heat and cold packs, may be used as well as splinting of joints when necessary.

Joint aspiration can be beneficial in relieving acute effusion. This is usually combined with local steroid injection. Ultimately, surgical joint replacement may become necessary to relieve irreversible joint damage.

Extra-articular manifestations

Systemic manifestations of RA occur to a variable extent in individual patients. When detected they may suggest a more severe condition warranting more aggressive therapy.

Rheumatoid nodules. Approximately 25% of patients with RA have rheumatoid nodules, which are thought to be a manifestation of previous vasculitic activity caused by immune complex deposition. In addition to the extensor surface of the forearm, they can be found in myocardium, pericardium, sclera, dura mater, spleen, larynx and synovium, where they may exert local effects.

Synovitis. Disease may extend from the joint to cause tendonitis and bursitis.

Muscle wasting. Although this is commonly secondary to disuse atrophy, it can also be caused by rheumatoid vasculitis.

Respiratory system. RA can affect the lungs, including pleural effusion, rheumatoid nodules, interstitial fibrosis and obliterative bronchiolitis.

Cardiac complications. These include pericarditis, effusion, myocarditis, rheumatoid granulomata and coronary arteritis. Most of these manifestations remain subclinical and are incidental postmortem findings; however, in patients with RA, the possibility of cardiac involvement must always be borne in mind.

Nervous system. Sensory or mixed sensory/motor peripheral neuropathy may occur in a classic glove and stocking distribution. Other causes of neuropathy in RA include nerve entrapment and mononeuritis multiplex. Cord damage may occur as a result of atlantoaxial subluxation or vertebral artery compression.

Amyloidosis. Although a common finding at postmortem, amyloidosis is rarely symptomatic. It may cause proteinuria, gastrointestinal malabsorption or organomegaly.

Vasculitis. This may manifest as mononeuritis multiplex, digital gangrene, subacute skin ulceration or a syndrome virtually indistinguishable from polyarteritis nodosa. A range of different vessel sizes is, therefore, affected in each presentation, from capillaries to large arteries.

The eye. Keratoconjunctivitis sicca, scleritis and uveitis can occur. Severe scleritis can cause scleromalacia, which can ultimately lead to perforation of the eye with extrusion of the vitreous (secleromalacia perforans). Drug side effects may also manifest in the eye and regular ophthalmologic assessment of patients with RA on therapy is advised.

Renal system. Although the kidney is usually not affected by RA, amyloidosis and gold therapy may cause proteinuria. More commonly, however, a tubulointerstitial nephropathy is induced by NSAIDs; therefore, renal function should be monitored during therapy.

Gastrointestinal system. Ulceration and haemorrhage may be secondary to NSAID or steroid use. The newer NSAIDs (COX-2 inhibitors) may reduce the frequency of this side effect. Gastrointestinal vasculitis may occur rarely and cause ischaemic colitis. Amyloidosis may cause malabsorption.

Felty's syndrome. The association of RA with splenomegaly and neutropenia is known as Felty's syndrome. Patients are usually seropositive but characteristically their synovitis may be relatively inactive. They are prone to recurrent bacterial infection and may develop lymphadenopathy with a form of lymphoma (large granulocytic lymphocytic lymphoma).

Sjögren's syndrome. This syndrome describes the development of keratoconjunctivitis sicca and/or xerostomia with RA or another connective tissue disease. There is usually the development of anti-Ro/anti-La antibodies, and patients with Sjögren's syndrome are at increased risk of developing lymphoma of the gut-associated lymphoid tissue.

Prognosis

RA is a potentially severe systemic disease; however, there is some heterogeneity in its clinical expression. Spontaneous remission may occur, usually within the first 2 years after onset. However, most patients have brief episodes of acute inflammatory activity interspersed with longer periods of remission or low-grade activity. A small percentage has a sustained progressive and severe form of the disease. A diagnosis of RA indicates significant morbidity and early mortality. Figures suggest that only 50% of patients will be in full-time employment 10 years after diagnosis, while 10% will be completely incapacitated by that stage. Median life expectancy for men with RA is reduced by up to 18 years and cardiovascular disease is the major determinant in this respect. Poor prognostic indicators are:

- diagnosis before the age of 30 years
- high-titre RF
- female gender
- joint erosions on radiography at presentation
- poor prognostic DR4 allele.

7.3 Spondarthropathies

Learning objectives

You should:
- know the common presenting features of connective tissue diseases that are seronegative
- understand the difficulties in diagnosis in some of these conditions
- be aware of the potential long-term complications
- be familiar with commonly used treatments.

Patients can present with clinical features of a connective tissue disease but with negative results for autoimmune serology. Some patients will develop a seropositive disease with time.

Ankylosing spondylitis

Ankylosing spondylitis typically presents in the late teens or twenties with back pain and morning stiffness. Radiographs of the spine and sacroiliac joints may be normal at presentation or show evidence of sacroileitis. As the disease progresses, the sacroiliac joints fuse, as do the lumbar vertebrae, giving the classic clinical picture of axial rigidity, which is confirmed radiologically as a 'bamboo spine'. Extra-articular features are common and include uveitis, pulmonary fibrosis, aortic valve disease and amyloidosis. Men are affected much more commonly than women. There is a well-known association with HLA-B27, as more than 90% of affected patients are positive. Testing for HLA-B27 is, however, of limited value as it is a common antigen in Caucasian populations and < 10% of HLA-B27-positive individuals will be affected by ankylosing spondylitis.

Psoriatic arthritis

Psoriatic arthritis presents in a number of distinct clinical patterns and in some cases can be difficult to distinguish from RA. The major presentations include:

- RA-like
- spondarthritis
- dactylitis
- distal interphalangeal joint arthritis
- arthritis mutilans.

The arthritis usually occurs in those with a well-documented history of psoriasis but may occasionally precede the rash. Nail pitting is usually associated with distal interphalangeal joint arthritis. Approximately 10% of patients with psoriasis will develop psoriatic arthritis.

Reiter's syndrome and reactive arthritis

Reiter's syndrome consists of a triad of arthritis, urethritis and conjunctivitis, and it is usually triggered by either genitourinary or gastrointestinal infection. The broader term **reactive arthritis** would include Reiter's syndrome after dysentery and any other non-septic arthritis associated with an episode of infection. The terms **sexually acquired reactive arthritis** and **enteric reactive arthritis** have recently been introduced. Typical pathogens implicated include *Shigella, Campylobacter, Salmonella, Yersinia, Giardia, Ureaplasma, Mycoplasma, Neisseria* spp. and *Escherichia coli*. The arthritis tends to affect large weight-bearing joints and may vary in its severity from a mild transient synovitis to a chronic destructive arthritis. Recurrent attacks are recognised in susceptible individu-

als and there are no specific laboratory tests. The ESR and CRP may be elevated. Treatment is with NSAIDs, sulfasalazine or direct injection of steroid into the joint.

Enteropathic arthropathy

Enteropathic arthropathy describes the arthropathy associated with ulcerative colitis and Crohn's disease. Typically it affects the axial skeleton, and patients may present with an intermittent synovitis of the weight-bearing joints or sacroileitis. In both forms of inflammatory bowel disease, the arthritis mirrors disease activity in the gut; panproctocolectomy is curative in ulcerative colitis.

Whipple's disease

The association of migratory arthritis with malabsorption should raise the possibility of Whipple's disease, which is caused by intestinal infection with *Tropheryma whippelii*. Bacilliform bodies may be seen on electron microscopy of small bowel and hypogammaglobulinaemia may occur. Treatment is with long-term antibiotics.

7.4 Juvenile idiopathic arthritis

Learning objectives

You should:
- know the diagnostic criteria for juvenile idiopathic arthritis
- know the three main patterns
- understand the management of juvenile idiopathic arthritis
- be aware of the potential long-term complications.

Juvenile idiopathic arthritis (JIA) is a generic term that covers several previous diagnostic categories. Three diagnostic criteria must be met:

- onset of arthritis before the age of 16 years
- arthritis for > 6 weeks
- exclusion of other diseases.

There are three main patterns of JIA.

Polyarticular JIA. This may occur at any age in childhood and makes up 30% of those with JIA. By definition, five or more joint groups are involved, the most common being the knees, wrists and ankles. There is a female predominance and older children tend to present with this form of JIA. There may occasionally be lymphadenopathy and fever, but systemic symptoms are uncommon. Most children are seronegative, but the seropositive subgroup is practically indistinguishable from those with adult RA. It is important to remember that RF occurs as a frequent non-specific finding after infection and for that reason it is important to ensure at least three positive RF tests over a 3-month period.

Oligoarticular JIA. Previously referred to as pauciarticular juvenile chronic arthritis, this is the most common type of JIA, accounting for over 50% of cases. The typical presentation is in preschool girls, the female to male ratio being 4:1. Ankle, elbow and knee joints are most commonly affected. RF is typically negative but anti-nuclear antibodies are detected in a subgroup. It is important to highlight the potential diagnosis of JIA to the immunology laboratory undertaking the autoimmune serology, as the titres of autoantibodies may be low (1:10–1:20) and many laboratories will routinely report such sera as negative. The most serious complication of this condition is uveitis, which tends to occur in the anti-nuclear antibodies-positive subgroup and affects both sexes equally. All children diagnosed with JIA should, therefore, have a slit lamp examination as part of their early assessment.

Systemic JIA. Fever and rash are the main clinical features of this, the least frequent category of JIA (formerly known as **Still's disease**). Presentation typically occurs before the age of 5 years, with boys and girls being equally affected. The fever is characteristic, with normal/subnormal temperature in the mornings, but fever of up to 40°C in the late afternoon. Approximately half the children develop a salmon-pink, evanescent rash, which often appears with the fever. Lymphadenopathy and hepatosplenomegaly may occur, as well as pericarditis and subcutaneous nodules. There may be no joint symptoms, or the development of polyarthralgia or polyarthritis. The diagnosis is entirely clinical.

Management

The drug management of JIA centres on the use of NSAIDs and where appropriate, intra-articular steroids. Methotrexate is proving useful in those children who fail to respond to NSAIDs. Aspirin is contraindicated in children because of the reported association with Reye's syndrome. The involvement of a multidisciplinary team with the whole family is essential for the successful management of JIA.

Adult Still's disease

Adult Still's disease is an unusual condition that presents with the same clinical features as systemic JIA in young adults. It is essential that infection and lymphoma are excluded. Symptoms should respond to oral salicylates but steroids may be required. The condition can become chronic.

7.5 Connective tissue diseases

Learning objectives

You should:
- know the clinical features and diagnostic criteria for the connective tissue diseases
- understand which organ systems can be affected
- know the investigations that should be undertaken if a connective tissue disease is suspected
- understand the management of each connective tissue disease
- be aware of the potential long-term complications.

Systemic lupus erythematosus

Systemic lupus erythematosus (SLE) is a multisystem disease that predominantly affects young women. The ratio of female to male patients is approximately 9:1 and certain ethnic groups are very commonly affected including Black and Chinese people. People with complement deficiencies (especially C2 or C4 deficiency) are also more commonly affected.

Clinical features

There is a wide spectrum of clinical features that may occur in SLE. In its most mild form, discoid lupus erythematosus, symptoms are restricted to a skin rash (Fig. 46). In the systemic form, the most common initial features are fatigue, fever, weight loss, joint pains and skin rash. Approximately 40–60% of patients will experience cardiac, respiratory, neurological or renal features at some stage in their illness. A brief description of the ways in which SLE affects these systems follows.

Musculoskeletal effects. Joint and muscle pain are common and may precede any of the other features. The small joints of the hands are often affected and these symptoms can be difficult to differentiate from early RA in some patients. There is usually synovitis, but pain may appear disproportionate to the degree of swelling; joint erosion is unusual.

Cutaneous features. The classical rash appears on sun-exposed areas. A butterfly rash is the description given to the erythematosus rash present on the nose, which spreads out to involve the cheeks. The scalp

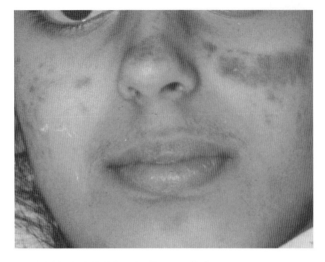

Fig. 46 Typical facial rash of systemic lupus erythematosus.

may be involved, causing patchy, permanent alopecia. Transient alopecia may also occur with flares in SLE activity. Photosensitivity is particularly noted in patients with anti-Ro antibodies. Biopsy is useful to confirm the diagnosis as there are characteristic immunoglobulin and complement deposits at the dermal–epidermal junction (Fig. 43).

Cardiovascular system. Pericarditis is thought to be very common in SLE but is often asymptomatic. Some estimate that as many as 10% of patients with SLE have evidence of pericardial effusion on investigation. Myocardial involvement can lead to conduction defects, arrhythmias and occasionally cardiac failure. The classical Libman–Sacks endocarditis most frequently affects the mitral valve, causing valvular incompetence. Hypertension is a common consequence of SLE-related renal disease. Vasculitis can occur as a secondary complication of SLE and can cause skin ulceration, myocardial infarction, scleritis, etc.

Respiratory system. Pleural effusion and pleurisy are common and pleuritic pain can be a persistent problem. Progressive reduction in lung volume can occur and is often referred to as the **shrinking lung syndrome**. There may be recurrent pneumonitis, and patients on long-term immunosuppressive therapy are especially prone to recurrent bacterial infections.

Neurological features. Neuropsychiatric symptoms are frequently reported and if present can cause diagnostic difficulty. It is thought that 50% of people with renal lupus also have central nervous system lupus. There are no specific tests that predict the development or confirm the presence of central nervous system lupus. The commonest of these symptoms are disordered mental ability and seizures, while cranial nerve palsies, headache, peripheral neuropathy and tremor, etc. are also reported. The basis of these symptoms is thought to be small-vessel vasculitis or specific anti-neuronal immunological activity.

Renal involvement. Renal involvement is a major factor in determining prognosis in SLE as 60% of patients develop renal disease, probably from immune complex deposition in the glomerulus. Direct immunofluorescent examination of renal biopsies usually confirms the presence of mesangial deposits of immunoglobulin and complement (Ch. 12). Proliferative glomerulonephritis is common and leads to nephrotic syndrome, hypertension and progressive renal failure. If untreated, mortality can be as high as 60% at 3 years.

Haematological features. Autoimmune haemolytic anaemia is a common presenting feature and usually responds well to treatment with corticosteroids. Other common manifestations include lymphopenia, neutropenia and thrombocytopenia. The last usually responds to splenectomy. Patients may have normochromic anaemia of chronic disease.

The anti-phospholipid syndrome. This occurs as a complication of lupus (but can also occur as a primary syndrome in non-lupus patients). The clinical features are

- recurrent thrombosis (arterial or venous)
- thrombocytopenia
- recurrent fetal loss (usually in the second trimester)
- heart valve lesions.

Patients have high-titre IgG anti-phospholipid autoantibodies and/or a related autoantibody, the **lupus anticoagulant**. Lupus anticoagulant is directed against factor X in the clotting cascade and paradoxically it causes prolongation of the clotting time *in vitro* but a tendency to thrombosis *in vivo*. Testing for the lupus anticoagulant is undertaken in coagulation laboratories.

Investigation

Immunological testing is considered very important in SLE, not least because it can contribute two out of the necessary four American College of Rheumatologists' criteria for diagnosis (Table 32). Anti-nuclear antibodies are present in most if not all patients with lupus. Most have anti-dsDNA antibodies and many will have positive tests for anti-ENA (Table 33). Serial measurement of complement components (C3 and C4) are of value in monitoring disease activity (Table 34). Typically, the ESR is elevated during acute flares of SLE; however, the CRP remains normal. This may reflect fundamental macrophage dysfunction in the condition. If the CRP is elevated, one should consider the possibilities of

Table 33 Nuclear antibody specificities

Specificity	Clinical association
Anti-double-stranded DNA	Systemic lupus erythematosus, chronic active hepatitis
Anti-nucleolus	Scleroderma
Anti-centromere	CREST variant of scleroderma
Anti-histone	Hydralazine-induced lupus
Anti-extractable nuclear antigens (ENA)	
Anti-Smith (Sm)	Systemic lupus erythematosus
Anti-ribonucleoprotein (RNP)	Mixed connective tissue disease
Anti-Ro	Sjögren's syndrome/systemic lupus erythematosus
Anti-La	Sjögren's syndrome

- infection
- serositis
- synovitis
- vasculitis.

Management

The management of SLE must be tailored to the individual patient's needs. Individual patients may be aware of particular factors that trigger relapse, such as exposure to sunlight, specific drugs and infection, and these should carefully be avoided. In mild forms of SLE, use of sun-blocking creams and NSAIDs can be adequate. Topical steroid creams can be used for the rashes. In patients in whom this is inadequate, hydroxychloroquinine salts are often used and can be very effective in the early stages of disease. This group of drugs can, however, cause retinal damage and regular ophthalmologic review is required for patients on long-term therapy.

As SLE is common in young women, the safety of the use of the oral contraceptive pill should be considered. It is contraindicated in those with SLE who also have migraine, hypertension, a history of thrombosis or high-titre anti-phospholipid antibodies.

For many patients, the mainstay of therapy is the use of oral prednisolone. The management of acute flares often requires high doses of prednisolone; however, the minimum dose required to control disease activity should be used for maintenance. Often the use of a second drug, a steroid-sparing agent, is required to allow the necessary reduction in prednisolone dose. Commonly used second drugs include azathioprine, mycophenolate mofetil and cyclophosphamide, and most clinicians aim to use a maintenance daily dose of prednisolone of < 10 mg. Appropriate bone protective therapy must be prescribed from the initiation of steroid therapy.

Prognosis

Prior to the advent of immunosuppressive therapy, SLE was a condition with a very high mortality. That situation has dramatically improved in the last 20 years and 5-year survival in SLE exceeds 90%, with 10-year survival of 80–90%. Renal disease remains the worst prognostic factor, but the advent of widespread renal-replacement therapy in the forms of dialysis or organ transplantation has greatly improved these patients' outlook. Recent advances in treatment include the use of the anti-B cell monoclonal antibody rituximab (Ch. 9).

Scleroderma (systemic sclerosis)

Scleroderma is a multisystem disorder that is characterised by fibrosis of connective tissue. The aetiology is unknown; however, it has an approximate 3:1 female to male predominance and the onset of the condition tends to be in the third and fifth decades of life. While **systemic sclerosis** probably best describes the condition, the term **scleroderma** is most commonly used as in practice it describes the visible and most common feature of the condition, the fibrosis and hardening of the skin, which can be very disfiguring.

Clinical features

There are three main phases of the skin changes
- oedema
- fibrosis and contraction
- atrophy.

Table 34 Patterns of autoantibody and immunochemical investigations in systemic lupus erythematosus

Anti-double-stranded DNA	C3	C4	C-reactive protein	Interpretation
High	Normal	Normal	Normal	Systemic lupus erythematosus active
Moderate	Low	Low	Normal	Systemic lupus erythematosus active
Low	Low	Low	Normal	? Renal disease
High	High	High	High	? Infection
High	Low	Low	High	? Serositis/vasculitis

There are also three main clinical presentations: morphoea, limited systemic sclerosis and diffuse systemic sclerosis.

Morphoea. This is a localised form of the condition with skin changes only.

Limited systemic sclerosis. This form is not usually associated with renal involvement; however, it is associated with pulmonary hypertension in a significant proportion. Patients need to be monitored carefully (including regular echocardiography) to exclude the development of this complication. Limited systemic sclerosis includes the variant formerly known as CREST syndrome. The acronym CREST comes from the combination of clinical features: *c*alcinosis, *R*aynaud's phenomenon, *o*esophageal immotility, *s*clerodactyly, *t*elangiectasia). Typically, antibodies against centromere are detected in patients with CREST.

Diffuse systemic sclerosis. The diffuse form is characterised by widespread pathological changes. The dermatological features may be very evident in the face and hands. These usually cause a progressive change in facial appearance characterised by tightened skin, pinched nose and difficulty opening the mouth (Fig. 47). The hands may develop flexion deformities and there may be intracutaneous and subcutaneous calcification. Renal involvement is characteristic of diffuse systemic sclerosis. The use of angiotensin-converting enzyme inhibitors is important in reducing the decline in renal function. Anti-SCL-70 autoantibodies can usually be detected in patients with this form of the condition.

Raynaud's phenomenon is an almost universal feature and may be the presenting feature. It may be severe, with development of digital gangrene in some cases.

Sjögren's syndrome

Sjögren's syndrome is a clinical triad of dry eyes (keratoconjunctivitis sicca), dry mouth (xerostomia) and an associated inflammatory arthritis. Patients with dry eyes and mouth in the absence of arthritis are said to have the **sicca complex**. This is common in the elderly (approximate prevalence 1%), but when it affects younger people it is thought that approximately 60% will go on to develop Sjögren's syndrome.

Sjögren's syndrome is a condition that mainly affects middle-aged women and is caused by a lymphocytic infiltrate of the lacrimal and salivary glands, which causes their destruction and failure of glandular secretion. Other exocrine glands in the pancreas, lungs and vagina may be affected, with local symptoms developing.

In addition to the ocular and oral features, patients often present with non-specific fatigue, dyspareunia and recurrent chest infection. Investigation usually identifies anti-nuclear antibodies with anti-Ro in 70% and anti-La in 40%. Of those with arthritis, 90% will be RF positive. The ESR is usually high and there may be anaemia of chronic disease. Measurement of serum immunoglobulins will often identify a polyclonal increase; however, because of an association with lymphoproliferative disease, paraprotein should be carefully sought. If there are appropriate suggestive clinical features, cryoglobulin testing should be undertaken (Chs 11 and 12).

There are clinical associations with autoimmune thyroid disease and the development of primary biliary cirrhosis (Ch. 6). Importantly, patients may go on to develop lymphoproliferative disease. This last complication may be difficult to diagnose, as the lymphoma may be initially restricted to mucosa-associated lym-

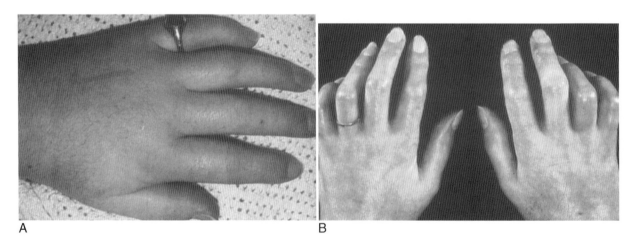

A   B

Fig. 47 Contrasting clinical features affecting the hands in connective tissue diseases: (a) typical sausage-shaped fingers of mixed connective tissue disease; (b) scleroderma causes narrowing of the fingers with flexural contractures of the fingers (sclerodactyly).

phoid tissue, but monitoring of the ESR, immunoglobulins and urine for free light-chain excretion is helpful.

Mixed connective tissue disease

Mixed connective tissue disease is a syndrome in which patients have clinical features of polymyositis, scleroderma and SLE. Serologically, the typical finding is a speckled anti-nuclear antibody with specificity for ribonucleoprotein (anti-RNP). This should be in the absence of other lupus associated autoantibodies or ENA specificities (e.g. anti-double-stranded DNA, anti-Sm). Complement levels are usually normal. Because of the ill-defined nature of the syndrome, some clinicians will refer to such patients as having **overlap syndromes** or **undifferentiated connective tissues disease**. In most patients the disease eventually follows a pattern more typical of either SLE or systemic sclerosis.

The features generally ascribed to mixed connective tissue disease include sclerodermatous changes in the skin, including classic 'sausage-shaped' fingers. There is often pulmonary involvement, including pulmonary fibrosis, hypertension or pleurisy. The prognosis in mixed connective tissue disease is better than in SLE because there is usually no renal or cerebral involvement. The response to oral corticosteroid therapy is usually good.

Polymyositis and dermatomyositis

Polymyositis and dermatomyositis are inflammatory conditions affecting muscle and skin. They may occur either alone or in combination with other connective tissue diseases or malignancy in a minority of patients. It is thought that polymyositis has a similar prevalence to systemic sclerosis. It is more common in women and in patients of African origin.

Clinical features

The major clinical symptom is progressive proximal muscle weakness, which may be insidious in onset. The condition can present both in childhood and adulthood (typically the fifth or sixth decade of life). Often patients will notice difficulty climbing stairs or weakness of the neck muscles. More acute presentations do occur and are typically associated with muscle pain (myalgia). Progression of the disease is indicated by difficulty swallowing or breathing and muscle contractures may develop. There may be arthralgia and fevers in some patients. Typical skin features include a lilac/heliotrope rash around the eyes and a generalised erythematous rash, which may be photosensitive and tends to occur on extensor surfaces. These are the characteristic features of dermatomyositis. Progressive involvement of the diaphragm leads to dyspnoea on lying flat. Although renal disease is not a primary feature, high levels of serum myoglobin may occur in active myositis, causing renal impairment. Up to 20% of adults will have an underlying malignancy, typically carcinoma of the lung, breast, stomach or ovary.

A subtype of polymyositis is the **anti-synthetase syndrome** in which patients develop thickened and cracked palmar skin, which is often associated with underlying pulmonary fibrosis.

Investigation

Serum muscle enzyme measurements, electromyography and muscle biopsy are the most important investigations. Creatine phosphokinase is the most sensitive marker of disease activity. Objective assessment of muscle strength and magnetic resonance scanning of muscle may also be helpful in long-term assessment. There is a weak association with HLA-B8 and HLA-DR3. Lung function tests and computed tomography are important to detect evidence of pulmonary fibrosis. A number of autoantibodies are reported to occur in polymyositis and dermatomyositis; however, anti-Jo-1 is the only one readily available in most diagnostic laboratories. Detection of anti-Jo-1 is associated with the anti-synthetase syndrome and, particularly, with pulmonary involvement.

Management

Oral prednisolone at a daily dose of approximately 40–60 mg/day is usually required to control the initial presentation of disease. The use of a second steroid-sparing agent usually allows this dose to be reduced to more acceptable long-term levels. Treatment may be required for many years. Patients with occult malignancy and pulmonary fibrosis tend to respond less well to treatment.

Self-assessment: questions

Multiple choice questions

1. The most specific autoantibodies for systemic lupus erythematosus (SLE) is:
   a. Anti-Ro
   b. Anti-La
   c. Anti-Sm (anti-Smith)
   d. Anti-double-stranded DNA (anti-dsDNA)
   e. Anti-ribonucleoprotein (anti-RNP)

2. The percentage of patients with rheumatoid arthritis and positive for rheumatoid factor is:
   a. 10%
   b. 25%
   c. 50%
   d. 75%
   e. 90%

3. In juvenile idiopathic arthritis it is most common for affected children to have:
   a. Five or more joints involved
   b. Rheumatoid factor positive
   c. Strongly positive anti-nuclear antibodies
   d. Characteristic butterfly rash
   e. Late development of classic rheumatoid arthritis

4. Rheumatoid factor (RF) is:
   a. A good prognostic indicator in rheumatoid arthritis
   b. An autoantibody directed against nuclear components
   c. Highly specific for rheumatoid arthritis
   d. Associated with cryoprotein formation
   e. A useful marker of disease activity in rheumatoid arthritis

5. In systemic lupus erythematosus (SLE):
   a. The female to male ratio is approximately 1:2
   b. Cardiac disease is the major cause of mortality
   c. Approximately 90% of patients develop end-stage renal failure after 5 years
   d. C-reactive protein is a useful marker of disease activity
   e. Type II hypersensitivity is the major immunopathogenetic mechanism

6. CREST syndrome is typically associated with:
   a. anti-Ro specific antibodies
   b. Progressive renal disease
   c. Dysphagia
   d. Cutaneous pathergy
   e. Raynaud's phenomenon

7. The patient's prognosis in systemic lupus erythematosus is:
   a. Worse in the presence of anti-Sm antibodies
   b. Better in the presence of anticardiolipin antibodies
   c. Worse in the presence of hypocomplementaemia
   d. Better in the presence of microscopic haematuria
   e. Worse in the absence of anti-dsDNA antibodies

Case history questions

History 1

A 14-year-old Pakistani girl presents with fever and increasing lethargy over the previous 3 weeks. On examination, she has raised red tender lesions over her cheeks and vascular lesions over the soles of her feet. Table 35 gives the results of the investigations.

Table 35 Results of the investigations in case history 1

Parameter	Value	Normal range
Haemoglobin (g/l)	85	130–180
Urea (mmol/l)	15.3	2.1–8.9
Creatinine (µmol/l)	210	53–133
Autoimmune screen		
Antinuclear antibody	1:320	
Anti-Sm	Positive	
C3 (g/l)	0.650	0.7–1.7
C4 (g/l)	0.11	0.13–0.43
Erythrocyte sedimentation rate (mm/h)	87	
C-reactive protein (mg/l)	120	0–10

1. The most likely diagnosis is:
   a. systemic lupus erythematosus (SLE)
   b. Wegener's granulomatosis
   c. Henoch–Schönlein purpura
   d. Typhoid fever
   e. Cryoglobulinaemia

History 2

A 64-year-old man with a 30-year history of rheumatoid arthritis attends your clinic for review. His arthritis has been effectively controlled on a combination of non-steroidal anti-inflammatory drugs and latterly gold therapy. He complains of recent weight loss (6 kg over 12 months) and episodic diarrhoea. There is also a history of recent dental infection, which required surgical drainage and antibiotic therapy. On examination, his joints are deformed but not actively inflamed. There is superficial furunculous over the back. Respiratory and cardiac examinations are unremarkable, although on abdominal examination a splenic edge is palpable. Investigations gave the results in Table 36.

Table 36 Results of the investigations in case history 2

Parameter	Value	Normal range
Haemoglobin (g/l)	95	130–180
Total white cell count ($\times 10^9$/l)	4.7	4–10
Lymphocytes ($\times 10^9$/l)	3.5	1.5–3.5
Neutrophils ($\times 10^9$/l)	0.5	2–7.5
Monocytes ($\times 10^9$/l)	0.35	0.2–0.8
Basophils ($\times 10^9$/l)	0.03	0.01–0.1
Erythrocyte sedimentation rate (mm/h)	66	
C-reactive protein (mg/l)	15	< 10
Autoimmune screen		
Antinuclear antibody	1:320	
Rheumatoid factor (IU/l)	70	< 20
C3 (g/l)	0.65	0.7–1.7
C4 (g/l)	0.04	0.13–0.43

1. Based on the clinical findings and investigative results, is there a unifying explanation?
2. Would any further investigations be helpful?

Table 37 Blood test results for data interpretation question 1

Parameter	Value	Normal range
Anti-nuclear antibody (IgG)	1:160	
Rheumatoid factor	Negative	
C3 (g/l)	1.08	0.7–1.7
C4 (g/l)	0.15	0.13–0.43
C-reactive protein (mg/l)	67	0–10

Data interpretation

1. A 23-year-old woman complains of joint pain and stiffness particularly first thing in the morning. Her GP has undertaken some blood tests, the results of which are given in Table 37.

   a. How would you interpret these results?
   b. What further tests (if any) would you advise?

2. The results in Table 38 were obtained from a 60-year-old female patient who recently attended the ophthalmology clinic. How would you interpret these?

Table 38 Blood test results for data interpretation question 2

Parameter	Value	Normal range
Anti-nuclear antibody (IgG)	1:2560	
Rheumatoid factor	Negative	
Extractable nuclear antigen screen		
Anti-Ro	Positive	
Anti-La	Positive	
Anti-RNP	Negative	
Anti-Sm	Negative	
C3 (g/l)	1.3	0.7–1.7
C4 (g/l)	0.26	0.13–0.43
IgG (g/l)	28.5	7–16
IgA (g/l)	4.8	0.8–4.7
IgM (g/l)	1.9	0.5–3.0

Self-assessment: answers

Multiple choice answers

1. a. **False.** Anti-Ro is typically found in primary and secondary Sjögren's syndrome.
   b. **False.** Anti-La is typically found in primary and secondary Sjögren's syndrome.
   c. **True.** Anti-Sm has high specificity for SLE but low sensitivity, being found in only < 30% patients.
   d. **False.** Anti-dsDNA is commonly detected in patients with SLE but is not specific for it, being commonly detected in other connective tissue diseases.
   e. **False.** Anti-RNP is found in patients with SLE, but when identified in the absence of antibodies against other extractable nuclear antigens is more suggestive of mixed connective tissue disorder.

2. a. **False.**
   b. **False.**
   c. **False.**
   d. **True.** Approximately 75% of patients with rheumatoid arthritis are positive for rheumatoid factor. This group are more prone to develop extra-articular complications of their disease compared with those negative for rheumatoid factor.
   e. **False.**

3. a. **True.** This is characteristic of juvenile idiopathic arthritis.
   b. **False.** Most children with juvenile idiopathic arthritis are negative for rheumatoid factor.
   c. **False.** Whilst the detection of anti-nuclear antibodies is important in the investigation of these children, autoantibody titres tend to be low (and therefore may be falsely reported as negative).
   d. **False.** Rash, when it occurs, does not have this distribution characteristically and can be fleeting.
   e. **True.** This is not true for the majority of children.

4. a. **False.** Patients with detectable serum RF are more likely to suffer complications of rheumatoid arthritis and therefore have worse prognosis.
   b. **False.** RF is an autoantibody directed against the Fc portion of IgG molecules.
   c. **False.** RF occurs in a wide range of infectious and inflammatory disorders.
   d. **False.** RF activity is characteristic of type II and III cryoprotein formation.

e. **False.** RF levels are not a useful marker of disease activity. Serial acute phase protein (e.g. C-reactive protein) should be used.

5. a. **False.** The female to male ratio is approx. 8:1.
   b. **False.** Cardiac disease is not the major cause of mortality; however, it is increasingly recognised as a problem for patients with SLE.
   c. **False.** Approximately 60% of patients develop renal disease, the prevalence and severity of which is influenced by the use of immunosuppressant therapy.
   d. **False.** C-reactive protein does not usually rise with flares of SLE activity, although a raised level may be a useful indicator of infection, vasculitis or serositis in patients with SLE.
   e. **False.** Type III hypersensitivity is thought to be the major immunopathogenic mechanism in SLE-related renal disease.

6. a. **False.** Anti-centromere antibodies are typical of CREST syndrome.
   b. **False.** Progressive renal disease is not a feature.
   c. **True.** Involvement of the oesophagus may lead to dysphagia.
   d. **False.**
   e. **True.** This is a typical feature.

7. a. **False.** Anti-Sm antibodies have diagnostic but not prognostic significance.
   b. **False.** Anti-cardiolipin antibodies are associated with thrombotic complications and, therefore, a worse prognosis.
   c. **True.** Hypocomplementaemia suggests active immune complex-mediated disease and a greater risk of sequelae such as renal disease.
   d. **False.** Microscopic haematuria implies renal involvement.
   e. **False.** Anti-dsDNA antibodies have diagnostic but not prognostic significance.

Case history answers

History 1

1. The most likely diagnosis in this case is SLE. The history suggests a relatively acute onset illness and the cutaneous features were typical of vasculitic lesions. The investigative results are strongly indicative of SLE with anaemia, impaired renal function and autoimmune serology specific for SLE. The erythrocyte sedimentation rate is

elevated, consistent with active disease and the raised C-reactive protein is consistent with active vasculitis. There are no historical features to suggest either Wegener's granulomatosis or typhoid fever. The distribution of rash is not typical of Henoch–Schönlein purpura and the serology suggests the alternative diagnosis of SLE. The description of the rash is not suggestive of cryoglobulinaemia, which is also virtually excluded by the relatively normal C4.

History 2

1. The presentation with weight loss and recurrent infections (dental, cutaneous and possibly gastro-intestinal) after a long history of rheumatoid arthritis would suggest that he has developed splenomegaly. Investigations indicate a mild anaemia with significant neutropenia. His auto-immune serology was consistent with rheumatoid arthritis and he had a notable low serum C4. The combination of neutropenia and splenic enlargement suggests Felty's syndrome as a possible cause for his recurrent infection. The low C4 is unusual and could represent an inherited defic-iency of C4, which would have predisposed him to the development of autoimmune disease.

2. Alternatively one could look for physical signs of cryoglobulinaemia and undertake appropriate test-ing. Very rarely, patients with Felty's syndrome may go on to develop a form of lymphoma (large granu-lar lymphocytosis) and, therefore, blood film should be examined for abnormal lymphocytes. Gold ther-apy is also a known cause of hypogammaglobuli-naemia and this possibility should be borne in mind and serum immunoglobulins measured.

Data interpretation

1. a. The results are suggestive of an underlying inflammatory process but are not at this stage diagnostic. An IgG anti-nuclear antibody titre of 1:160 suggests the possibility of an autoimmune process and, in the context of the clinical histo-ry, early systemic lupus erythematosus or rheumatoid arthritis would be the two diag-noses that one would wish to exclude initially. The negative rheumatoid factor does not exclude rheumatoid arthritis as it is positive in only approximately 60% of patients. The raised C-reactive protein is of interest as this marker is not usually raised in systemic lupus erythe-matosus and this would, therefore, be more in favour of a diagnosis of rheumatoid arthritis.

   b. Serial measurements of C-reactive protein would be useful if there is clinical evidence of synovitis as it may prove a useful indicator of disease activity and response to therapy. Ultrasound or magnetic resonance imaging of joints would be useful to look for evidence of early erosions. Further characterisation of the anti-nuclear antibody would be helpful and, therefore, anti-nuclear antibody specificity and tests for anti-double-stranded DNA should be requested.

2. The results indicate a strongly positive anti-nuclear antibody with positive anti-Ro and anti-La speci-ficity. There is also a polyclonal increase in total serum immunoglobulins. The only clinical details are that this lady has attended the eye clinic. The serology and immunochemistry would be entirely consistent with Sjögren's syndrome and it is likely that her attendance at the eye clinic may have been with xerophthalmia (dry eyes). The ophthal-mologist should have undertaken a Schirmer's test to confirm a failure of tear production. Long-term follow up of patients with Sjögren's syndrome is recommended as in addition to their problematic symptoms related to dryness, they are at risk of developing lymphoma.

8 Vasculitis

Chapter overview

Vasculitis, or the inflammation of blood vessels, can occur as a result of infection, trauma, autoimmunity or localised inflammation. In this chapter, however, we will focus on a group of clinical conditions that are characterised by systemic vasculitis — inflammation of blood vessels throughout the body — which are thought to be autoimmune in origin. These conditions differ from each other in their clinical presentation and ultimate outcome, but share the common pathological process of vascular inflammation. The disorders are traditionally classified by the size of vessel affected (small, medium or large) and whether there is granuloma formation. In some of these conditions, characteristic autoantibodies (anti-neutrophil cytoplasmic antibodies (ANCA)) are detected and these can be helpful in diagnosis and disease classification.

8.1 Introduction

Learning objectives

You should:
- be familiar with the classification of primary vasculitides.

Primary vasculitides are a group of disorders characterised by inflammation of blood vessels. The traditional classification of these conditions is based on vessel size and the presence or absence of granuloma (Table 39).

The American College of Rheumatology published diagnostic criteria that assist in the differentiation of vasculitic conditions from one another; these are listed in Table 40. The majority of these conditions are relapsing and remitting in nature and, therefore, patients are prone to acute relapse if therapy is not adequately maintained.

8.2 Large-vessel diseases

Learning objectives

You should:
- understand what diseases affect large vessels
- know the typical clinical presentations
- understand the management of the conditions
- be familiar with the long-term complications of each condition.

Takayasu's arteritis

Takayasu's arteritis is a granulomatous inflammatory disorder that affects the aorta. It is also known as 'pulseless disease' because affected individuals often have impalpable radial arterial pulses at presentation.

Clinical features

Takayasu's arteritis typically affects young women in the second and third decade of life. The female to male ratio is approximately 8:1. There may initially be symptoms of fever, fatigue and arthralgia, reflecting the systemic inflammatory process. After a variable time period, usually several years, the condition enters a chronic phase that is characterised by the symptoms caused by vascular stenoses. These symptoms may include poor circulation in the cerebral or upper limb vessels or occasionally renal ischaemia.

Patients affected by Takayasu's arteritis may have no obvious symptomatic early phase but may be diagnosed during investigation for hypertension, heart failure, visual symptoms or the incidental finding of vascular bruits. Hypertension is caused by the aortic stenotic lesions, which often causes blood pressure to be unequal in the arms, and also by renal artery stenosis.

Table 39 Histological classification system for vasculitic disorders

Vessel size	Granuloma positive	Granuloma negative
Large	Takayasu's arteritis	Giant cell arteritis
Medium		PAN, Kawasaki disease
Small	Churg–Strauss syndrome, Wegener's granulomatosis	Microscopic polyangiitis, Henoch–Schönlein purpura, cryoglobulinaemia, cutaneous leukocytoclastic vasculitis

Investigation

There are no 'diagnostic' blood tests for Takayasu's arteritis, the diagnosis is largely based on clinical presentation and radiological imaging findings. High-quality imaging of the aorta is essential in the initial assessment and monitoring of this condition. The use of contrast angiography or magnetic resonance imaging allows the identification of stenotic lesions. Serial imaging assists in monitoring the response to medical therapy and determining where and if surgical intervention is indicated.

The condition is classified into three subtypes (Fig. 48):

- type I involves the aortic arch and the major vessels arising from it
- type II involves the descending aorta often affecting the renal arteries
- type III is a combination of types I and II.

Serum inflammatory markers (e.g. C-reactive protein (CRP)) are often moderately increased in the acute phase (50–100 mg/l) and monitoring of CRP is helpful in the assessment of the response to medical therapy in some patients.

Management

Use of corticosteroids is indicated in the acute phase, usually in combination with a second steroid-sparing agent such as azathioprine. Response to treatment is usually monitored by a combination of symptoms and acute phase proteins. Immunosuppression is usually continued for up to 2 years, and in the long term antiplatelet agents including aspirin may be beneficial. Given the critical sites of vascular inflammation in Takayasu's arteritis and the uncertainty in assessment of disease activity, it can be difficult to decide with confidence when therapy can be safely withdrawn.

The major factors associated with morbidity in Takayasu's arteritis are hypertension, cerebrovascular occlusion and cardiac failure. It is, therefore, essential that a multidisciplinary team including cardiologists, vascular surgeons and immunologists is involved in the management of this condition.

Giant cell arteritis

Giant cell arteritis is a granulomatous inflammatory disorder that usually affects the carotid artery or its extracranial branches. It typically affects elderly people and in approximately 50% of cases is associated with polymyalgia rheumatica.

Clinical features

Patients often present with headache, which may be associated with scalp tenderness and a palpable temporal artery. Facial pain also occurs, sometimes associated with chewing (jaw claudication) and there may be other manifestations of vascular insufficiency including loss or alteration of sensation or taste. There is a risk of sudden blindness, caused by arteritis affecting the ophthalmic arteries; to prevent this, early diagnosis and treatment are essential. Giant cell arteritis can occasionally affect the aorta and its abdominal branches, and in such cases is difficult to differentiate from Takayasu's arteritis.

Investigation

The most characteristic abnormality in giant cell arteritis is an elevation of the erythrocyte sedimentation rate

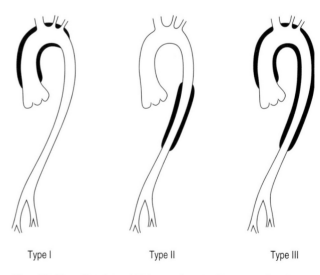

Type I   Type II   Type III

Fig. 48 Classification of Takayasu's arteritis according to disease extent.

Table 40 American College of Rheumatology 1990 criteria for the diagnosis of vasculitis disorders

Criteria for disorder	Description
Takayasu's arteritis[a]	
1. Age at disease onset < 40 years	Development of symptoms or findings related to Takayasu's arteritis at age < 40 years
2. Claudication of extremities	Development and worsening of fatigue and discomfort in muscles of one or more extremity while in use, especially the upper extremities
3. Decreased brachial artery pulse	Decreased pulsation of one or both brachial arteries
4. BP difference > 10 mmHg	Difference of > 10 mmHg in systolic blood pressure between arms
5. Bruit over subclavian arteries or aorta	Bruit audible on auscultation over one or both subclavian arteries or abdominal aorta
6. Arteriogram abnormality	Arteriographic narrowing or occlusion of the entire aorta, its primary branches, or large arteries in the proximal upper or lower extremities, not due to arteriosclerosis, fibromuscular dysplasia, or similar causes; changes usually focal or segmental
Giant cell (temporal) arteritis[b]	
1. Age at disease onset ≥ 50 years	Development of symptoms or findings beginning at age 50 or older
2. New headache	New onset of or new type of localised pain in the head
3. Temporal artery abnormality	Temporal artery tenderness to palpation or decreased pulsation, unrelated to arteriosclerosis of cervical arteries
4. Elevated erythrocyte sedimentation rate	Erythrocyte sedimentation rate ≥ 50 mm/h by the Westergren method
5. Abnormal artery biopsy	Biopsy specimen with artery showing vasculitis characterised by a predominance of mononuclear cell infiltration or granulomatous inflammation, usually with multinucleated giant cells
Polyarteritis nodosa[c]	
1. Weight loss ≥ 4 kg	Loss of 4 kg or more of body weight since illness began, not caused by dieting or other factors
2. Livedo reticularis	Mottled reticular pattern over the skin or portions of the extremities or torso
3. Testicular pain or tenderness	Pain or tenderness of the testicles, not caused by infection, trauma or other causes
4. Myalgias, weakness or leg tenderness	Diffuse myalgias (excluding shoulder and hip girdle) or weakness of muscles or tenderness of leg muscles
5. Mononeuropathy or polyneuropathy	Development of mononeuropathy, multiple mononeuropathies or polyneuropathy
6. Diastolic BP > 90 mmHg	Development of hypertension with diastolic BP > 90 mmHg
7. Elevated BUN or creatinine	Elevation of BUN > 400 mg/l or creatinine > 15 mg/l, not a result of dehydration or obstruction
8. Hepatitis B virus	Presence of hepatitis B surface antigen or antibody in serum
9. Arteriographic abnormality	Arteriogram showing aneurysms or occlusions of the visceral arteries, not due to arteriosclerosis, fibromuscular dysplasia or other non-inflammatory causes
10. Biopsy of small or medium-sized artery containing PMN	Histological changes showing the presence of granulocytes or granulocytes and mononuclear leukocytes in the artery wall
Churg–Strauss syndrome[d]	
1. Asthma	
2. Eosinophilia > 10%	
3. Neuropathy, mono or poly	
4. Pulmonary infiltrates, non-fixed	
5. Paranasal sinus abnormality	
6. Extravascular eosinophils	

Continued

Table 40 American College of Rheumatology 1990 criteria for the diagnosis of vasculitis disorders — cont'd

Criteria for disorder	Description
Wegener's granulomatosis[e]	
1. Nasal or oral inflammation	Development of painful or painless oral ulcers or purulent or bloody nasal discharge
2. Abnormal chest radiograph	Chest radiograph showing the presence of nodules, fixed infiltrates or cavities
3. Urinary sediment	Microhaematuria (> 5 red blood cells per high power field) or red cell casts in urine sediment
4. Granulomatous inflammation on biopsy	Histological changes showing granulomatous inflammation within the wall of an artery or in the perivascular or extravascular area (artery or arteriole)
Henoch-Schönlein purpura[f]	
1. Palpable purpura	Slightly raised 'palpable' haemorrhagic skin lesions, not related to thrombocytopenia
2. Age ≤ 20 at disease onset	Patient 20 years or younger at onset of first symptoms
3. Bowel angina	Diffuse abdominal pain, worse after meals, or the diagnosis of bowel ischaemia, usually including bloody diarrhoea
4. Wall granulocytes on biopsy	Histologic changes showing granulocytes in the walls of arterioles or venules

BP, blood pressure (systolic; difference between arms); BUN, blood urea nitrogen; PMN, polymorphonuclear neutrophils.
[a]At least three of these six criteria are present; the presence of any three or more criteria yields a sensitivity of 90.5% and a specificity of 97.8%.
[b]At least three of these five criteria are present; the presence of any three or more criteria yields a sensitivity of 93.5% and a specificity of 91.2%.
[c]At least three of these ten criteria are present; the presence of any three or more criteria yields a sensitivity of 82.2% and a specificity of 86.6%.
[d]At least four of these six criteria are present; the presence of any four or more of the six criteria yields a sensitivity of 85% and a specificity of 99.7%.
[e]At least two of these four criteria are present; the presence of any two or more criteria yields a sensitivity of 88.2% and a specificity of 92.0%.
[f]At least two of these four criteria are present; the presence of any two or more criteria yields a sensitivity of 87.1% and a specificity of 87.7%.

(ESR), often > 100 mm/h. Temporal artery biopsy can be useful to confirm the diagnosis, but the inflammation is characteristically patchy and, therefore, a normal biopsy does not rule out the diagnosis. Treatment should not be delayed while awaiting a biopsy.

Treatment

Oral corticosteroids are the mainstay of treatment, and the condition characteristically responds rapidly to relatively low doses of oral prednisolone (e.g. 40 mg daily). Once the disease is brought under control, the dose of prednisolone should be reduced to the minimum compatible with clinical remission. This should then be continued for at least 2 years and sometimes up to 5 years. In those requiring prolonged therapy or in whom it is not possible to reduce the prednisolone dose sufficiently, steroid-sparing agents should be considered. Bone-protective therapy is particularly important in such patients.

8.3 Medium-vessel disease

Learning objectives

You should:
- understand what diseases affect medium vessels
- know the typical clinical presentations
- understand the management of the conditions
- be familiar with the long-term complications of each condition.

Polyarteritis nodosa

Clinical features

Polyarteritis nodosa is a systemic necrotising arteritis that affects medium-size arteries. Typical symptoms and signs include fever, weight loss, myalgia, subcutaneous nodules, purpura, abdominal and testicular pain, and mononeuritis multiplex. Men are more frequently affected than women and the symptoms relate to the anatomical distribution of the affected vessels. Commonly, the skin, kidneys, gastrointestinal tract, nervous system and heart are affected.

Renal involvement may manifest as hypertension, haematuria and acute or chronic renal failure. The occurrence of glomerulonephritis should raise the pos-sibility of microscopic polyangiitis, which is considered a separate condition (see below).

Investigation

Patients are often anaemic, with a leukocytosis and raised ESR. Coeliac and renal angiography will usually demonstrate multiple small aneurysms (Fig. 49). Interventional radiological techniques may be used to stop such aneurysms bleeding. Renal, rectal and sural nerve biopsies may also reveal arteritis.

Churg–Strauss syndrome

Clinical features

Churg–Strauss syndrome has many similarities to polyarteritis nodosa; however, there are characteristic differences in the clinical presentation and prognosis.

Churg–Strauss syndrome is usually distinguished by

- a history of adult-onset asthma
- peripheral blood eosinophilia
- absent/mild renal disease.

The major pathological difference from polyarteritis nodosa is that the majority of patients with Churg–Strauss syndrome have pulmonary vasculitis. The better prognosis in Churg–Strauss syndrome compared with polyarteritis nodosa is because of the lack of renal disease in the former.

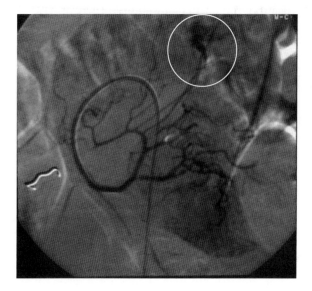

Fig. 49 Angiography from a patient with polyarteritis nodosa demonstrate active bleeding from an aneurysm (circled).

Management

The principal medical management of both poly-arteritis nodosa and Churg–Strauss syndrome is by the use of combination immunosuppressive therapy. An induction phase lasting up to 2 years usually includes continuous-oral/pulsed-intravenous cortico-steroids in combination with cyclophosphamide. Thereafter, maintenance oral corticosteroid with a steroid-sparing drug such as azathioprine or metho-trexate is indicated.

A number of patients with occult Churg–Strauss syndrome have been identified when patients with adult-onset asthma were commenced on leukotriene receptor antagonist drugs. The improved asthma control in these patients allowed a reduction in oral corticosteroid dose that then 'unmasked' other, previously unrecognised, vasculitic features.

Kawasaki disease

Kawasaki disease, also known as **mucocutaneous lymph node syndrome**, is an acute, usually self-limiting disease of early childhood.

Clinical features

Kawasaki disease is characterised by fever, exanthematous rash, mucous membrane involvement, conjunctival injection and cervical lymphadenopathy. There is an underlying necrotising arteritis that affects the coronary arteries in up to 60%. In such cases, sudden death may occur from coronary artery occlusion, myocarditis or aneurysm rupture. There is also the potential for late mortality several years after the acute illness, again caused by aneurysm rupture.

Investigation

The diagnosis is largely based on recognition of the clinical features; however, a marked elevation of ESR and CRP is characteristic and a thrombocytosis forms part of the diagnostic criteria (Table 40).

Treatment

Treatment with high-dose intravenous immunoglobulin (ivIg) in the acute phase of the illness has been proven to prevent the coronary complications. A dose of 2 g/kg body weight ivIg is given as either a single dose or divided into four or five doses given on successive days. It appears that ivIg must be administered within the first 10 days of the illness in order to be effective.

8.4 Small-vessel disease

Learning objectives

You should:

- understand what diseases affect small vessels
- know the typical clinical presentations
- understand the contribution of anti-neutrophil cytoplasmic antibody (ANCA) testing to diagnosis
- understand the management of the conditions
- be familiar with the long-term complications of each condition.

Microscopic polyangiitis

Clinical features

The presentation of microscopic polyangiitis can be very similar to polyarteritis nodosa; however, as small arteries are chiefly affected, renal involvement is common and this often dominates the clinical presentation. Rapidly progressive glomerulonephritis (RPGN) can be the only presenting feature of microscopic polyangiitis or it may occur in combination with pulmonary haemorrhage (pulmonary renal syndrome). An important differential diagnosis of pulmonary renal syndrome is Goodpasture's syndrome (Ch. 6).

Investigation

Patients with microscopic polyangiitis typically have perinuclear anti-neutrophil cytoplasmic antibodies (p-ANCA; Fig. 50) detectable in their serum and these are usually confirmed as anti-myeloperoxidase specificity (MPO-ANCA). The diagnostic use of ANCA test-

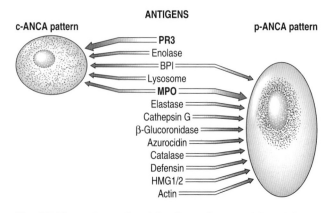

Fig. 50 The pattern of staining for anti-neutrophil cytoplasmic antibodies (ANCA), either in the cytoplasm (c) or around the nucleus (perinuclear).

ing is further discussed in Chapter 12. The indications for ANCA testing are:

- glomerulonephritis (especially RPGN)
- pulmonary haemorrhage
- cutaneous vasculitis with systemic features
- multiple lung nodules
- chronic destructive disease of the upper airways
- long-standing sinusitis/otitis
- subglottic tracheal stenosis
- mononeuritis multiplex or other peripheral neuropathy
- retroorbital mass.

It is important to emphasise here that a negative p-ANCA does not exclude microscopic polyangiitis and that p-ANCA may be detected in a range of other clinical conditions including infections and connective tissue disorders. Tissue diagnosis should be obtained whenever possible. Monitoring of patients with microscopic polyangiitis should include serial measurements of CRP to assess vasculitic activity as well as assessment of renal function.

Management

As with large- and medium-vessel vasculitides, combination immunosuppressive therapy must be instituted to achieve remission and maintain the condition under control. The predilection to cause RPGN indicates that close monitoring of renal function is essential and supportive renal-replacement therapy (haemodialysis or peritoneal dialysis) may be required. Pulmonary haemorrhage can be mild, moderate or severe, and mechanical ventilation may be required during the acute phase of the illness.

Wegener's granulomatosis

Wegener's granulomatosis is the most common of the primary small-vessel vasculitides. It is characterised histologically by necrotising granulomata, which typically affect the upper or lower airways or the kidneys.

Clinical features

Wegener's granulomatosis is a disorder that primarily affects middle-aged men. The disease may be limited to the upper respiratory tract, patients presenting with symptoms of chronic sinusitis or recurrent epistaxis caused by nasal mucosal ulceration. Increasing breathlessness and haemoptysis are common presenting features in those with pulmonary involvement, but in contrast to polyarteritis nodosa, blood pressure is usually normal. Renal involvement is present in approximately 85% of patients and this may have a major prognostic significance.

Investigations

The diagnosis is clinical but investigations can be helpful. The ESR and CRP are usually raised. Chest radiograph may show diffuse infiltrates, nodules or cavitating lesions: but hilar adenopathy is unusual. Biopsy is advised wherever possible, either of the upper airway, lung or kidney. Patients with Wegener's granulomatosis typically have cytoplasmic ANCA (c-ANCA) detectable in their serum and these are usually confirmed as anti-proteinase 3 specificity (PR3-ANCA). The diagnostic use of ANCA testing is further discussed in Chapter 12; however, detection of c-ANCA is relatively specific for Wegener's granulomatosis, particularly for active systemic disease. As in microscopic polyangiitis, it is important to emphasise that a negative c-ANCA does not exclude the diagnosis of Wegener's granulomatosis.

Management

The principles are similar to those for microscopic polyangiitis. It is important that the multisystem nature of Wegener's granulomatosis is taken into account when planning the management of affected patients. The involvement of renal, respiratory, rheumatology, immunology and ear/nose/throat specialists may all be required.

Cryoglobulinaemia

Cryoglobulinaemia is an important cause of secondary small-vessel vasculitis. It is associated with a range of conditions, from the benign to malignant. The recognition of cryoglobulinaemia and its correct classification can be very useful in identifying important underlying disorders.

Cryoglobulins are abnormal immunoglobulins that precipitate in the circulation when they are cooled. There are three main subtypes (Table 41):

- type I are monoclonal proteins that are associated with underlying lymphoproliferative disease and usually do not cause vasculitis
- type II have a monoclonal component, but also rheumatoid factor activity and, therefore, form immune complexes; they may be associated with lymphoproliferative or autoimmune disease
- type III is polyclonal, has rheumatoid factor activity and forms immune complex.

Types II and III, through their formation of immune complex, are thus able to activate the complement system and cause inflammation, which usually manifests as small-vessel vasculitis.

Table 41 Classification of cryoglobulins

Type	Immunoglobulin	Rheumatoid factor	Associated conditions
I Monoclonal cryoglobulin	IgM	No	Myeloma, Waldenstrom's macroglobulinaemia, chronic lymphocytic leukaemia
	IgG	No	
	IgA	No	
	Free light chain	No	
II Mixed cryoglobulin	IgM–IgG	Yes	Myeloma, Waldenstrom's macroglobulinaemia, chronic lymphocytic leukaemia, rheumatoid arthritis, Sjögren's syndrome
	IgG–IgG	Yes	
	IgA–IgG	Yes	
III Mixed polyclonal cryoglobulinaemia	IgM–IgG	Yes	Systemic lupus erythematosus, rheumatoid arthritis, Sjögren's syndrome, Epstein–Barr virus, cytomegalovirus, viral hepatitis, chronic active hepatitis, primary biliary cirrhosis, post-streptococcal glomerulonephritis, infectious endocarditis, leprosy, kala-azar, tropical splenomegaly
	IgM–IgG–IgA	Yes	

Clinical features

The presenting symptoms may be palpable purpura affecting the lower legs (Fig. 51), fatigue, arthralgia and haematuria. The dominant symptoms may be those of the underlying disorder.

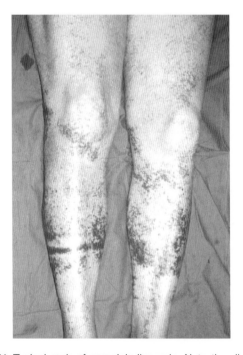

Fig. 51 Typical rash of cryoglobulinaemia. Note the distribution over the lower legs with sparing of the skin where the patient has been wearing socks.

Investigation

If cryoglobulinaemia is suspected, it is essential to liaise with the local immunology laboratory to ensure that appropriate blood samples are taken and analysed. For successful cryoglobulin detection, it is essential that the blood sample is not allowed to cool below 37°C from the moment the sample is drawn until it reaches the laboratory for analysis. Therefore, appropriately warmed syringes and sample bottles must be used and the sample transported to the laboratory in a warmed flask. Failure to follow appropriate sample collection procedures will result in the cryoglobulin precipitating with the clot in the sample tube and remaining undetected.

A useful clue to the presence of cryoglobulin may, however, be obtained by the measurement of complement components C3 and C4 in a routinely collected blood sample. Typically, there is a low level of C4 with normal level of C3. This is because cryoglobulins cause inefficient complement activation (in the fluid phase) by the classical pathway. There is, therefore, consumption of the early classical components (C1, C2, C4) but the C3 convertase is not efficiently formed and C3 is, therefore, relatively spared. A similar pattern of C3 and C4 levels is also seen in patients' C1 esterase inhibitor deficiency (Ch. 4).

Once a cryoglobulin is detected, it is essential that thorough investigation identifies the underlying cause of the cryoglobulinaemia (Table 41). It was previously thought that many type II cryoglobulins were idiopathic (**mixed essential cryoglobulinaemia**); however, it is now recognised that up to 90% of such cases are associated with hepatitis C infection.

Table 42 International Study Group diagnostic criteria for Behçet's disease

Symptoms	Requirement
Must have	
Mouth ulcers	Any shape, size or number at least three times in any 12 months
Plus two of the four 'hallmark' symptoms	
Genital ulcers	Including anal ulcers and spots in the genital region and swollen testicles or epididymitis in men
Skin lesions	Papulopustules, folliculitis, erythema nodosum, acne in post-adolescents not taking corticosteroids
Eye inflammation	Iritis, uveitis, retinal vasculitis, cells in the vitreous
Pathergy reaction	Papule > 2 mm diameter 24–48 hours or more after needleprick

Management

Treatment of the underlying condition is essential; however, in managing the symptoms of the cryoglobulinaemia, simple measures including thermal underwear and socks can reduce the development of purpura. Neurological or renal disease requires the use of corticosteroids and cyclophosphamide therapy. Recently there are reports of clinical response to the anti B-cell monoclonal antibody Rituximab.

Henoch–Schönlein purpura (HSP)

Henoch–Schönlein purpura is usually a disease of children.

Clinical features

The typical presentation is of a purpuric rash over the buttocks and extensor aspect of the lower limbs. Often the appearance of the rash is preceded by a viral upper respiratory infection and there may be associated arthralgia and proteinuria and/or haematuria. Focal glomerulonephritis occurs in approximately 50% of cases. The disease is normally self-limiting and requires symptomatic treatment only; however, in a minority renal failure develops. When Henoch–Schönlein purpura occurs in adults, it tends to be a more severe condition that can be difficult to differentiate from microscopic polyangiitis.

Investigation

There are no specific diagnostic tests for Henoch–Schönlein purpura, but acute phase proteins are raised; skin biopsy may indicate IgA and complement in blood vessel walls.

Behçet's disease

Behçet's disease is characterised by a clinical triad of aphthous-type oral and genital ulcers, and iritis.

There are no pathognomonic clinical signs and the diagnosis can, therefore, be very difficult to make with certainty. The international Behçet's Disease Study Group diagnostic criteria are said to be 95% sensitive and 100% specific for the diagnosis (Table 42). Pathergy is a phenomenon described in Behçet's disease but is actually very rare in patients in the UK. It is an excessive inflammatory (chiefly neutrophilic) response to minor injury that may manifest as mouth ulcers triggered by dental procedures or the formation of 'sterile pustules' after minor trauma such as venepuncture.

The underlying pathogenesis of Behçet's disease is a venulitis, and large-vessel thrombosis can occur with serious consequences (e.g. stroke). Neuro-Behçet's disease may also manifest as meningitic or brainstem symptoms. Gastrointestinal Behçet's disease may be clinically indistinguishable from Crohn's disease; however, histological examination of the bowel wall should identify characteristic deep ulceration in Behçet's disease. Ocular involvement can cause iritis and retinal vasculitis, and blindness is a frequent outcome. Arthritis occurs in approximately 60% of patients and typically affects the large weight-bearing joints. There are no diagnostic laboratory tests and the reported association with HLA-B5 is not usually helpful in the diagnostic process. Treatment is tailored to the individual patient. Oral ulceration responds to colchicine or thalidomide. The latter should not be prescribed for women of child-bearing potential without detailed discussion of the teratogenic risks and need for effective contraceptive strategies. Baseline and annual nerve conduction velocity studies are also recommended during thalidomide treatment. Ciclosporin is effective in controlling eye disease.

Self-assessment: questions

Multiple choice questions

1. Takayasu's arteritis is:
   a. Primarily a disorder of middle-aged men
   b. Characterised by inflammation limited to the vascular endothelium
   c. A cause of systemic hypertension
   d. Specifically associated with anti-neutrophil cytoplasmic antibodies (ANCA)
   e. Associated with a 5-year mortality of > 75%

2. Type III Takayasu's arteritis involves:
   a. Aortic root only
   b. Aortic arch only
   c. Descending aorta only
   d. Aortic arch and descending aorta
   e. Renal arteries only

3. Typical presenting features of polyarteritis nodosa include:
   a. Butterfly rash
   b. Subcutaneous nodules
   c. Testicular pain
   d. Fever
   e. Neurological symptoms

4. Microscopic polyangiitis is typically associated with:
   a. Microscopic haematuria
   b. Positive c-ANCA (anti-neutrophil cytoplasmic antibodies)
   c. Joint pains
   d. Hepatic impairment
   e. Hair loss

5. Type I cryoglobulinaemia is associated with:
   a. Hepatitis C infection
   b. Systemic lupus erythematosus
   c. False-positive rheumatoid factor
   d. Lymphoproliferative disease
   e. Polyclonal increase in serum immunoglobulins

6. Indications for ANCA (anti-neutrophil cytoplasmic antibody) testing include:
   a. Unexplained arthropathy
   b. Impaired renal function
   c. Purpuric rash
   d. Pulmonary haemorrhage
   e. Stridor

7. Typical features of Behçet's disease include:
   a. Superficial oral ulceration
   b. Association with HLA-B5
   c. Iritis
   d. Arthritis affecting large joints
   e. Urethritis

Case history questions

History 1

A 22-year-old woman has been referred to hospital for investigation and management of hypertension. Her blood pressure was recorded at 180/110 mmHg. Investigations indicated:

- serum urea and electrolytes: normal
- full blood count: normal
- ESR 96 mm/h
- fasting lipids normal
- anti-nuclear antibody negative
- anti-neutrophil cytoplasmic antibodies (ANCA) negative.

She was commenced on combination therapy with atenolol 50 mg daily and nifedipine 60 mg daily and had a good response with blood pressure falling to 124/84 mmHg at review 3 months later. In the interim, ultrasound of abdomen suggested an enlarged left kidney. Angiography of the renal arteries indicated a stenosis of the left renal artery with 30% reduction in diameter. The right renal artery had a high-grade stenosis. The right kidney was non-functional. Renal vein sampling indicated high renin values on the right side. Right renal artery stenosis was diagnosed and right nephrectomy performed.

Blood pressure control improved after surgery and antihypertensive medication was withdrawn. Three years after surgery she was re-referred because of headache, occasional shortness of breath and paraesthesia in the left arm. Her ESR was noted to be persistently high (100 mm/h) but no cause was identified. Six years after nephrectomy, she was referred with persisting paraesthesia in the left arm and a reduction in the left radial pulse pressure. Angiography of the aortic arch revealed significant stenosis affecting the left subclavian and vertebral arteries and both carotid arteries; ESR was 80 mm/h and C-reactive protein 30 mg/l. A diagnosis of Takayasu's arteritis was made and combination therapy with prednisolone and methotrexate commenced.

1. During the initial investigation of this lady, the ANCA test was negative: did this rule out a vasculitic disorder at the time?
2. With hindsight, how might you explain the paraesthesia affecting the left arm?
3. What is the likelihood of reversing the stenosis identified using combination immunosuppressive therapy?
4. What investigations (if any) would be helpful in monitoring disease activity in this lady?
5. How would you modify treatment if this lady were planning to become pregnant?
6. For how long should immunosuppression be continued?
7. What other treatment modalities might be considered?

History 2

A 50-year-old nursing sister presented with a purpuric rash over the lower legs. There is a previous history of tonsillitis occurring 2 weeks prior to the development of the rash. A diagnosis of postviral thrombocytopenia is made and symptoms resolve over a 4-week period. Four months later she presented with numbness and weakness of her hands and feet with a recurrence of the purpuric rash. Table 43 shows the results of the investigations.

1. What is the differential diagnosis?
2. What further investigations might be helpful?
3. What therapeutic options might be considered and how would you assess response to treatment?

History 3

A 5-year-old girl presents with a febrile illness that has lasted for 6 days. On examination, there is marked cervical lymphadenopathy and conjunctivitis. Tonsils were not clearly visualised. Respiratory examination revealed no added sounds. There had been no reduction in temperature despite oral antibiotic treatment. Table 44 shows the results of the investigations.

1. What is the most likely diagnosis?
2. What treatment if any would you institute?
3. What is the long-term prognosis?

Table 44 Results of the investigations in case history 3

Parameter	Value	Normal range
Haemoglobin (g/l)	105	130–180
Total white cell count (× 10⁹/l)	Normal	4–10
Platelets (× 10⁹/l)	500	150–450
C-reactive protein (mg/l)	150	0–10

Table 43 Investigation in case history 2

Parameter	Value	Normal range
Haemoglobin (g/l)	125	130–180
Total white cell count (× 10⁹/l)	8	4–10
Erythrocyte sedimentation rate (mm/h)	80	
Urea (mmol/l)	7.0	2.1–8.9
Creatinine (µmol/l)	105	53–133
Alanine aminotransferase (U/l)	17	< 45
Aspartate aminotransferase (U/l)	26	< 41
C-reactive protein (mg/l)	145	0–10
Platelets (× 10⁹/l)	120	150–450
Perinuclear anti-neutrophil cytoplasmic antibody (p-ANCA)	Positive (1:160)	
Anti-neutrophil cytoplasmic antibody (MPO-ANCA) (U/l)	15	< 5
Chest X-ray	Normal lung fields	
Urine microscopy	No white cells/casts	

Self-assessment: answers

Multiple choice answers

1. a. **False.** It is a disorder chiefly affecting young women.
   b. **False.** Granulomatous inflammation affects the vessel wall.
   c. **True.** Hypertension may be a presenting feature and is associated with mortality.
   d. **False.** ANCA are typically negative in Takayasu's arteritis.
   e. **False.** However, it does lead to hypertension and cerebrovascular occlusion.

2. a. **False.**
   b. **False.** Type I involves the aortic arch only.
   c. **False.** Type II involves the descending aorta only.
   d. **True.** Both arch and descending aorta are involved in type III.
   e. **False.** Renal artery involvement occurs in types II and III.

3. a. **False.** This is not a feature.
   b. **True.** This is typical.
   c. **True.** This is typical.
   d. **True.** This is typical.
   e. **True.** Typically mononeuritis multiplex.

4. a. **True.** Microscopic haematuria is commonly detected.
   b. **False.** c-ANCA is typically associated with Wegener's granulomatosis.
   c. **True.** Small joint pains are common.
   d. **False.** Hepatic impairment is not a common feature.
   e. **False.** Hair loss is not a feature.

5. a. **False.** Hepatitis C infection is associated with type III cryoglobulinaemia.
   b. **False.** Systemic lupus erythematosus can be associated with types II and III.
   c. **False.** Rheumatoid factor is negative ion type I cryoglobulinaemia.
   d. **True.** Lymphoproliferative disease is usually associated with type I cryoglobulinaemia.
   e. **False.** The increase in serum immunoglobulins is monoclonal.

6. a. **False.**
   b. **True.**
   c. **True.** Purpuric rash is an indication for testing if it is non-thrombocytopenic and there are other features to suggest vasculitis.

d. **True.**
   e. **True.** In some cases stridor could indicate sub-glottic stenosis.

6. a. **False.** Ulcers are typically deep and painful.
   b. **True.** Although this is rarely useful in diagnosis.
   c. **True.** Iritis is a characteristic feature of Behçet's disease.
   d. **True.** Arthritis typically affects large weight-bearing joints in Behçet's disease.
   e. **False.** Urethritis is not a typical feature.

Case history answers

History 1

1. No; ANCA are useful tests for vasculitic disorders that affect small vessels (e.g. Wegener's granulomatosis and microscopic polyangiitis) but are not found in large vessel vasculitis.
2. The symptoms in the left arm are likely to have been a consequence of impaired blood flow caused by stenosis of the left subclavian artery.
3. The stenoses are very unlikely to change as a consequence of immunosuppression. The purpose of medical therapy is to control inflammatory disease activity and prevent new stenoses occurring. This emphasises the difference between vasculitis *activity* (potentially controlled by medical therapy) and vasculitis *damage* (irreversible).
4. As already stated, ANCA is not useful in the diagnosis or monitoring of Takayasu's arteritis. In this case, both ESR and C-reactive protein were elevated and both fell to normal levels after immunosuppression was commenced. Both were, therefore, thought to reflect underlying disease activity and continue to be monitored in this case.
5. Methotrexate is teratogenic and, therefore, contraindicated in pregnancy. It is recommended that if a man or woman has been taking methotrexate, they should continue with effective contraception for at least 3 months after therapy is stopped. This lady did wish to start a family during her period of treatment and she was changed to azathioprine. This was an effective therapeutic alternative and there were no adverse effects on the pregnancy.
6. This is a difficult question to answer. It is anticipated that Takayasu's disease usually 'burns out' after about 5 years. This case, however, illustrates some of the difficulties in determining the duration of therapy, including the definition of when the condition first appeared. It is virtually certain

that the initial diagnosis of renal artery stenosis was, in fact, a manifestation of Takayasu's as her ESR was very high at the time. Her subsequent referral 6 years later with paraesthesia and persistently elevated inflammatory indicators indicated that her condition was still active. Other factors that should be considered include the critical sites of disease and also age. Continuing immunosuppression for inappropriately long periods increases the risk of therapy-associated side effects. In most of those with Takayasu's arteritis, immunosuppression would be continued for between 3 and 5 years, after which it would be gradually reduced with close monitoring of clinical condition and inflammatory markers.

7. Surgical intervention is an important part of the management of this condition, especially to treat symptoms caused by critical vascular stenoses. Surgical intervention is, therefore, used to address vasculitis *damage* rather than *activity*.

History 2

1. The initial clinical diagnosis of postviral thrombocytopenia is not supported by the investigations, which indicate a normal platelet count. Functional platelet abnormality might be considered, but this is unlikely to explain the development of neurological symptoms. The combination of rash and neurological symptoms is suggestive of a small-vessel vasculitis and the finding of a high C-reactive protein is consistent with that and indicates a significant acute phase response. The two main differentials would be Henoch–Schönlein purpura and microscopic polyangiitis. The absence of haematuria and the development of neuropathy would be against the former. The clinical features and the identification of a positive p-ANCA supports the latter.

2. In suspected vasculitic disorders it is always desirable to have a tissue diagnosis if possible. Skin biopsy was, therefore, undertaken, which confirmed vasculitis affecting small vessels. Had there been evidence of microscopic haematuria and impaired renal function, renal biopsy would be considered.

3. In this lady, oral prednisolone at a dose of 30 mg/day was commenced and her symptoms of rash and impaired sensation resolved over a 10-day period. She did not regain all her sensory function. Thus, clinical monitoring confirmed a therapeutic response. Biochemically, this was confirmed by a fall in C-reactive protein to normal levels. As long-term steroid therapy was anticipated, a baseline bone scan was undertaken and bisphosphonate therapy commenced. A steroid-sparing agent, azathioprine, was required and, therefore, regular full blood count was required.

History 3

1. The differential diagnosis in this case must include a wide range of infective causes for these symptoms. Viral upper respiratory tract infection would be the most common cause; however, the very high C-reactive protein level virtually excludes this. An acute tonsillar abscess should be considered, although the absence of tonsillar enlargement and localised swelling make this unlikely. Acute onset of a juvenile connective tissue disorder should be considered, but the clinical presentation is not particularly typical and the findings of thrombocytosis and very high C-reactive protein would be unusual. The unremitting nature of the fever is unusual and the single diagnosis that explains all the findings is Kawasaki disease.

2. Treatment should be instituted as soon as the diagnosis is considered likely. Intravenous immunoglobulin (2 g/kg body weight) should be given either as a single dose or divided over 4 days. It appears that this therapy must be instituted within 10 days of the onset of symptoms if it is to be effective in preventing the long-term complication of coronary artery aneurysm. Aspirin therapy is also indicated because of the thrombocytosis.

3. The long-term prognosis is good if the diagnosis is made early and appropriate therapy as above instituted. If the diagnosis is delayed however, there is a high incidence of coronary artery aneurysm and late sudden death can occur.

9 Immunological therapies

Chapter overview

The recognition of immunologically mediated diseases has led clinicians to use a wide range of therapies to modify or suppress the immune system in the hope of altering the course of the disease. This is an area of constant change and advancement, from the relatively simple antihistamine, through a range of immunosuppressant agents, to immune-modifying therapies, including desensitisation, intravenous immunoglobulin and the latest range of biological therapies. This chapter describes these therapies in terms of their mode of action, clinical indications, side effect profile and known interactions. Dosage information is not provided except in general terms; for this information you should consult current formularies (e.g. British National Formulary (BNF), MIMS, etc.).

9.1 Introduction

Learning objectives

You should:
- be familiar with a wide range of immunological therapies
- be aware of important/common side effects of each therapy
- understand their basic scientific modes of action.

Common immune-mediated conditions such as hay fever and eczema are treated with drugs that are immunosuppressive and anti-inflammatory. The more common occurrence of immunodeficiency caused by disease and treatment has also stimulated a range of immune therapies. Immune components such as cytokines are now being used in therapy and monoclonal antibodies are used to target specific cells or molecules.

9.2 Antihistamines

Learning objectives

You should:
- know the indications for use of antihistamines
- understand their mode of their action
- know their contraindications and side effects.

Antihistamines work by blocking histamine H_1 receptors, thus preventing the symptoms normally associated with histamine release in allergic reactions (rhinorrhoea, itch, wheeze, etc.). Generally, these drugs are taken orally although topical antihistamine creams, nasal sprays and eye drops are also used. The first-generation antihistamine drugs (e.g. hydroxizine, chlorphenamine) were relatively short acting, requiring regular dose intervals during the day and were associated with significant side effects. The newer antihistamines (e.g. acrivastine, cetirizine, desloratidine, fexofenadine) have fewer side effects and are longer acting, which allows once daily dosage.

Indications

Antihistamines are widely available both as 'over the counter' and prescription medications. They are widely used for the symptomatic relief of common allergic disorders including allergic rhinitis, urticaria and relief of the itch associated with eczema. They are also an important part of the emergency medical kit prescribed for people with food allergies.

The pharmacological actions of individual antihistamines do differ and patients may respond better to one antihistamine rather than another. It is, therefore, worth trying several alternatives if symptomatic response to the first prescribed drug is inadequate. In some chronic conditions (e.g. chronic idiopathic urticaria), it can be beneficial to combine the use of a sedating antihistamine at night with a non-sedating antihistamine in the morning.

Adverse effects

The adverse effects of antihistamines are divided into *central* and *peripheral*.

The central side effects are caused by the drugs crossing the blood–brain barrier and they include depressive (sedation, ataxia, fatigue, dizziness), stimulatory (seizures, insomnia, headaches, tremors) and neuropsychiatric (anxiety, depression, psychosis, hallucinations) effects. The newer generation of antihistamines do not cross the blood–brain barrier to the same extent and are, therefore, associated with fewer central side effects.

The peripheral effects include

- anticholinergic effects (blurred vision, dilated pupils, dry mouth, urinary retention)
- potentiation of the effects of alcohol and benzodiazepines
- cardiotoxicity: prolongation of QTc interval on electrocardiography (terfenadine and astemizole were both withdrawn from the market because of this cardiac risk).

9.3 Epinephrine (adrenaline)

Learning objectives

You should:
- know the use of epinephrine (adrenaline) to treat medical emergencies including anaphylactic reactions
- understand the indications for its use
- know its adverse effects.

Epinephrine (adrenaline) is a naturally occurring hormone that is used in therapeutic preparations to treat medical emergencies including anaphylactic reactions and some cardiac emergencies. It exerts much of its therapeutic effect via stimulation of β_2-adrenoceptors, causing increased heart rate, blood pressure and smooth muscle relaxation. The drug form is known as epinephrine (adrenaline is still added after it to ensure that there

is no doubt about what the drug is). Self-administration kits are now frequently prescribed for adults and children with severe food allergy (usually peanut allergy) or insect venom allergy. The kits usually come in the form of preloaded syringes (Min-i-jet, Aurum) or spring-loaded autoinjectors (Epi-pen, Ana-pen) and are designed for intramuscular administration. Auto-injectors are most frequently prescribed, as they are simple to use in an emergency and do not require any assembly at the time of use. They come in standard adult and paediatric doses (e.g. 0.3 mg for adult and 0.15 mg for a child weighing < 30 kg) and patients need to be instructed in when and how to use them.

Immunological indications

Not everyone with a food allergy needs an epinephrine (adrenaline) kit. These should be prescribed only after careful individual assessment of the patient. Factors in the history that would favour the prescription of an epinephrine (adrenaline) self-administration kit include

- systemic anaphylactic reactions
- laryngeal oedema causing respiratory obstruction
- severe allergic reaction after indirect or very limited allergen exposure
- associated asthma.

Limited angioedema (e.g. affecting only the lips or peripheries) is generally not an indication for the use of epinephrine (adrenaline) and such symptoms normally respond satisfactorily to oral antihistamines.

Adverse effects

In otherwise healthy children and young adults, the use of epinephrine (adrenaline) as emergency treatment of allergic reactions is usually well tolerated. There is, however, a particular risk of adverse reaction if the drug is incorrectly administered. Epinephrine (adrenaline) should be given *intramuscularly*. If given *intravenously*, there is a risk of potentially fatal cardiac arrhythmia.

Because of the cardiac stimulatory effects, however, use of epinephrine (adrenaline) in adults, even by the appropriate route (*intramuscular*) is associated with higher risk. In a small number of patients, use of epinephrine (adrenaline) has precipitated angina attacks and cerebral haemorrhage, probably by unmasking previously unrecognised cardiovascular disease. For this reason, the potential risks and benefits of treatment must be considered and explained to the patient prior to prescription.

9.4 Desensitisation

Learning objectives

You should:
- know what is meant by desensitisation
- understand the indications for its use
- know the adverse reactions.

Desensitisation is the term used to describe the therapeutic reversal of allergic sensitisation to environmental allergens. Desensitisation typically involves a series of subcutaneous injections of allergen, which may be administered over a short or relatively prolonged period of time.

Indications

In the UK, desensitisation is generally restricted to patients suffering from seasonal allergic rhinitis caused by pollens. Some specialist centres undertake desensitisation to house dust mite and some animal allergens (e.g. cat dander). In the USA and mainland Europe, immunotherapy is much more widely available.

Typically, for grass pollen desensitisation, a series of weekly injections of grass pollen is given for 6–8 weeks prior to the grass pollen season. For venom allergy (wasp and bee venom), the course is usually much longer, with a weekly induction phase lasting several months followed by monthly maintenance doses usually for a minimum of 3 years. Rush desensitisation is a modification of the technique, whereby the incremental doses are given over a very short period (typically 24–48 hours) under supervision in hospital. In some centres, this technique is used for grass pollen and venom desensitisation; however, it is very labour intensive and is most often reserved for rare cases of life-threatening drug allergy (e.g. penicillin allergy) where rapid response is required.

Adverse reactions

Adverse reactions during immunotherapy are common. Approximately 70% of people undergoing venom desensitisation will experience an adverse reaction during therapy. These range from the mild (local erythema and swelling at the injection site) through to major anaphylactic reactions. Most reactions are of minor or moderate severity; however, major reactions can occur at any stage in the treatment course. The majority of reactions occur in the first 30 minutes after injection and, for that reason, close observation of the patient for 1 hour is recommended on each occasion.

The occurrence of adverse reactions is the major reason for the cautious approach to immunotherapy in the UK. A significant number of deaths occurred during immunotherapy during the 1980s, at which time treatment was being administered in the primary care setting. Desensitisation should now only be administered in specialist hospital based units with full resuscitation facilities available.

9.5 Corticosteroids

Learning objectives

You should:
- be aware of the range of corticosteroid drugs, their potencies and their mode of administration
- know their mechanism of action
- understand the indications for their use
- know their adverse effects.

Corticosteroids are a family of drugs that have broad immunosuppressive and anti-inflammatory actions. They are available in topical, oral or parenteral forms and are used in a wide range of clinical conditions, a comprehensive description of which is beyond the scope of the chapter. The anti-inflammatory activity of different types of orally administered corticosteroids is indicated in Table 45.

Mechanisms of action

Corticosteroids may affect many cell types within the body to exert their immunosuppressant and anti-inflammatory actions. The anti-inflammatory potency is related to the glucocorticoid activity of the corticosteroid, assuming there is low intrinsic mineralocorticoid activity. The effect of these drugs also depends on the dose used and the route of administration. Broadly speaking, the major mechanism of action in humans is an inhibitory effect on monocytes and macrophages,

Table 45 Equivalent anti-inflammatory activity of corticosteroid preparations

Corticosteroid	Dose equivalent to 5 mg oral prednisolone (mg)
Betamethasone	0.75 (750 µg)
Cortisone acetate	25
Deflazacort	6
Dexamethasone	0.75 (750 µg)
Hydrocortisone	20
Methylprednisolone	4
Triamcinolone	4

with reduced phagocytic function and diminished interleukin IL-1 secretion. In animals, corticosteroids have a marked lymphocytotoxic effect, but in humans this is only significant against abnormal lymphocytes, for example in lymphoproliferative disorders, and also when corticosteroids are used at very high doses, typically intravenously.

Adverse reactions

Corticosteroids are potent immunosuppressants but their major disadvantage is their multiple side effects; these include weight gain, hirsutism, hypertension, acne, diabetes mellitus, recurrent infection, growth retardation, osteoporosis and reduced physiological response to stress, because of adrenal suppression.

The appropriate dose of corticosteroid varies greatly from one condition and patient to the next. In the acute management of autoimmune haemolytic anaemia, acute glomerulonephritis or immune thrombocytopenic purpura, 1–2 mg/kg methylprednisolone daily is indicated. In severe life-threatening situations, such as systemic vasculitis, pulsed high-dose regimens of 10 mg/kg are used (maximum dose 1000 mg). In the long-term control of autoimmune disorders, however, the minimum practical dose is used (e.g. an oral dose of < 7.5 mg daily of prednisolone) in order to minimise drug side effects. Often a second immunosuppressant drug is used (as a *steroid-sparing agent*) in order to reduce the oral steroid requirement.

Topical corticosteroids are important drugs in the control of atopic eczema but the side effects of steroid creams include thinning of the skin and the development of striae. In order to minimise such local effects, it is crucial to use the minimum appropriate dose of topical steroids and to understand the relevant 'strengths' of the commonly available preparations (Table 46).

Prevention of steroid-associated osteoporosis and adrenal suppression has received much attention recently. It is now recommended that appropriate bone-protective therapy (e.g. bisphosphonates, calcium and vitamin D supplements) is commenced as soon as chronic oral steroid therapy is started, and regular bone density scanning should be undertaken. The adrenal suppressive effect of inhaled steroids is also now recognised and it is essential that the minimum inhaled dose of steroids necessary to control symptoms is maintained. An important factor in ensuring maximum efficacy of inhaled steroid use is correct instruction in inhaler technique and selection of the most appropriate type of inhaler for the individual patient (dry powder, aerosol, etc.). With regard to nasal inhalers, the position of the head is crucial to ensure maximum delivery of the spray to the nasal mucosa. Recommended positions for the use of nasal inhalers are indicated in Figure 52.

9.6 Immunosuppressive drugs

Learning objectives

You should:
- know the range of actions of the non-corticosteroid immunosuppressive drugs
- understand their role in transplantation
- understand their other indications
- understand their modes of action
- know their adverse effects.

Table 46 Potency of topical corticosteroid preparations: the least potent drug that is effective is the drug of choice

Potency	Examples
Mild	Hydrocortisone 1%
Moderate	Clobetasone butyrate 1%
Potent	Betamethasone (0.1%), hydrocortisone butyrate
Very potent	Clobetasol propionate (0.05%)

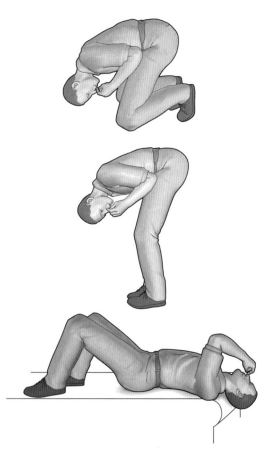

Fig. 52 Recommended positions to adopt when using a nasal inhaler.

The non-corticosteroid drugs commonly used to suppress the immune system include those with the following properties:

- cytotoxic
- antimetabolite
- antiproliferative
- anti-T cell activation.

These groups of drugs were introduced to the management of patients undergoing transplantation and autoimmunity because of their ability to suppress the immune response. Usually, the management of these conditions requires therapy at lower dosage and is associated with fewer side effects than occurs in the treatment of malignancy. Their use in combination with corticosteroids enables significant reductions in the doses of corticosteroids required (in this context they are often referred to as *steroid-sparing agents*). The major complication of long-term use is myelosuppression and immunosuppression, with a long-term increase in susceptibility to malignancies (e.g. lymphoma).

Drug development in this area has been focused on developing ever more specific therapies, to interact with identified components of the immune system and deliver targeted immunosuppression with an improved side effect profile. This increased specificity of immunosuppressive strategies is demonstrated in the following section as examples of each type of therapy are discussed.

Cytotoxic drugs

Cytotoxic drugs were originally introduced for the treatment of a range of cancers and, as the name suggests, their major effect is to kill cells capable of self-replication.

Cyclophosphamide

Cyclophosphamide is one of the most widely used cytotoxic drugs in chemotherapy for cancer and it is frequently used in combination with corticosteroids in the management of severe autoimmune conditions, especially systemic vasculitis. As an alkylating agent it acts by cross-linking DNA strands, thus preventing normal mitosis. It is particularly toxic to B cells. Side effects include a dose-dependent neutropenia and lymphopenia, alopecia, infertility (especially in males) and, infrequently, haemorrhagic cystitis (these complications should not occur at low dose). Dosage is determined by disease severity and according to renal function, bone marrow function and the patient's age.

Antimetabolite drugs

Methotrexate

Methotrexate is used in maintenance treatment of childhood leukaemias but it is increasingly used in the control of a number of inflammatory diseases including rheumatoid arthritis, poliomyelitis, psoriasis, Reiter's syndrome and graft-versus-host disease following bone marrow transplantation. It also appears to have a role in steroid-dependent asthma although the exact mode of action in this condition is unclear. Methotrexate inhibits dihydrofolate reductase, thus preventing the conversion of folic acid to its active form, tetrahydrofolate. This prevents normal thymidine synthesis and cell division. Side effects include bone marrow suppression, megaloblastic anaemia, pneumonitis and mucositis. Long-term drug toxicity is increased in hepatic impairment. Acute side effects are partially reversible by the administration of folinic acid.

Antiproliferative drugs

The antiproliferative drugs act to block some steps required for cell multiplication, such as DNA synthesis, and are used for treatment of tumours and in conditions where a cell type is overproduced, such as lymphocytes.

Azathioprine

Azathioprine is an analogue of the cytotoxic drug 6 mercaptopurine (both are thiopurines) and was originally introduced in the 1950s for renal transplant recipients. It is now frequently used as a steroid-sparing agent in the management of many autimmune disorders. Thiopurines block the synthesis of inosinic acid, the precursor of adenylic and guanylic acid, and thus impair DNA synthesis. Their major effect is on developing T and natural killer cells and, consequently, there is a delay before clinical onset of action. The most important side effect is bone marrow suppression. Weekly monitoring of full blood count is advised during induction, with measurements every 3 months during maintenance therapy. The patient must be warned of increased susceptibility to infection, and any unexplained illness occurring while on therapy requires thorough investigation and potentially withdrawal of treatment if infection is suspected. The usual maintenance dose range is 1–3 mg/kg daily.

Mycophenolate mofetil

Mycophenolate mofetil is a relatively recently introduced prodrug that is used in combination with corticosteroids and ciclosporin in the prophylaxis of renal transplant rejection. Mycophenolic acid is the active metabolite and is rapidly produced by hydrolysis after ingestion of the drug. Mycophenolic acid selectively inhibits inosine monophosphate dehydrogenase, which prevents lymphocyte purine biosynthesis. The inhibition of this enzyme causes a depletion of guanine nucleotides, inhibition of DNA synthesis and prevents clonal expansion of both T and B cells. Close monitoring is necessary with weekly full blood counts for the first month of treatment, every 2 weeks for the next month and monthly for the first year of treatment. Its use is mainly limited to specialist transplantation units, although it is beginning to impact on the management of autoimmune disorders and severe atopic eczema.

Anti-T cell activation

T cell activation is a problem after transplantation and in some autoimmune disorders.

Ciclosporin

Ciclosporin has revolutionised the management of patients after transplantation and it is also finding a place in the management of some autoimmune disorders in both systemic and topical preparations.

Ciclosporin is a fungal metabolite with a cyclic undecapeptide structure; it acts selectively to inhibit T cell activation. The drug combines with cytosolic proteins called **cyclophilins**, which inhibit **calcineurin** and prevents the calcium-dependent activation of the gene for IL-2. The transcription of this gene is a crucial event in T cell activation and, therefore, ciclosporin is a relatively selective T cell immunosuppressant.

Ciclosporin does not cause myelotoxicity but it does cause a dose-dependent reduction in renal function that must be carefully monitored and differentiated from organ transplant failure or rejection. Monitoring of trough plasma levels is essential. Other side effects include hirsutism, gingival hyperplasia and seizures. In common with other immunosuppressants, there is an increased long-term risk of lymphoma and skin neoplasm.

Tacrolimus (FK506)

Tacrolimus is a macrolide that is not chemically related to ciclosporin but has a similar mode of action. Its use is currently limited to patients receiving hepatic and renal transplantations, although there is evidence to suggest it will have significant clinical impact in autoimmunity. In topical form, it is increasingly being used for severe atopic eczema. Tacrolimus binds to the cytosolic FK506-binding protein (FKBP), preventing

activation of the gene for IL-2. It has a similar range of side effects to ciclosporin.

9.7 Other immunosuppressive strategies

Learning objectives

You should:
- be aware of the non-pharmacological and novel biological immunosuppressive strategies that exist
- understand the use of plasma and immunoglobulin replacement
- understand how monoclonal antibodies are produced and their nomenclature system
- understand the use of recombinant cytokines
- know the use and limitations of such therapies.

In addition to the pharmacological immunosuppressive drugs discussed above, a number of non-pharmacological and novel biological therapies have been utilised and are emerging in clinical practice. These include

- plasma exchange
- immunoglobulin-replacement therapy
- monoclonal antibody therapy
- cytokines and anti-cytokines.

Plasma exchange

Plasma exchange is a process that replaces the patient's serum with a physiologically balanced fluid. The basis of treatment is that circulating factors (e.g. autoantibodies) are removed from the circulation and this has a beneficial effect on acute disease. In practice, treatment is normally provided as a day case in hospital. The patient is linked to a plasma-exchange machine for several hours by intravenous lines. Whole blood flows into the machine, where serum is separated off. The cellular components of blood are then resuspended in physiological fluids and reinfused into the patient. Plasma exchange has been available for many years and continues to be of value in the acute management of some severe autoimmune conditions including Goodpasture's syndrome, myasthenia gravis or Rhesus disease, in which autoantibodies are known to be pathogenic (primary autoantibodies). Plasma exchange allows removal of these autoantibodies acutely but has no proven role in the long-term management of these conditions.

Immunoglobulin-replacement therapy

Immunoglobulin-replacement therapy is indicated for patients with proven primary immunodeficiency

(Ch. 4), antibody-deficiency syndromes and severe combined immunodeficiency and in some patients with secondary immunodeficiency (e.g. in some B cell chronic lymphocytic leukaemia or multiple myeloma). Immunoglobulin-replacement therapy was originally given as weekly intramuscular injections; however, as the quality of manufacturing improved, intravenous administration became possible. The vast majority of immunoglobulin-replacement therapy is given as intravenous immunoglobulin (ivIg), although for very small children and adults with poor venous access, subcutaneous immunoglobulin therapy is increasingly used. It is likely that the use of the subcutaneous route will increase because of the ease of such administration. There are a number of commercially available immunoglobulin preparations, all of which are made from pooled blood donations from a minimum of 1000 donors. As immunoglobulins are derived from human blood donations, the risk of viral transmission must be considered. Each manufacturer includes a different set of antiviral 'steps' in the manufacturing process and it is important to be aware of the differences between products before deciding which one to prescribe. Antiviral steps include low pH, treatment by solvent–detergent, nanofiltration and pasteurisation.

Intravenous immunoglobulin is extremely effective in preventing infections and lung damage and improving quality of life. The usual immunoglobulin dosage is 400 mg/kg given every 3 weeks. Regular preinfusion serum IgG levels are measured and should be maintained within the physiological range (usually > 8 g/l). Patients must be weighed regularly and appropriate increments in ivIg dosage made because growth (in children) and weight (in adults) often increases significantly after the initial diagnosis and treatment. Various ivIg preparations differ in their content. Once a patient is established on a particular product, it must not be changed without clear clinical indications.

Adverse reactions

The main potential side effect of treatment is reaction to the infusions. This may be related to infusion rate, intercurrent infection or anti-IgA antibodies in IgA-deficient patients. Transmission of viral infection is now a very small risk because of careful viral screening and new antiviral steps in the production of ivIg from pooled donor sera. Recent advances include self-administration of ivIg at home and the development of subcutaneous administration, which is of particular value in the very young. Although immunoglobulin replacement is the mainstay of treatment for antibody deficiency, there are other aspects of therapy.

High-dose intravenous immunoglobulin therapy

High-dose ivIg therapy (1–2 g/kg) is of proven benefit in autoimmune thrombocytopenia, Kawasaki disease and Guillain–Barré syndrome. The mode of action is incompletely understood, but it may involve blockade of Fc receptors, disturbance of anti-idiotypic networks or suppression of macrophage and/or T cell activation. This therapy has specific side effects, including aseptic meningitis, acute haemolysis (when ivIg is not cross-matched) and acute deterioration in renal function. It should, therefore, only be used for those conditions in which clinical benefit is proven by properly controlled studies.

Monoclonal antibodies and anti-cytokines

Monoclonal antibodies are synthetic immunoglobulin molecules manufactured to have a single antigen-binding specificity. Commonly, this specificity will be directed at surface molecules of T, B, antigen-presenting cells or cytokines, with the aim of modulating undesirable aspects of the immune response. There is a standardised nomenclature for monoclonal antibodies that indicates the target of the antibody and its source (Table 47). Each name should have four syllables. For example, Rituximab has the unique prefix *Ri*, followed by *tu* (indicating tumour target) followed by *xi* (indicating it is a chimeric antibody) and a common suffix *mab* (indicating a monoclonal antibody). In addition to *mab*, other suffixes may be used to indicate different properties including *tox* (monoclonal antibody

Table 47 Examples of nomenclature for therapeutic monoclonal antibodies

Unique prefix	Target	Source	Compound name	Target
Ri	Tum (tumour)	Xi (chimera)	Ri-tu-xi-mab	CD20 (B cells)
Inf	Lim (immune modulator)	Xi (chimera)	Inf-li-xi-mab	Tumour necrosis factor-α
Bi	Cir (cardiovascular)	O (mouse)	Bi-cir-o-mab	Fibrin (for imaging)
Se	Vir (viral)	U (human)	Se-vir-u-mab	Cytomegalovirus
Dac	Lim (immune modulator)	Zu (humanised)	Dac-li-zu-mab	CD25 (activated T cells)
Ne	Bac (bacteria)	U (human)	Ne-bac-u-mab	Gram-negative organisms

conjugated to a toxin), *pegol* (monoclonal antibody conjugated to polyethylene glycol) or *cept* (monoclonal antibody fused to another protein). A number of monoclonal antibodies have anti-cytokine properties and so examples of monoclonal antibodies and anti-cytokines are discussed together.

Infliximab

Infliximab inhibits the activity of tumour necrosis factor-α (TNF-α) and is indicated in severe rheumatoid arthritis. It is increasingly being used in other severe inflammatory conditions but should only be prescribed by appropriate specialists. Infliximab is administered by intravenous infusion. An increasingly recognised adverse effect is infection, with both tuberculosis and septicaemia being reported. Appropriate screening should be undertaken before therapy and institution of antituberculous chemoprophylaxis may be necessary. Hypersensitivity reactions also occur, with the development of human anti-chimeric antibodies (HACA). For this reason, coadministration with another immunosuppressant (e.g. methotrexate) is usually recommended.

Etanercept

Etanercept is also an anti-TNF-α agent. However, as its name indicates, it is a fusion protein consisting of a TNF-α receptor joined to an IgG molecule. Etanercept is administered subcutaneously and so there are no infusion-associated side effects. It is, however, associated with an increased risk of infection as above, with a particular susceptibility to herpes zoster virus being reported.

Rituximab

Rituximab is directed against CD20, which is a surface marker on mature B cells. It causes lysis of B cells and is used for the treatment of advanced follicular and some other lymphomas. Rituximab is administered intravenously and is associated with significant side effects, including cardiac arrhythmias, heart failure and cytokine release syndrome. This last syndrome may be mild, moderate or severe, and death has been reported after rituximab infusion. Premedication with antihistamines, analgesics and corticosteroids should, therefore,

be considered and treatment with rituximab should only be undertaken by specialist teams.

Cytokines

Recombinant cytokines are used in a number of clinical areas both to potentiate the immune response to infectious agents and for their antitumour properties. A number of examples are briefly discussed.

Interferon-α

Interferon-α has been used for its antitumour effect in some lymphomas, leukaemias, AIDS-related Kaposi's sarcoma and renal cell carcinoma. It is most commonly used in the management of chronic hepatitis B and hepatitis C infections. Interferon-α is administered subcutaneously and common side effects include influenza-like symptoms. Bone marrow suppression, hepatic and renal toxicity are also reported.

Interferon-β

Interferon-β is used for its immunomodulatory properties. The main indication is in patients who have **relapsing, remitting multiple sclerosis**. However, not all patients respond to therapy and deterioration is reported in some. Benefit from the use of interferon-β in other forms of multiple sclerosis is not proven. Adverse effects of therapy include local irritation at injection sites, influenza-like symptoms and occasionally hypersensitivity reactions, including anaphylaxis and urticaria.

Interferon-γ

Interferon-γ is specifically used in patients with chronic granulomatous disease and some other primary immunodeficiencies (Ch. 4) to assist in the immunological response to intracellular microorganisms (e.g. mycobacteria and salmonella). It has been used in some cases of multidrug-resistant tuberculosis. Interferon-γ is administered subcutaneously, usually three times weekly and the dose is calculated according to body surface area. As with the other interferons, influenza-like symptoms may be a problem; anaemia and disturbed liver and kidney biochemistry can also occur.

Self-assessment: questions

Multiple choice questions

1. Which one of the following drugs is most likely to be associated with excessive drowsiness?
   a. Acrivastine
   b. Cetirizine
   c. Desloratidine
   d. Hydroxizine
   e. Fexofenadine

2. Which one of the following drugs specifically inhibits calcineurin?
   a. Azathioprine
   b. Ciclosporin
   c. Cyclophosphamide
   d. Methotrexate
   e. Mycophenolate mofetil

3. Which one of the following drugs can cause cough?
   a. Ciclosporin
   b. Tacrolimus
   c. Methotrexate
   d. Cyclophosphamide
   e. Azathioprine

4. Which one of the following drugs is an alkylating agent?
   a. Azathioprine
   b. Ciclosporin
   c. Cyclophosphamide
   d. Methotrexate
   e. Mycophenolate mofetil

5. Which of the following drugs prevents normal purine synthesis?
   a. Azathioprine
   b. Ciclosporin
   c. Cyclophosphamide
   d. Methotrexate
   e. Mycophenolate mofetil

6. Which one of the following drugs inhibits the enzyme dihydrofolate reductase?
   a. Azathioprine
   b. Ciclosporin
   c. Cyclophosphamide
   d. Methotrexate
   e. Mycophenolate mofetil

7. Intravenous immunoglobulin (ivIg) therapy:
   a. Is of proven value in chronic granulomatous disease
   b. Must only be administered in the hospital environment
   c. Has now been superseded by monoclonal antibody therapy
   d. Is proven to prevent lung damage in antibody-deficiency syndromes
   e. Is useful in the treatment of severe allergy

8. Which one of the following require regular monitoring of drug levels?
   a. Cyclophosphamide
   b. Methotrexate
   c. Ciclosporin
   d. Azathioprine
   e. Methylprednisolone

9. Which one of the following monoclonal antibodies specifically binds to T cells?
   a. Basiliximab
   b. Alemtuzumab
   c. Infliximab
   d. Rituximab
   e. Trastuzumab

10. Wasp venom desensitisation is:
    a. Only indicated if there is a history of two or more anaphylactic reactions to wasp stings
    b. Recommended for all patients with a history of allergic reactions to wasp stings
    c. Associated with side effects in less than 30% of patients
    d. Effective after a 6-week course of injections
    e. Suitable for use in primary care

11. Self-administration of epinephrine is:
    a. The treatment of choice for idiopathic angioedema
    b. Equally safe in all age groups
    c. Associated with a risk of cardiac arrhythmia
    d. Associated with a risk of stroke
    e. Frequently required in nut-allergic individuals

12. In a patient prescribed oral prednisolone therapy:
    a. Bisphosphonate should only be prescribed after 6 months' treatment
    b. A maintenance dose of 15 mg/day is not associated with long-term side effects
    c. Acne is a recognised side effect
    d. Monthly full blood count is required
    e. Coadministration of a histamine H_2 antagonist may be required

13. Interferon-γ therapy is effective in:
    a. Relapsing/remitting multiple sclerosis
    b. Multidrug-resistant tuberculosis
    c. Laryngeal papillomatosis
    d. Hepatitis C infection
    e. Kaposi's sarcoma

14. Which of the following topical steroid preparations is most potent?
    a. Hydrocortisone
    b. Clobetasol proprionate
    c. Betamethasone
    d. Clobetasone
    e. Hydrocortisone butyrate

Case history questions

History 1

A 14-year-old male had attended his GP complaining of headache. This was mainly frontal in distribution and was sometimes associated with a 'runny nose' and itchy eyes. His symptoms were present throughout the year. His GP had diagnosed allergic rhinitis. He had initially prescribed oral antihistamines and subsequently the boy's mother had bought him a topical nasal decongestant. Despite initial symptomatic improvement, he developed a dry mouth at night and difficulty breathing through his nose. Three months later, his symptoms were more severe than at presentation.

1. From the clinical details given, what is the most likely allergen that is affecting him?
2. Give two reasons why he might have developed a dry mouth and difficulty breathing through his nose.
3. Why might his symptoms now be worse than at presentation?

Self-assessment: answers

Multiple choice answers

1. a. **False.** Acrivastine is non-sedating.
   b. **False.** Cetirizine is non-sedating.
   c. **False.** Desloratidine is non-sedating.
   d. **True.** Hydroxizine is an older, sedating antihistamine.
   e. **False.** Fexofenadine is non-sedating.

2. a. **False.** Azathioprine inhibits normal purine synthesis.
   b. **True.** The drug bound to a cyclophilin inhibits calcium-dependent activation of the gene for interleukin-2.
   c. **False.** Cyclophosphamide is an alkylating agent.
   d. **False.** Methotrexate inhibits dihydrofolate reductase.
   e. **False.** Mycophenolate mofetil selectively inhibits inosine monophosphate dehydrogenase.

3. a. **False.**
   b. **False.**
   c. **True.** This is a recognised side effect of methotrexate.
   d. **False.**
   e. **False.**

4. a. **False.** Azathioprine inhibits normal purine synthesis.
   b. **False.** Ciclosporin inhibits calcineurin.
   c. **True.** It acts by cross-linking DNA strands, thus preventing normal mitosis. It is particularly toxic to B cells.
   d. **False.** Methotrexate inhibits dihydrofolate reductase.
   e. **False.** Mycophenolate mofetil selectively inhibits inosine monophosphate dehydrogenase.

5. a. **True.** Azathioprine inhibits normal purine synthesis.
   b. **False.** Ciclosporin inhibits calcineurin.
   c. **False.** Cyclophosphamide is an alkylating agent.
   d. **False.** Methotrexate inhibits dihydrofolate reductase.
   e. **True.** Mycophenolate mofetil selectively inhibits inosine monophosphate.

6. a. **False.** Azathioprine inhibits normal purine synthesis.
   b. **False.** Ciclosporin inhibits calcineurin.
   c. **False.** Cyclophosphamide is an alkylating agent.
   d. **True.** Methotrexate inhibits dihydrofolate reductase.
   e. **False.** Mycophenolate mofetil selectively inhibits inosine monophosphate.

7. a. **False.** This is not indicated in chronic granulomatous disease.
   b. **False.** Home therapy programmes are well established.
   c. **False.** Monoclonal antibodies are not effective in preventing infection.
   d. **True.** Immunoglobulin replacement therapy is indicated for patients with proven primary immunodeficiency.
   e. **False.** IvIg is not indicated in allergy.

8. a. **False.** Regular full blood count is required.
   b. **False.** Regular liver and lung function tests are required.
   c. **True.** Ciclosporin causes a dose-dependent reduction in renal function and so therapeutic plasma levels must be carefully monitored.
   d. **False.** Regular full blood count is required.
   e. **False.**

9. a. **True.** Basiliximab binds to CD25, which is expressed on activated T cells.
   b. **False.** Alemtuzumab binds CD52, which is expressed on a wide range of cells including lymphocytes and monocytes.
   c. **False.** Infliximab binds to tumour necrosis factor.
   d. **False.** Rituximab binds to CD20 expressed on B cells.
   e. **False.** Trastuzumab binds to the human epidermal growth factor receptor 2.

10. a. **False.** It is indicated for patients with a history of anaphylactic reaction, but most would also require a high risk of subsequent stings as well (e.g. forestry workers, etc.).
    b. **False.** Recommended for those with severe systemic and not just localised/limited reactions.
    c. **False.** Approximately 70% of patients experience side effects.
    d. **False.** Treatment for several years is usually required although shorter (rush) regimens are used in some centres.
    e. **False.** Desensitisation should only be undertaken in specialised units.

11. a. **False.** Antihistamines are the treatment of choice for idiopathic angioedema.
    b. **False.** There are increased risks in the elderly.
    c. **True.** Cardiac arrhythmia is a particular risk in those with preexisting cardiac disease.
    d. **True.** There are reports of stroke occurring after self-administration of epinephrine.
    e. **False.** Epinephrine should not be required frequently; if it were it would suggest a failure of dietary avoidance of nuts.

12. a. **False.** Bisphosphonate therapy should be commenced early to prevent bone density loss.
    b. **False.** A dose of 15 mg/day is high and would be associated with side effects. Maintenance should aim to be < 7.5 mg/day in an adult.
    c. **True.**
    d. **False.**
    e. **True.** Coadministration may be required to prevent gastric side effects.

13. a. **False.** Interferon-β is indicated in relapsing/remitting multiple sclerosis.
    b. **True.** Interferon-γ is effective in multidrug-resistant tuberculosis.
    c. **False.** Interferon-α is effective in laryngeal papillomatosis.
    d. **False.** Interferon-α is effective in hepatitis C infection.
    e. **False.** Interferon-α is effective in Kaposi's sarcoma.

14. a. **False.** Hydrocortisone 1% is mild (see Table 46).
    b. **True.** Clobetasol propionate (0.05%) is very potent.

c. **False.** See Table 46.
d. **False.** See Table 46.
e. **False.** See Table 46.

Case history answers

History 1

1. The clinical details are limited, but it appears likely that he is allergic to at least one aeroallergen; because his symptoms are present all year, it is unlikely to be any of the pollens as these produce seasonal symptoms. He could be allergic to a domestic pet, but no information is provided regarding pets at home; assuming there are none, the most likely allergen is house dust mite.

2. These symptoms may be as a result of disease or treatment! If he were prescribed a sedating antihistamine, this could have been the cause of the dry mouth. Alternatively, if his rhinitis was severe enough to cause nasal obstruction (as suggested by difficulty breathing through the nose) he may have been mouth breathing at night, which also would cause a dry mouth.

3. The use of a topical decongestant is probably implicated here. Whilst these provide short-term relief, they should not be used for more than a few days. If they are used for longer, there tends to be diminishing effect (tachyphylaxis) and also worsening of symptoms (rebound) on withdrawal of treatment. If antihistamines alone are inadequate to control symptoms, then a nasal steroid inhaler should be prescribed.

10 Transplantation

Chapter overview

Solid organ and bone marrow transplantation were both successfully developed in the second half of the 20th century. The list of organs that have been successfully transplanted continues to grow, with kidney, liver, lung, heart and corneal transplants occurring routinely in specialist centres. It was the development of our understanding of the ABO blood group system and later the human leukocyte antigen (HLA)/major histocompatibility complex (MHC) along with the mechanisms of experimental transplant rejection that allowed us to define different mechanisms of transplant rejection. The development of tissue-typing techniques allowed the best matching of donors with recipients and a reduction in rejection episodes. This chapter will describe the basic mechanisms of graft rejection, the principles of tissue typing and some specific aspects of solid organ and bone marrow transplantation.

10.1 General principles

Learning objectives

You should:
• be familiar with the role of the ABO blood group and human leukocyte antigen (HLA)/major histocompatibility complex (MHC) systems in transplantation
• understand the mechanisms of hyperacute, acute and chronic graft rejection
• know the principles of tissue typing.

Transplantation of organs from cadaver or live donors has become commonplace in clinical practice. Successful transplantation is dependent on *matching* a range of blood group and tissue antigens between the donor and recipient. This requires careful clinical and laboratory assessment of the patient prior to selection for transplantation. In addition, advances in surgical technique, immunosuppressive drug therapy and treatment of post-transplantation complications have all played a crucial role in the development of this treatment strategy. From the early successes of kidney transplantation in the 1960s, we have seen the widespread development of this technique as the definitive renal-replacement therapy for a wide range of disorders. Bone marrow transplantation, originally developed as treatment for acute leukaemia, is also now widely applied for a range of haematological and other disorders including immunological conditions. Other solid organ transplantations were developed in the 1980s and 1990s, including heart, heart–lung, liver, pancreas and cornea. Transplantation of each of these organs presents unique challenges which require different management strategies.

Many patients previously thought not to be candidates now fall within the groups who should be considered for transplantation; therefore, it is important to be familiar with the indications for and processes involved in their assessment. Equally important, there is an ever-increasing population of transplant recipients who present in diverse clinical situations and may develop some of the late complications identified.

The ABO system

The blood group antigens of the ABO system are crucial in solid organ transplantation because this system is associated with antibodies to the non-expressed ABO antigens. The *rules* for transplantation and blood transfusion across the ABO system are the same (Table 48). ABO antigens are expressed not only on erythrocytes but also on vascular endothelium. Therefore, if a solid organ is transplanted to an ABO-incompatible recipient, the recipient will have preformed antibodies (isohaemagglutinins) that will react with the donor endothelium once the organ is perfused with blood. This would result in vascular coagulation and immediate graft failure.

Table 48 The ABO system and transplantation

Recipient ABO group	Isohaemag-glutinins present	Suitable donor	Comment
O	Anti-A, Anti-B	Type O	Universal donor
A	Anti-B	Type A or type O	
B	Anti-A	Type B or type O	
AB	None	Type A, type B or type O	Universal recipient

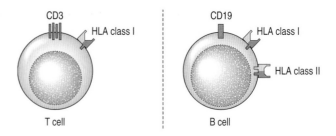

Fig. 53 Expression of HLA molecules on T and B cells. T cells, like all nucleated cells in the body, express HLA class I molecules but do not constitutively express class II molecules. In contrast, B cells express both class I and class II molecules constitutively; therefore, in the cytotoxicity or cross-match tests, antibodies to class I and class II molecules can be distinguished.

The human leukocyte antigen/major histocompatibility complex

The HLA system is a set of leukocyte surface antigens termed HLA-A, HLA-B, HLA-C and HLA-D (subdivided into HLA-DP, HLA-DQ and HLA-DR). The HLA molecules are encoded by a group of genes that lie on the short arm of chromosome 6, known as the MHC. The terms HLA and MHC are, therefore, often used interchangeably. The genes of the MHC are grouped in two major sets, referred to as class I and class II (Ch. 1 and Fig. 7, p. 9). Each set contains three genetic loci that have a large number of alleles coding for HLA antigens. The genes for some complement components and cytokines also lie within the MHC (in the class III region), but their products are quite unrelated to class I and class II molecules.

Class I. HLA-A, HLA-B and HLA-C are the class I molecules and are expressed on all nucleated cells of the body. Their structure comprises a large α-chain, and a small β-chain known as β_2-microglobulin. The latter is encoded on a different chromosome and shows no sequence variability. Class I antigens (i.e. from alleles at the A, B and C loci) are expressed on all nucleated cells (two from each locus on diploid cells).

Class II. Class II HLA molecules are two-chain (α and β) structures, both chains are encoded in the HLA locus and are polymorphic. Class II antigens (from alleles at the DP, DQ and DR loci) are expressed on a more limited range of cells: classical antigen-presenting cells, B lymphocytes and activated T lymphocytes (Fig. 53).

As was noted in Chapter 1, class I and II antigens are central to antigen presentation and the generation of an effective immune response; however, they also play key roles in transplant rejection.

HLA class I molecules express endogenously produced peptide fragments in their peptide-binding groove and thus allow T cells to recognise 'foreign' peptides (e.g. viral antigens). Should an unmatched organ be transplanted, the immune system would rapidly recognise this tissue as foreign and a range of immunological effector mechanisms, including antibody, complement and cellular components, would be activated; this would result in organ damage and *rejection*. There are several classical patterns of organ rejection that are described here.

Mechanisms of graft rejection

Hyperacute reactions

Hyperacute graft rejection typically occurs if there is a mismatch between donor and recipient in the MHC class I or ABO systems. MHC class I mismatch results in preformed antibody in the recipient binding to MHC class I antigens in the donor organ. Similarly, in ABO mismatch preformed isohaemagglutinins related to the ABO system (Table 48) bind to the vascular endothelium of the transplanted organ (see above). Such antibody binding initiates activation of the complement and clotting cascades, which results in localised inflammation and thrombosis. This leads to ischaemia and necrosis of the graft and occurs rapidly, within minutes to hours of organ transplantation. There may be symptoms and signs of inflammation including fever, tenderness and swelling of the transplanted organ, haematuria and tubular cells within the urine. Once initiated, there is no effective means of preventing hyperacute rejection. The emphasis is, therefore, on prevention of this complication, by close attention to MHC and ABO typing and monitoring of patients for ABO and donor-specific sensitisation prior to transplantation (see below).

Acute reactions

Acute rejection usually occurs from 1 week to 3 months after transplantation and its onset can be insidious. The main clinical feature is a rising serum creatinine and it is important to exclude other causes for this, including surgical complications or infection. Acute rejection is not primarily antibody mediated but is associated with a lymphocytic infiltrate of the transplanted organ. The mechanisms of immune activation in acute rejection probably include both antigen-presenting cells carried within the donated organ ('passenger' antigen-presenting cells) and recipient antigen-presenting cells processing and presenting MHC class I and II molecules from the organ. This results in $CD4^+$ and $CD8^+$ T cell activation, causing both a cytotoxic response and the stimulation of antibody directed against the donor antigens. Hence cell-mediated mechanisms predominate but secondary antibody-dependent cell-mediated cytotoxicity also occurs. There is loss of graft function and there may be swelling and fever. Acute rejection can be controlled if it is recognised early and immunosuppressive therapy commenced (usually with high-dose corticosteroids, anti-T cell globulin or anti-CD3 monoclonal antibodies). The condition may relapse and lead eventually to chronic rejection.

Chronic rejection

Chronic rejection usually occurs months to years after transplantation. The exact pathogenetic mechanisms are not known but it is characterised histologically by progressive fibrosis. Vascular narrowing is also seen and endothelial proliferation is thought to be responsible. Depending on the organ transplanted, chronic rejection leads to glomerular or bile duct loss or coronary artery occlusion. Multiple immunological mechanisms probably underlie chronic graft rejection. In some cases, it follows from acute rejection, but in others there is no prior history. Chronic rejection is usually unresponsive to immunosuppressive therapy and leads to progressive graft failure.

10.2 Kidney (renal) transplantation

Learning objectives

You should:
- know the principles of renal transplantation
- be aware of the use of tissue typing
- understand the problems associated with differing sources of kidney.

Kidney transplantation is the treatment of choice for end-stage renal disease. The increased availability of haemodialysis and peritoneal dialysis means that many more patients now survive long enough, in good health, to be suitable for transplantation. There are few contraindications to transplantation but included would be an unacceptably high risk in undergoing anaesthesia, surgery or immunosuppressive therapy. Examples would include severe cardiopulmonary disease, malignancy or ongoing infection.

There are two potential sources of donor organs: living related donors and cadaveric organs.

Assessment of patients prior to transplantation

Irrespective of the source of the organ, the donor and recipient must be ABO compatible. HLA matching should be as close as possible (including HLA-A, HLA-B, HLA-C and HLA-D loci) and patients' serum must be cross-matched to ensure there are no preformed antibodies to donor antigens that might trigger hyperacute rejection (see below).

Tissue typing

Tissue typing describes the process of establishing the HLA antigens expressed by the patient. Once it is decided that a patient requires renal transplantation, they undergo tissue typing using a series of serological, cellular and, increasingly, molecular tests.

The details of their HLA class I and II antigen expression is then usually entered onto one or more national databases of patients awaiting transplant. This ensures that, in the event of a cadaveric donor organ becoming available, it is transplanted into an immunologically suitable recipient. This may involve the transportation of the donor kidney over great distances. In cases where living related donors are considered, there is a 1:4 chance that there will be a **haplotype match**. HLA genes are closely located together on chromosome 6 and, therefore, are inherited in **haplotypes** (Fig. 54). Siblings may have zero, one or two haplotype matches. It was noted early on that the

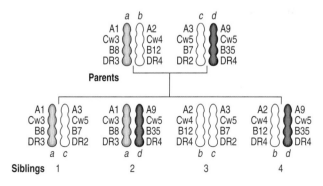

Fig. 54 Haplotype inheritance in the HLA system.

greater the haplotype match the better the chances of organ survival. In fact, with improved immuno-suppression, family members with zero haplotype matches can achieve 90% organ survival at 1 year. In renal transplantation, it appears that matching at the HLA-DR locus has a greater influence on graft survival than matching at HLA class I loci.

Panel reactive antibodies/presensitisation

Patients awaiting transplantation are also assessed for the presence of antibodies directed against transplantation antigens. A broad *panel* of cells expressing a very wide range of HLA antigens is used to identify these antibodies. The stimulus to form such antibodies may have been that a previous kidney was rejected, or multiple pregnancies or blood transfusions. However, they may also occur in patients with none of these histories; therefore, all patients must be screened. High-titre panel reactive antibodies are associated with a poorer graft outcome and a greater risk of graft rejection. Samples for presensitisation testing are usually collected on a monthly basis from all patients awaiting transplantation. In this way, a longitudinal picture is established of the degree of presensitisation of each patient and these samples are also used in the later cross-matching process when a potential donor becomes available (see below).

Cross-matching

Cross-matching is the process of identifying whether a potential recipient has preformed antibodies specific to the donor (Table 49 and Fig. 55). Donor lymphocytes and recipient serum are used to identify antibody against class I or class II antigens. A positive cross-match to class I antigens is a contraindication to transplantation as hyperacute rejection is highly likely. Interestingly, the detection of antibodies against donor

class II antigens is not a contraindication to proceed and may, in fact, confer a graft-survival advantage. This may reflect the fact that class II antigens are expressed on only a limited range of cells within the body.

Blood transfusion

Chronic renal disease is often associated with anaemia and it has been noted for many years that patients who had received multiple blood transfusions prior to transplantation appeared to have better long-term graft survival. In the past, multiple planned transfusions were prescribed to benefit the patient from this effect. The immunological mechanism has not been fully clarified; however, it is likely that multiple transfusions cause presensitisation in susceptible individuals and thus prevent those receiving organs to which they might otherwise be reactive. It is also possible that other immunological mechanisms including some form of 'post-transfusion immunosuppression' may be involved. Advances in immunosuppressive therapy since the early 1990s mean that any additional advantage provided by transfusion programmes is now difficult to demonstrate.

Donor selection

In the UK, cadaveric renal transplantation is much more common than living related donation; however, limitation in the supply of cadaveric organs has dictated a continued need for living related donation.

Living related donor transplantation

Living related donor transplantation raises a number of issues that should be fully considered, in addition to the simple 'matching' process. It is essential that such a donor has two functioning kidneys and is otherwise healthy. In particular, donors are assessed for heart disease, malignancy, chronic infection and diabetes. The psychological impact, both of donating and receiving a relative's organ, need to be considered and formal psychological assessment is necessary. If the patient suffers from a renal condition that has a potentially hereditary component, the risk that the donor might subsequently develop renal disease should also be considered.

Cadaveric transplantation

Organ donation is not considered from patients with transmissible infections, renal disease, malignancy or systemic diseases known to impair renal function. Once appropriate consent has been obtained for the removal of organs from a suitable cadaver, a number of procedures must be undertaken. ABO and HLA typing is performed and a sample of lymph node or

Table 49 Cross-matching in renal transplantation

Serum source	Donor cells used (% cells killed after incubation)		Interpretation
	T cells	B cells	
Negative control	< 10	< 10	Test system satisfactory
Positive control	> 90	> 90	Test system satisfactory
Recipient A	< 10	< 10	No antibodies: proceed
Recipient B	> 90	> 90	Antibodies to class I: do not proceed
Recipient C	< 10	> 90	Antibodies to class II: proceed

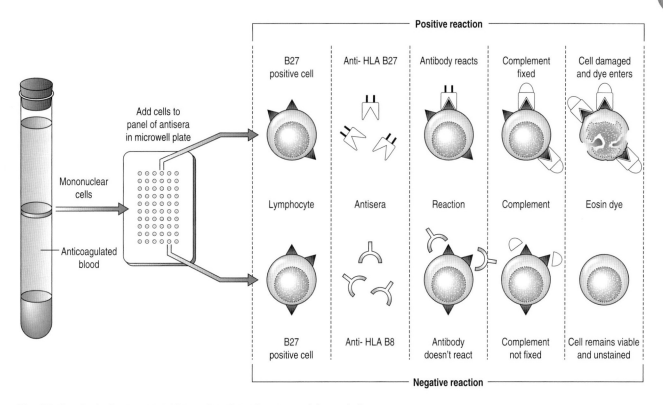

Fig. 55 Serological cross-matching using the microcytotoxicity technique.

spleen is obtained as a source of lymphocytes for cross-matching purposes. Patients on the waiting list with compatible ABO groups and the highest number of HLA matches are identified. Their most recent serum sample and their most reactive serum obtained within the previous 2 years are both tested against the donor lymphocytes in a cross-match system (Table 49). The potential pool of recipients is thus reduced by excluding those with positive cross-matches and positively identifying those with the best HLA match. Once these histocompatibility factors have been fully explored, other factors including urgency of transplant, length of time on dialysis and so on may be taken into account.

There is a significant time factor that must also be considered. Once the kidneys are removed from the body, they are perfused with specialised preservation fluids and kept cool. The **warm ischaemia time**, the interval between cessation of blood flow and commencement of mechanical perfusion, should be less than 30 minutes. The **cold ischaemia time**, the duration of mechanical perfusion prior to vascular anastamosis in the recipient, should be less than 48 hours. Ischaemic time should be kept to a minimum to ensure the best possible outcome.

Post-transplantation care

Close monitoring is essential after transplantation, both for signs of acute or chronic rejection (Figs 56 and 57)

and also other complications including infection, haemorrhage or acute tubular necrosis. In the face of unexpected deterioration of renal function, core biopsy or fine-needle aspiration may be required.

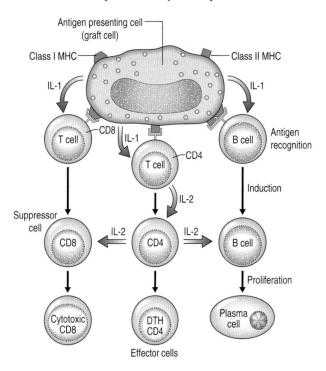

Fig. 56 Immunological sensitisation to graft antigens: primary allograft rejection. IL, interleukin.

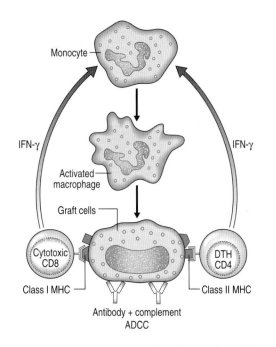

Fig. 57 Immunological effectors of graft rejection. IFN, interferon; ADCC, antibody-dependent cell-mediated cytotoxicity.

Immunosuppressive therapy is essential to prevent graft rejection. The use of prednisolone in combination with azathioprine allowed early success in the development of renal transplantation. The advent of new immunosuppressant drugs in the 1980s and 1990s, including ciclosporin, tacrolimus and mycophenolate mofetil, has allowed further development of immunosuppressive regimens. In general, most centres use a combination of three immunosuppressive drugs for the first 6 months after a transplantion and this is subsequently reduced to two drugs thereafter. Episodes of acute rejection are usually treated with intravenous methylprednisolone (1 g daily for 3 days). If repeated episodes of acute rejection occur, anti-thymocyte globulin or anti-CD3 monoclonal antibodies may be used to target T cells while anti-CD25 monoclonal antibodies may be used to specifically target activated T cells.

These powerful immunosuppressant agents are all associated with particular acute side effects (Ch. 9). The need for significant immunosuppression renders the recipient secondarily immunocompromised and vulnerable to infection. If an organ infected with cytomegalovirus (CMV) is transplanted into a recipient who is not immune to CMV, acute CMV infection can occur. Epstein–Barr virus, which grows in B cells, can become activated in the immunosuppressed patient and cause a lymphoproliferative disorder known as **post-transplant lymphoproliferative disorder**. In both this and acute CMV infection, a difficult judgement has to be made regarding a reduction in immunosuppression, which is likely to allow the recipient's immune system to respond to the viral infection but risks loss of the graft. With these combination drug regimens, there is also an increased risk of lymphoma occurring many years later, particularly if anti-thymocyte globulin has been used.

Of particular importance in this context is that ciclosporin is nephrotoxic and blood levels should be monitored. Most regimens suggest that ciclosporin should be stopped after 9 months to prevent long-term nephrotoxicity. Azathioprine can also cause marrow suppression and rarely, in some patients, a significant secondary antibody deficiency requiring intravenous immunoglobulin-replacement therapy.

Graft survival

Initial studies indicated that matching at HLA-DR was a particularly important predictor of renal graft survival. With the advent of triple drug immunosuppressive regimens, this effect is no longer significant for first transplants; however, HLA-DR-matched grafts undergo fewer episodes of acute rejection. Subsequent graft survival is beneficially influenced by DR matching.

10.3 Other solid organ transplantation

Learning objectives

You should:

- be aware of spectrum of solid organ transplantation commonly undertaken
- understand the particular problems with each organ.

Heart

Indications for heart transplantation include advanced coronary artery disease, dilated cardiomyopathy and, in children, complex congenital cardiac defects otherwise unamenable to surgery. Drug regimens developed in the renal transplant programmes have allowed much better survival of cardiac grafts. There are a number of key differences that distinguish the process of cardiac from renal transplantation. Like kidney donation, the heart is perfused with preservation fluid; however, the allowable cold ischaemia time is probably only 4–6 hours. This dictates important limitations both on the laboratory assessment of donor and recipient and also on the distances over which a donor organ can be safely transported. In most centres, therefore, HLA matching is not undertaken. ABO compatibility is necessary and patients awaiting transplant are regularly assessed for presensitisation and are cross-matched once a donor organ is available. Rejection of a cardiac graft can be difficult to diagnose and may become manifest through changes in the electrocardiograph or signs on endomyocardial biopsy. Acute rejection episodes occur frequently and are treated aggressively with the drug regimens described for renal rejection. Failure to control acute rejection carries a much poorer prognosis in cardiac transplantation as there is no alternative life-support system other than retransplantation. Overall survival rates are thought to be as good as for renal transplantation, with 1- and 5-year survival rates of 80% and 70%, respectively.

Heart and lung

Combined heart and lung transplantation is undertaken for patients with advanced cardiopulmonary disease, although early mortality is high. Single lung transplantation has also been shown to be effective treatment for end-stage cystic fibrosis, bronchiectasis, pulmonary hypertension, pulmonary fibrosis or emphysema caused by α_1-antitrypsin deficiency. Lung transplant recipients can be monitored using bronchoalveolar lavage to identify rejection or infection.

Liver

Liver transplantation is now indicated for a range of conditions including primary biliary atresia, primary biliary cirrhosis, primary sclerosing cholangitis, post-hepatic cirrhosis, alcoholic liver disease, hepatocellular carcinoma, autoimmune liver disease and acute liver failure, including drug-induced causes such as paracetamol poisoning. Transplantation is usually only considered if survival beyond 18 months is otherwise deemed unlikely. Donor and recipient must be ABO compatible, but HLA matching is not required. The physical size of the donated organ is a factor in determining a suitable recipient and some centres use partial liver grafts for small recipients. This may mean in some situations that a single donor can provide a liver transplant for more than one patient. Overall survival rates are now very good with 90–95% 1-year survival reported for patients transplanted for primary biliary cirrhosis.

Cornea

Corneal transplants are unique in the sense that there is no need for HLA typing or systemic immunosuppression. As the cornea is avascular, it is considered an *immunologically privileged* site. In corneal grafts that become vascularised however, HLA matching does improve survival and local application of steroid drops can control acute inflammatory episodes.

10.4 Bone marrow transplantation

Learning objectives

You should:

- know the principles of bone marrow transplantation
- know the indications for bone marrow transplantation
- understand the problem of graft-versus-host disease.

The first successful bone marrow transplantation (BMT) was for severe combined immune deficiency (SCID; Ch. 4) in 1968. In that case, the donated bone marrow was taken from one of the child's parents. BMT was subsequently developed in the 1970s and 1980s as treatment for haematological and immunological conditions. For malignant conditions, the patient was usually treated with total body irradiation and high-dose chemotherapy to eradicate tumour cells, followed by BMT from a suitable donor. Originally, most donors were identical twins (**syngeneic**) or genotypically HLA-identical individuals (**allogeneic**). However, as an HLA-identical donor was available for only a minority of patients, partially matched related or phenotypically matched related and unrelated donors increasingly became used. For conditions where the disease process did not always affect the marrow (e.g. Hodgkin's and non-Hodgkin's lymphoma), **autologous BMT** (reinfusion of the patient's own marrow) also became a useful therapeutic option. More recently, however, autologous transplantation has largely been superseded by autologous **peripheral blood stem cell transplantation** (PBSCT). This technique developed from the observation that high numbers of haemopoietic stem cells (found in the fraction of CD34+ cells) were identified in peripheral blood after chemotherapy and appropriate growth factor treatment. These cells could then be harvested by leukopheresis and subsequently be reinfused as an alternative to BMT. Hence high-dose chemo- and radiotherapy followed by PBSCT has become a therapeutic option in a wider range of conditions than originally treated by conventional BMT. The common indications for bone marrow transplantation and PBSCT are summarised in Table 50.

Patient selection and preparation

Donor and recipient do not have to be ABO compatible and HLA identical. The latter criterion is difficult to fulfil and, furthermore, the use of immunosuppressant drugs now allows successful transplantation using donors with one haplotype mismatch (e.g. parents of children with SCID).

Table 50 Common indications for bone marrow transplantation

Disease	Allogeneic/ syngeneic	Autologous peripheral blood stem cell transplant
Aplastic anaemia	Yes	No
Leukaemia		
Acute myeloid leukaemia	Yes	Yes
Acute lymphoblastic leukaemia	Yes	Yes
Chronic myeloid leukaemia	Yes	No
Myelodysplasia	Yes	No
Multiple myeloma	Yes	Yes
Non-Hodgkin's lymphoma	Yes	Yes
Hodgkin's disease	Yes	Yes
Immunodeficiency		
Severe combined immunodeficiency	Yes	No
Wiskott–Aldrich syndrome	Yes	No
Chronic granulomatous disease	Yes	No
X-linked hyper-IgM syndrome (CD40 ligand deficiency)	Yes	No
Osteopetrosis	Yes	No
Solid tumours[a]		
Breast	No	Yes
Lung	No	Yes
Ovary	No	Yes
Testis	No	Yes

[a]Allogeneic and autologous bone marrow transplantation remains experimental in solid tumours but has been used where indicated.

Bone marrow donor

The process of bone marrow donation differs from other organ donation in that probably less than 5% of the donor marrow is taken and this regenerates in approximately 8 weeks. The donor, therefore, suffers no long-term haematological or immunological deficiency as a result of the process. Bone marrow is usually aspirated from the iliac crests and sometimes the sternum of the donor under anaesthesia. The aspirated marrow is stored in anticoagulant and filtered to ensure a single cell suspension, free of bony spicules. The cellular infusion is then administered to the recipient intravenously and the infused cells then repopulate the bone marrow. Where there is an ABO mismatch, the marrow is depleted of red cells prior to reinfusion. The recipient's blood counts are expected to return to normal over the next 3–6 weeks.

Recipient

Patients undergoing BMT for malignant disease require a potent antineoplastic regimen and supralethal ablation of the bone marrow. This is typically achieved by a combination of intravenous cyclophosphamide (50–60 mg/kg body weight for 2–4 days) plus total body irradiation (1000–1400 cGy over 3–5 days). At this stage, depending on underlying disease, prophylactic methotrexate and ciclosporin may be given to prevent GvHD. Patients undergoing BMT for primary immunodeficiency disorders do not require such potent treatment, although some 'conditioning' chemotherapy is used, depending on the nature of underlying disorder.

Transplantation procedure

Donor bone marrow is infused intravenously at a dose of approximately 3×10^8 nucleated cells/kg body weight. In some patients, the marrow is T cell depleted to reduce the risk of GvHD; however, that carries the risk of less effective outcome because of the absence of a graft versus leukaemia effect (GVL: see below).

Following the preparatory treatment and prior to successful engraftment of donor marrow, the patient is very vulnerable to infection. The patient is nursed under barrier precautions and broad spectrum antimicrobial prophylaxis to prevent bacterial, fungal, viral and protozoal infection is instituted. The role of co-trimoxazole and antifungal agents in preventing *Pneumocystis carinii pneumonia* and candidal infection, respectively, is particularly important. Patients are also at risk of bleeding due to thrombocytopenia and regular platelet infusions are given to maintain a platelet count > 15 000/μl. Anaemia may also develop requiring blood transfusion. It is crucial that any blood products given are cytomegalovirus (CMV) negative where donor and recipient are both CMV negative. Irradiation with X-rays (25 Gy/unit) is also required to prevent infusion of immunocompetent lymphocytes that could cause transfusion associated GvHD. Following the recovery of blood counts, patients at risk of CMV infection (CMV-positive donor, recipient or both) are monitored using the polymerase chain reaction to detect CMV. Preemptive treatment with ganciclovir has largely abolished death from CMV infection after BMT.

Response to treatment

Successful engraftment is heralded by a rising peripheral blood white cell count and the identification of mature neutrophils in the circulation, usually 2-4 weeks after transplantation. Once neutrophil numbers are above 500/μl, the greatest risk of bacterial infection has passed; however, there remains a significant risk of viral and fungal infection as lymphocyte responses are immature. The rate of recovery of peripheral blood white cell counts is the main influence on the necessary duration of barrier nursing and antimicrobial prophylaxis. Hospitalisation would be expected to last from weeks to several months and close clinical follow up is essential for the first 3 to 6 months. Tolerance of the new bone marrow is usually achieved by approximately 6 months, at which time immunosuppressive therapy is slowly withdrawn. In terms of immunity, the post-BMT patient is very similar to a neonate and a full primary course of immunisations is required.

Complications

The three major initial complications include

- failure of engraftment
- infection
- graft-versus-host disease (GvHD).

Failure of engraftment

Failure of the expected rise in peripheral blood white cell count may indicate a failure of bone marrow engraftment that may be due to either an inadequate infusion of cells or rejection by residual activity of the recipients' immune system. If an inadequate infused dose is thought to be the problem, further infusion is possible.

The conditioning regimens of high-dose chemo- and radiotherapy should ensure ablation of the recipients' immune system; however, where milder conditioning has been used (e.g. in primary immunodeficiency) some residual immune activity may cause rejection. Some degree of conditioning is, therefore, considered essential in most BMT. Where an unrelated donor provides the bone marrow, some of the recipient's own bone marrow is stored so that, in the event of failed engraftment for whatever reason, the patient can be reinfused with their own marrow.

Infection

Susceptibility to infection has been discussed above; however, the status of both donor and recipient for CMV exposure is important. In a patient previously exposed to CMV (the majority of adults), virus can become reactivated once the patient has become immunosuppressed.

It is also possible that BMT engraftment may be incomplete and the patient may be left with a degree of secondary immunodeficiency. In such patients regular ivIg maintenance therapy as in primary antibody deficiency (see Ch. 4) may be required.

Graft-versus-host disease

BMT is associated with the unique complication of GvHD in which the transplanted marrow recognises the recipient's tissues as 'foreign' and attacks them immunologically. Acute GvHD typically occurs around the time of haematological regeneration and manifests as a triad of maculopapular rash, mainly affecting the palms and soles, disturbed liver function and diarrhoea. The clinical grading of acute GvHD is summarised in Table 51. Acute GvHD is usually treated by high-dose intravenous methylprednisolone or occasionally by anti-lymphocyte globulin. Grade III–IV GvHD is a life-threatening complication after BMT. Interestingly, early BMT studies in patients with haematological malignancy indicated a better outcome for those who had a degree of acute GvHD. Hence the concept of *graft versus leukaemia* was developed. The theory is that a limited degree of GvHD serves to eradicate residual malignant cells that might otherwise remain untreated and ultimately cause disease relapse.

Chronic GvHD may develop after day 100 post-BMT and is not necessarily preceded by the acute form. It can cause a progressive sclerodermatous-like change in the skin, intestinal malabsorption and obstructive liver disease. Good results can be obtained with combination immunosuppression (e.g. prednisolone and mycophenolate mofetil) in limited chronic GvHD. Skin manifestations can improve with thalidomide or psoralen plus longwave ultraviolet radiation (PUVA). Extensive chronic GvHD carries a poor prognosis, with infection being a major problem.

Table 51 Clinical staging of graft-versus-host disease (GvHD)

Stage	Skin	Serum bilirubin (mg/l)	Volume diarrhoea (ml/day)
1	Maculopapular rash < 25% body surface	20–30	500–1000
2	Maculopapular rash 25–50% body surface	30–60	1000–1500
3	Generalised erythroderma	60–150	> 1500
4	Generalised erythroderma plus bullous formation and desquamation	> 150	> 1500 plus severe abdominal pain; with or without ileus

Self-assessment: questions

Multiple choice questions

1. What are the main effector cells in acute organ rejection?
   a. Donor B cells
   b. Donor T cells
   c. Recipient B cells
   d. Recipient T cells
   e. Recipient T and B cells

2. In hyperacute rejection, which of the following hypersensitivity mechanisms is implicated?
   a. Type I
   b. Type II
   c. Type III
   d. Type IV
   e. Type V

3. Which one of the following antigens is the major target of hyperacute rejection?
   a. B cell receptor
   b. HLA class I
   c. HLA class II
   d. Interleukin-2 receptor (CD25)
   e. T cell receptor

4. In renal transplantation, matching at which of the following loci has the greatest influence on ensuring graft survival?
   a. HLA-A
   b. HLA-B
   c. HLA-C
   d. HLA-D
   e. HLA-G

5. The monoclonal antibody anti-CD25 (Basiliximab) is increasingly being used in the treatment of transplant rejection. Which cells are targeted by this treatment?
   a. B cells
   b. Dendritic cells
   c. Macrophages
   d. Natural killer cells
   e. T cells

6. Which of the following laboratory findings are typical of acute graft-versus-host disease?
   a. Increased serum aspartate aminotransferase (AST)
   b. Increased serum urea
   c. Low platelet count
   d. Raised total white cell count
   e. Low haemoglobin

7. How long does it usually take for a bone marrow donor to regenerate their donated marrow?
   a. 1 week
   b. 2 weeks
   c. 1 month
   d. 2 months
   e. 6 months

8. Following bone marrow transplantation, regular platelet transfusions are required to keep threshold platelet levels above:
   a. $5 \times 10^9/l$
   b. $15 \times 10^9/l$
   c. $50 \times 10^9/l$
   d. $75 \times 10^9/l$
   e. $100 \times 10^9/l$

9. Allogeneic bone marrow transplantation is of proven benefit in which of the following disorders?
   a. Wiskott–Aldrich syndrome
   b. Acute myeloid leukaemia
   c. Myasthenia gravis
   d. Aplastic anaemia
   e. Breast cancer

10. Peripheral blood stem cell transplantation (PBSCT) is of proven benefit in which of the following disorders?
    a. Wiskott–Aldrich syndrome
    b. Acute myeloid leukaemia
    c. Myasthenia gravis
    d. Aplastic anaemia
    e. Breast cancer

Case history questions

History 1

A 16-year-old male who underwent renal transplantation 6 months previously presented at clinic, acutely unwell. He had been maintained on oral prednisolone, azathioprine and ciclosporin since his transplant. On examination his temperature was 38.7˚C and he had generalised lymphadenopathy and hepatosplenomegaly. Lymph node biopsy findings were suggestive of B cell lymphoma.

1. What is the most likely diagnosis?
2. What additional tests would be required?
3. If clonality studies were undertaken on the biopsy tissue (immunoglobulin gene rearrangement studies), what results might you expect?

4. What therapeutic intervention is likely to be helpful?

Self-assessment: answers

Multiple choice answers

1. a. **False.** Antigen-presenting cells carried within the donated organ are partly involved.
   b. **False.** See (a).
   c. **False.**
   d. **True.** Recipient CD4$^+$ and CD8$^+$ T cells are the main effectors although antibody molecules are also implicated.
   e. **False.**

2. a. **False.** Type I hypersensitivity involves IgE and mast cells and is not implicated in transplant rejection.
   b. **True.** Type II reactions involves the interaction of preformed antibody (IgG/IgM) with cell-surface bound antigens.
   c. **False.** Immune complex formation is not the significant mechanism in hyperacute rejection.
   d. **False.** Type IV mechanisms dominate in acute and chronic rejection.
   e. **False.** Type V was a description used to describe type II reactions involving endocrine organs, but it is no longer a widely used term.

3. a. **False.**
   b. **True.** Preformed antibodies directed against HLA class I or the ABO system are the cause of hyperacute rejection.
   c. **False.**
   d. **False.**
   e. **False.**

4. a. **False.** However, HLA matching should be as close as possible (including HLA-A, HLA-B, HLA-C and HLA-D loci).
   b. **False.** See (a).
   c. **False.** See (a).
   d. **True.** Matching at the HLA-D locus appears to have the greatest influence on graft survival.
   e. **False.** See (a).

5. a. **False.** CD25 is specific for T cells.
   b. **False.**
   c. **False.**
   d. **False.**
   e. **True.** CD25 is the interleukin-2 receptor, which is expressed on activated T cells.

6. a. **True.** Increased serum AST is typical of graft-versus-host disease along with a typical rash and diarrhoea.
   b. **False.**
   c. **False.**
   d. **False.** The peripheral blood white cell count would be expected to decrease after bone marrow engraftment.
   e. **False.**

7. a. **False.**
   b. **False.** However, the first signs of a successful engraftment are seen after 2–4 weeks: rising peripheral blood white cell count and the identification of mature neutrophils in the circulation.
   c. **False.** See (b).
   d. **True.** Although quite variable, 2 months is thought to be the average recovery time.
   e. **False.** Tolerance of the new bone marrow is usually achieved by approximately 6 months, at which time immunosuppressive therapy is slowly withdrawn.

8. a. **False.** The risk of haemorrhage would be very high with platelet levels of $5 \times 10^9/l$.
   b. **True.** A commonly accepted threshold level is $15 \times 10^9/l$.
   c. **False.** Platelet transfusion would not normally be required with levels of $50 \times 10^9/l$ and above.
   d. **False.** See (c).
   e. **False.** See (c).

9. a. **True.** Patients with Wiskott–Aldrich syndrome are typically undergoing bone marrow transplantation before 5 years of age.
   b. **True.** See Table 50.
   c. **False.** Myasthenia gravis is caused by anti-acetylcholine receptor antibodies: primary autoantibodies directly interfering with neuro-muscular signal transmission.
   d. **True.** See Table 50.
   e. **False.** See Table 50.

10. a. **False.** See Table 50.
    b. **True.** See Table 50.
    c. **False.** Myasthenia gravis is caused by anti-acetylcholine receptor antibodies: primary

autoantibodies directly interfering with neuro-muscular signal transmission.

   d. **False.** See Table 50.

   e. **True.** A number of solid tumours are now being treated by PBSCT.

Case history answers

History 1

1. The history of lymphadenopathy occurring after transplantation is very suggestive of post-transplantation lymphoproliferative disease (PTLD). However, this patient is on potent immunosuppression and other causes of widespread lymphadenopathy including disseminated infection must be considered and excluded.

2. It would be essential to have a chest radiograph and cultures of blood, urine and sputum if available. Screening for viral infection would also be important, particularly Epstein–Barr virus and cytomegalovirus. It is likely that this is PTLD and, therefore, polymerase chain reaction analysis for Epstein–Barr virus in the biopsy would be essential.

3. Interestingly, PTLD is not usually a clonal disorder and this distinguishes it from other types of lymphoma. The lymphoid hyperplasia is thought to be driven by uncontrolled proliferation of Epstein–Barr virus and the B cells are polyclonal. Immunoglobulin gene rearrangement studies would not be expected to identify a monoclonal rearrangement.

4. This patient has been maintained on triple immunosuppression for 6 months and it is likely that a reduction in the number of agents and/or dose of the drugs would result in adequate restoration of immune function to regain control of the Epstein–Barr virus proliferation. This clearly carries the risk of transplant rejection, but is a necessary step.

11 Lymphoproliferative diseases

Chapter overview

Malignant transformation of lymphoid cells results in a number of lymphoproliferative disorders. This group of conditions includes chronic lymphocytic leukaemia, lymphomas, multiple myeloma, Waldenstrom's macroglobulinaemia and some types of cryoglobulinaemia. These disorders have a wide range of clinical presentations and widely differing prognosis; however, the common feature they share is the monoclonal proliferation of lymphoid cells (i.e. they originate from a single clone of cells that has undergone malignant transformation). This chapter describes the clinical features of these conditions, which affect both adults and children, and focuses on their investigation and principles of management. The use of immunochemical investigation is of particular importance in the investigation of suspected lymphoproliferative disease and this chapter is closely cross-referenced to the relevant sections of Chapter 12. The clinical management of the majority of these conditions is undertaken by haematologists and is, therefore, beyond the scope of this chapter.

11.1 Introduction

Learning objectives

You should:
- understand the distinction between leukaemias and lymphomas
- be aware of the range of lymphoproliferative disorders
- understand the use of laboratory tests to confirm a suspected diagnosis.

The traditionally understood difference between leukaemias and lymphomas is that in the former abnormal leukocytes are detectable in the peripheral blood and bone marrow and in the latter the abnormal cells are confined to the tissues (mainly lymph nodes and spleen). There is, however, overlap between the conditions in terms of the cells of origin (Fig. 58) and in a number of their clinical features. In some cases traditional histological and morphological diagnostic techniques may be inadequate to differentiate one condition from another. Furthermore, with modern highly sensitive detection systems, abnormal cells can be detected in the peripheral blood of up to 50% of patients with non-Hodgkin's lymphoma. Therefore, a combination of clinical, morphological and immunological features is used to differentiate and classify these conditions, the major features of which are summarised in this chapter. Chronic lymphocytic leukaemia is included in this chapter on lymphoproliferative diseases because of its close relationship to lymphomas. To learn about the acute leukaemias, the reader is referred to the Haematology volume in the Master Medicine series.

11.2 Specific conditions

Learning objectives

You should:
- understand the cell type affected and the effects this will have
- know the common presenting features of these conditions
- know the laboratory tests suitable to confirm a suspected diagnosis
- understand the major principles of management.

Chronic lymphocytic leukaemia

Chronic lymphocytic leukaemia (CLL) is a condition that typically occurs in the older age group and affects men twice as frequently as women. In approximately 25%, the diagnosis is discovered incidentally, the patient being asymptomatic. In other cases the patient may

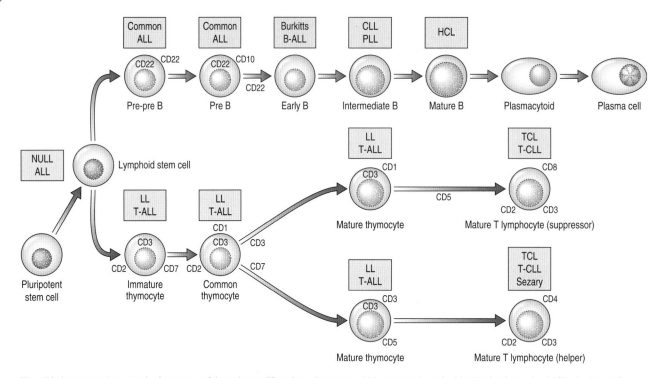

Fig. 58 Immunophenotypic features of lymphoproliferative diseases. ALL, acute lymphoblastic leukaemia; HCL, hairy cell leukaemia; LL, lymphoblastic lymphoma; TCL, T cell lymphoma; CLL, chronic lymphocytic leukaemia; PLL, prolymphocytic leukaemia;

present with symptoms such as lymphadenopathy, purpuric rash, weight loss, night sweats, recurrent chest infections or symptoms attributable to anaemia (pallor, fatigue, breathlessness). Rarely there is an acute presentation with symptoms of severe anaemia and thrombocytopenia. Although classified as a leukaemia, many of its features are more typical of lymphoma and CLL is included in some classifications of lymphoma.

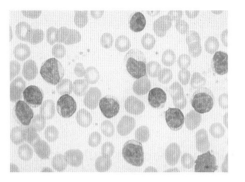

Fig. 59 Peripheral blood film from a patient with B-CLL. Note that multiple, well-differentiated small lymphocytes are present in the blood film. Immunophenotyping of these cells confirms they are of B cell origin and monoclonal (either kappa or lambda light chain positive).

Investigation

The lymphocyte count is raised but can vary from just above normal ($> 15 \times 10^9/l$) up to $300 \times 10^9/l$. Morphologically, the lymphocytes are typically well-differentiated small lymphocytes (Fig. 59), indicating their mature stage of development (Fig. 58); in approximately 95% of cases they will be of B cell origin (B-CLL). A useful confirmatory test is **lymphocyte phenotyping** (Ch. 12) in which large numbers of cells can be analysed rapidly to establish their expression of cell-surface antigens/markers (CD antigens). Typical lymphocyte phenotype profiles are indicated in Figure 59. A characteristic finding in B-CLL is that the abnormal B cells aberrantly express CD5, which is normally a pan-T antigen. Therefore, the finding of B cells carrying this pan-T marker (CD19$^+$CD5$^+$ cells) is considered confirmatory evidence of B-CLL if there is the appropriate clinical presentation. Small percentages of CD19$^+$CD5$^+$ cells may also be found in neonates and patients with some autoimmune disorders; however, these are distinct from B-CLL cells.

Lymph node biopsy is rarely required but if undertaken, a low-grade, diffuse lymphocytic lymphoma pattern is identified. Approximately 30% of patients with B-CLL will develop hypogammaglobulinaemia during the course of their illness and total serum immunoglobulins should, therefore, be measured at presentation and regularly throughout treatment.

Management

As CLL can be asymptomatic and run a relatively benign course, treatment is not always necessary. However, if the patient is symptomatic or has evidence of secondary organ failure, then treatment should be commenced. The usual first-line therapy is chlorambucil (2–10 mg/day); if there is a good response, treatment may be discontinued. The occurrence of autoimmune haemolytic anaemia or thrombocytopenia is commonly treated with oral prednisolone (initially 50–100 mg/day). If this is a persisting problem, splenectomy may be considered; however, this would depend on the general health of the individual patient.

A small percentage of patients with B-CLL develop significant secondary immunodeficiency related to their hypogammaglobulinaemia and present with recurrent chest and upper airway infection. If this is a significant clinical problem, then intravenous immunoglobulin (ivIg) therapy should be considered (Ch. 4). However, ivIg should only be prescribed if there is a history of infection, not simply on the basis of low serum immunoglobulin levels.

Prognosis

The prognosis in B-CLL is very variable and depends on the stage of disease at diagnosis. The majority of patients survive > 5 years, and the condition can be compatible with much longer survival; however, occasionally there may be a more aggressive course. A related disease, prolymphocytic leukemia, occurs in which the abnormal cells are prolymphocytes (Fig. 58); there is usually massive splenomegaly and the prognosis in this type of disease is poor.

Hairy cell leukaemia

Hairy cell leukaemia is another chronic B cell lymphoproliferative disorder. It tends to present in the elderly, and men are more frequently affected than women (4:1).

Clinical features

Presenting features tend to be non-specific fatigue and possibly abdominal discomfort related to splenomegaly. Lymphadenopathy is uncommon but infection may be a major clinical problem.

Investigations

There is often a pancytopenia and the lymphoid cells have a 'hairy' appearance, caused by multiple fine cytoplasmic projections. There may be fibrosis of the bone marrow causing a dry 'tap' on bone marrow aspirate. Lymphocyte phenotyping reveals a characteristic phenotype with abnormal expression of the adhesion molecule CD11c.

Treatment and prognosis

Treatment is with deoxycoformycin or 2-chlorodeoxyadenosine and prolonged remissions are possible. Interferon-α may be effective in non-responders. For those individuals with grossly enlarged spleens, splenectomy may provide symptomatic relief and, if there is little bone marrow involvement, may contribute to disease control.

Hodgkin's lymphoma

Hodgkin's lymphoma (also known as Hodgkin's disease) is a condition that typically affects young adults; however, there is a bimodal age distribution, with a second peak of incidence occurring in older adults.

Clinical features

Hodgkin's lymphoma usually presents with otherwise unexplained lymphadenopathy, often in the cervical region. Systemic itch is also a common presenting symptom and, therefore, Hodgkin's lymphoma should always be considered when a young adult presents with unexplained itch. Systemic symptoms of fever, night sweats and weight loss are also common, particularly in older patients, and their occurrence is important in the clinical staging of the condition (see below). Anaemia, when it occurs, tends to suggest relatively advanced disease. Once a diagnosis of Hodgkin's lymphoma is established, it is important to determine how many groups of lymph nodes are affected as disease extent at presentation is related to ultimate prognosis.

Investigation

Lymph node biopsy is essential and the cardinal histological feature is the detection of the Reed–Sternberg cell (Fig. 60). These are large binucleate cells that have eosinophilic nucleoli. Otherwise, there is a mixed cellular background in the nodes. The condition is subclassified histologically according to the predominant cell types identified and other histological features such as sclerosis (Table 52).

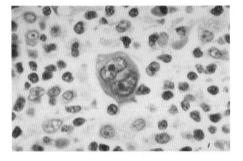

Fig. 60 The Reed–Sternberg cell is identified in the centre of this microscopic field of a lymph node section. It is a large binucleate cell with eosinophilic nucleoli. It is considered pathognomonic of Hodgkin's lymphoma.

Table 53 Staging of Hodgkin's lymphoma

Stage	Features
I	Single lymph node region involved, sometimes with local spread to extra-lymphatic tissue **(IE)**
II	Involvement of two or more node regions on the same side of the diaphragm, sometimes with local spread to extra-lymphatic tissue **(IIE)**
III	Involvement of nodes on both sides of the diaphragm (The spleen is considered as a 'node')
IV	Diffuse or disseminated involvement of one or more extralymphatic organs

Each stage is also divided into A or B according to absence or presence of systemic symptoms; these include a sustained fever (> 38˚C), weight loss (more than 10% of body weight in 6 months) and night sweats, but not pruritus.

Apart from classification of the condition, staging of the disease is required at presentation in order to guide therapeutic decisions and give prognostic information. Staging involves a combination of physical examination and imaging techniques to identify all the enlarged lymph node groups and any evidence of organomegaly (Table 53). Chest radiograph and computed tomographic scan of chest and abdomen are usually required.

In addition to advanced staging, other poor prognostic factors include

- serum albumin < 40 g/l
- haemoglobin < 105 g/l
- male gender
- age > 45 years
- white cell count > 15×10^9/l
- lymphocyte count < 0.6×10^9/l.

Management

For localised disease with or without systemic symptoms (stages IA and IB), radiotherapy directed at the affected and adjacent nodes is adequate. Radiotherapy may also be used in stage IIA disease, in which two or more node regions are involved on the same side of the diaphragm. Clinical trials are currently evaluating the role of chemotherapy in this stage of disease. For more extensive disease, combination chemotherapy is required. Autologous periph-

Table 52 Classification of Hodgkin's lymphoma

Nodular lymphocyte-predominant Hodgkin's lymphoma (HL)
Classical HL
Nodularsclerosis HL (grades 1 and 2)
Lymphocyte-rich classic HL
Mixed cellularity HL
Lymphocyte depletion

eral blood stem cell transplant is usually reserved for those patients who have relapsed after chemotherapy and required a second chemotherapy regimen. Overall, the 10-year survival for Hodgkin's lymphoma is reported as approximately 80%; however, the factors indicative of a poor prognosis mentioned above must be taken into account when advising individual patients. Age is a particularly important factor; patients over 50 years of age have a much worse prognosis.

Non-Hodgkin's lymphoma

Non-Hodgkin's lymphoma (NHL) is most common in the elderly although it can occur in children and adolescents.

Clinical features

Most patients present with lymphadenopathy, but this tends to affect multiple lymph node groups, unlike the often localised presentation of Hodgkin's lymphoma. Symptoms may be quite varied, with systemic symptoms including fever, weight loss and night sweats but also local symptoms attributable to lymph node enlargement. NHL can also occur as a primary tumour affecting the brain, gastrointestinal tract, skin, thyroid, bone or testes.

Investigation

As with Hodgkin's lymphoma, histological examination of lymph node tissue is essential to confirm the diagnosis and classify the lymphoma. The classification of NHL is related to the cell of origin (B or T cell) and the apparent stage of maturity of the cells (Fig. 58).

There are a number of different classification systems for NHL and the World Health Organization classification scheme is shown (Table 54).

Management

As there is a wide spectrum of severity associated with the different grades of NHL, so there is a wide spectrum of therapy available. Low-grade lymphomas are treated in much the same way as B-CLL. Radiotherapy does have a valuable role particularly in the treatment of follicular lymphomas that may be highly localised. Where there is diffuse disease, however, careful clinical consideration needs to be given to the benefits of therapy. Cure is unlikely in low-grade disease and, therefore, most treatment is palliative. It is important that the side effects of treatment should not be worse than the condition itself. For high-grade lymphoma, cure is possible and combination chemotherapy is usually indicated. The traditional regimen CHOP (cyclophosphamide, doxorubicin, vincristine, prednisolone) has been updated with the addition of rituximab (R-CHOP).

Mycosis fungoides

Mycosis fungoides is a cutaneous T cell lymphoma that typically affects middle-aged men. The malignant cell is a $CD4^+$ T cell, the nucleus of which has an unusual convoluted appearance. The clinical identification of malignant transformation may be difficult. The cutaneous lesions develop from plaques into tumours and fungating ulcers. By definition, mycosis fungoides is limited to the skin, but it can develop into a systemic disorder characterised by lymphadenopathy, splenomegaly and leukaemia. This is termed **Sézary's syndrome**.

Management

Topical steroids, cytotoxic drugs, and psoralens with ultraviolet light (PUVA) treatment may all be effective for mycosis fungoides. When systemic disease occurs, cytotoxic therapy is required. Prognosis is very variable, with median survival of 5 years. Survival figures are much better if the disease is diagnosed early.

Angioimmunoblastic lymphoma

Patients with angioimmunoblastic lymphoma typically present with fever, and on examination are found to have lymphadenopathy and hepatosplenomegaly. Investigation often reveals autoimmune haemolytic anaemia with hypergammaglobulinaemia. Histology of lymph nodes indicates a mixed lymphoid infiltrate with small blood vessel formation. Early presentation may be responsive to oral corticosteroids; however, a malignant T cell lymphoma usually emerges.

Adult T cell lymphoma/leukaemia

Adult T cell lymphoma/leukaemia is common in the Caribbean and Japan and is caused by infection with human T cell lymphotropic virus type 1. The phenotype is characteristic, with proliferation of $CD4^+$ cells intensely expressing CD25. There is usually widespread visceral involvement and hypercalcaemia is common. Response to chemotherapy is usually poor but encouraging remissions are reported after cytotoxic

Table 54 WHO classification of non-Hodgkin's lymphoma

B cell	T cell	Grade
B cell chronic lymphocytic leukaemia		Low
Extranodal marginal-zone B cell lymphoma of MALT type		Low
Follicular lymphoma		Low
Mantle cell lymphoma		Variable
Diffuse large B cell lymphoma		High
	Anaplastic large cell lymphoma (T/null)	High
	Peripheral T cell lymphoma, not otherwise characterised	High
	Rarer entities (< 5% of all lymphomas)	
Burkitt's lymphoma		High, with marked risk of CNS disease
	Precursor T cell lymphoblastic lymphoma	High, with marked risk of CNS disease
	Mycosis fungoides/Sézary's syndrome	Variable
	Angioimmunoblastic lymphoma	High
	Adult T cell lymphoma/leukaemia	High, with marked risk of CNS disease

therapy followed by combination antiretroviral and interferon-α therapy.

Multiple myeloma

The peak incidence of myeloma is in the seventh decade of life and men are affected more often than women.

Clinical features

The majority of patients present with typical disease features (Table 55) although approximately 10% of patients are thought to be identified from the incidental finding of an abnormal blood test (e.g. erythrocyte sedimentation rate (ESR) > 100 mm/h or paraprotein identified). Symptoms of anaemia and hypercalcaemia are common. Some patients will present with solitary lytic lesions of bone or mass lesions in other soft tissues (**plasmacytoma**).

Investigation

The diagnosis usually rests on demonstrating two out of three investigative criteria (Table 56). A serum paraprotein is detected in the vast majority. This is an abnormal immunoglobulin protein produced by the malignant clone of B cells; it appears as a band on serum protein electrophoresis (Fig. 61). In the UK, IgG myeloma is the most common type (57%) with IgA myeloma the second most common (27%). IgD (1.5%), IgM (0.2%) and IgE (0.1%) myeloma are all rare but free light-chain myeloma (with no heavy chain detected) accounts for approximately 13% of cases (kappa 7% and lambda 6%). Non-secretory variants of myeloma (no paraprotein/free light chains detected) account for 1.2% of cases.

Table 55 Typical features in myeloma

Organ/system	Symptoms/signs
Bone	Skeletal pain/pathological fractures (60%); hypercalcaemia with normal alkaline phosphatase (30%)
Renal	Impaired renal function; nephrotic syndrome
Haematological	Anaemia; high erythrocyte sedimentation rate (> 100 mm/h); rouleaux formation on blood film; thrombocytopenia; hyperviscosity
Neurological	Mental impairment; peripheral neuropathy; carpal tunnel syndrome; spastic paraparesis
Immune	Infection: related to immune paresis/neutropenia

Table 56 Laboratory investigations in the diagnosis of myeloma

Test	Features
Serum and urine electrophoresis	Identification of discrete paraprotein
Bone marrow examination	Increased percentage (> 20%) of plasma cells, ± abnormal morphology
Skeletal X-ray survey	Identification of typical 'punched-out' lytic lesions

Usually two out of three criteria are required for the diagnosis of myeloma.

Paraproteins

Not all paraproteins are associated with malignancy (see below) but three characteristics are important in identifying a malignant paraprotein.

Quantity. There is no absolute level of paraprotein, above which all paraproteins are malignant and below which they are not. Nonetheless, paraproteins of > 10 g/l are likely to be associated with malignancy; this probability increases with higher levels (> 30 g/l). Not all patients with myeloma have a high paraprotein level at presentation.

Immunoparesis. Immunoparesis is a phenomenon associated with malignant paraproteins. It is present if the non-paraprotein isotype(s) levels are < 50% of the lower limit of the age-related normal range. Therefore, if an IgG paraprotein is detected, the total serum levels of IgA and IgM should be examined.

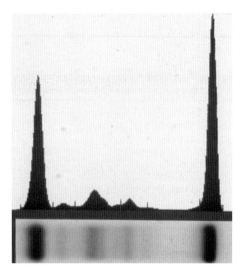

Fig. 61 Serum protein electrophoresis. The electrophoretic strip is at the bottom of the figure with the densitometric trace above it. There is an abnormal paraprotein peak identified in the mid-gamma region. Further investigation confirmed this as an IgG kappa paraprotein consistent with the diagnosis of multiple myeloma.

Monoclonal free light chains in the urine. Detection of free monoclonal free light chains in urine is highly suggestive of B cell malignancy.

Monitoring of myeloma

The prognosis in myeloma is variable and is dependent on a number of factors including tumour mass, renal function and age. Renal function at presentation is an important prognostic marker, but tumour mass is difficult to assess. Interestingly, the initial level of serum paraprotein does not appear to be a good prognostic indicator. A high level of urinary free light-chain excretion is associated with worse long-term survival, but this appears to reflect the association with poor renal function. Changes in paraprotein concentration are, however, useful in monitoring response to therapy, achievement of plateau phase and for disease progression. Some centres also now measure serum levels of free light chains. Serum β_2-microglobulin is a soluble surrogate marker of cellular turnover and is thought to be the best independent predictor of ultimate outcome as it also reflects the degree of renal failure. Overall survival is related both to age and the achievement of plateau phase, which is defined as

- asymptomatic/minimal symptoms attributable to myelomatosis
- stable haemoglobin level
- serum paraprotein, urinary free light-chain excretion and serum β_2-microglobulin levels stable in two samples taken 3 months apart.

Monoclonal gammopathy of uncertain significance

Monoclonal gammopathy of uncertain significance (MGUS) is the term used to describe a paraprotein that does not have the characteristics of a malignant paraprotein (defined above). In the past, these were described as 'benign paraproteins'; however, the observation that a percentage of patients eventually developed malignant features led to the reclassification as MGUS. The term benign paraprotein is now considered misleading and should not be used.

Clinical features

There are no specific clinical features to define patients with MGUS. Such patients are usually detected incidentally while the patient is being investigated for a wide range of physical symptoms, and this protein abnormality is not usually considered to cause symptoms.

MGUS is, however, common. A study of 856 patients with detectable serum paraproteins indicated that 541 (63%) were considered to have MGUS. Data indicate that MGUS is more frequent in the elderly and is found in approximately 3% of the population over the age of 70 years. The same authors studied 241 patients with MGUS and found that 33% of patients were over 70 years of age, with only 4% under 40 years. Patients were followed for a median of 22 years:

- in 19% there was no change in paraprotein level
- in 10%, the paraprotein had increased to > 30 g/l
- 24% had developed myeloma/amyloidosis/ Waldenstrom's macroglobulinaemia or other lymphoid malignancy
- 47% had died of an unrelated cause.

Detection of MGUS may be associated with underlying infective, inflammatory or indeed malignant conditions. It is thought that chronic immune stimulation in these conditions leads to the selective proliferation of a clone of B cells that gives rise to the MGUS. Long-term follow up is, therefore, essential and the paraprotein may disappear if the associated inflammatory condition is either cured or controlled. In contrast, an increasing absolute level of MGUS with the development of immune paresis or urinary free light chains should suggest malignant transformation.

Waldenstrom's macroglobulinaemia

Waldenstrom's macroglobulinaemia is a disease that is classically described in elderly men, in the eighth or ninth decade of life. It is, however, increasingly diagnosed in younger people.

Clinical features

Waldenstrom's macroglobulinaemia is characterised by the development of IgM paraprotein and symptoms are often related to the physical effects of the paraprotein on circulation. Symptoms can, therefore, appear non-specific and are related to hyperviscosity or the coexistence of cryoglobulinaemia. Typical features include visual disturbance, neurological symptoms (confusion, strokes), cardiac failure and Raynaud's phenomenon. On examination, there may be no abnormal physical findings, or there may be hepatosplenomegaly, fundal haemorrhage or lymphadenopathy. Because of the non-specific nature of symptoms and signs, this is a diagnosis that can be delayed or overlooked in an aged population who are prone to much other pathology and in whom some of the symptoms may be mistakenly regarded as an inevitable consequence of ageing. Typical laboratory features are:

- anaemia
- clotting disorders

- monoclonal IgM paraprotein on serum electrophoresis
- hyperviscosity
- excess lymphoplasmacytoid cells on bone marrow biopsy.

Investigation

In addition to the detection of an IgM paraprotein, it is necessary to measure plasma viscosity and test for cryoglobulins in these patients. It is essential that these complications of IgM paraproteins are considered and investigated, as correct identification and treatment will produce significant symptomatic relief for the patient. Plasma exchange is considered only when acute hyperviscosity syndrome occurs.

Cryoproteinaemia

Cryoproteins (including cryoglobulins and cryofibrinogens) are abnormal serum proteins that precipitate when cooled below a critical temperature. These proteins then form immune complexes and partially activate the classical complement pathway. Detection of low serum C4 with relatively normal C3 is typical of cryoproteinaemia and is caused by the inefficient classical pathway activation that occurs in the fluid phase. The incidental finding of this pattern of C3 and C4 should alert one to the possibility of underlying cryoproteinaemia (as well as C1 esterase deficiency and genetic deficiency of C4). Type I cryoglobulins are classically associated with lymphoproliferative disease while types II and III have both autoimmune and infectious associations (Ch. 8). Cryofibrinogenaemia is often associated with underlying malignancy. Full characterisation of cryoproteins is, therefore, essential in guiding the clinician to the correct diagnosis and most appropriate therapy. The management of a patient with cryoglobulinaemia should include appropriate therapy for the underlying disorder, and symptomatic relief with thermal clothing.

Self-assessment: questions

Multiple choice questions

1. In chronic lymphocytic leukaemia (CLL), the clonally expanded cells are most commonly derived from:
   a. B cells
   b. Dendritic cells
   c. Macrophages
   d. Natural killer cells
   e. T cells

2. A malignant paraprotein is suggested by:
   a. IgA isotype
   b. Level > 20 g/l
   c. Level < 10 g/l
   d. Low levels of other serum isotypes
   e. High levels of other serum isotypes

3. In monoclonal gammopathy of uncertain significance (MGUS):
   a. Bone marrow examination is always indicated
   b. In those affected, 75% progress to malignant paraproteins
   c. There is typically a serum level of > 10 g/l paraproteins
   d. There is an association with a monoclonal expansion of B cells
   e. There is an association with urinary free light chains

4. Typical features of hairy cell leukaemia include:
   a. Skin infiltration by CD4⁺ T cells
   b. Presentation in middle age
   c. Abnormal lymphocyte expression of CD11c
   d. Female to male ratio of 4:1
   e. Clonal expansion of B cells

5. A bad prognostic feature in Hodgkin's disease is:
   a. Haemoglobin of 90 g/l
   b. Male gender
   c. Lymphocyte count of $1 \times 10^9/l$
   d. Age 25 at presentation
   e. Raised liver function tests

Case history questions

History 1

A 78-year-old man is admitted to hospital with haematemesis. He has suffered from increasing confusion and loss of balance over the previous 6 months but otherwise was previously well. On examination he was thin and had several ulcers over the lower legs. He had signs suggestive of mild left ventricular failure and a moderately enlarged spleen. Investigations indicated the results in Table 57. The chest radiograph showed some blunting of costophrenic angles. Protein electrophoresis showed a discrete band in the mid-gamma region.

Table 57 Results for case history 1

Parameter	Value	Normal range
Haemoglobin (g/l)	100	130–180
Differential white cell count	Normal	
Urea (mmol/l)	12.0	2.1–8.9
Creatinine (µmol/l)	130	53–133
Alanine aminotransferase (U/l)	24	< 45
Aspartate aminotransferase (U/l)	35	< 41
C3 (g/l)	1.0	0.7–1.7
C4 (g/l)	0.2	0.13–0.43
IgG (g/l)	6.0	7–16
IgA (g/l)	2.0	0.8–4.7
IgM (g/l)	9.0	0.5–3.0

1. Which of the following investigations would be useful in confirming the likely clinical diagnosis?

   a. Indium-labelled white cell scan
   b. Anti-neutrophil cytoplasmic antibody (ANCA)
   c. Bone marrow examination
   d. Plasma viscosity
   e. Cryoglobulin analysis

2. What is likely to be the cause of his increasing confusion?

   a. Alzheimer's disease
   b. Anaemia
   c. Urinary infection
   d. Hypoxia
   e. Hyperviscosity

History 2

A 70-year-old male who is diagnosed with chronic lymphatic leukaemia (CLL) and has had several courses of chemotherapy, is admitted to hospital with bilateral pneumonia. History reveals that he has been suffering from frequent respiratory infections over the previous 6 months. Chest radiograph showed bilateral consolidation of lung bases; protein electrophoresis showed no paraprotein. Other results are shown in Table 58.

Table 58 Results for case history 2

Parameter	Value	Normal range
Haemoglobin (g/l)	115	130–180
Differential white cell count	70% lymphocytes	
Alanine aminotransferase (U/l)	24	< 45
Aspartate aminotransferase (U/l)	35	< 41
Complement (CH100)	Normal	
IgG (g/l)	5.0	7–16
IgA (g/l)	2.0	0.8–4.7
IgM (g/l)	2.5	0.5–3.0

1. Which lymphocyte subset is likely to predominate in the phenotypic analysis: CD3+CD4+, CD3+CD8+, CD19+CD5+, CD16+CD56+ or CD4+CD8+?
2. Which component of his immune system is likely to be defective: complement, T cells, B cells, natural killer cells and/or macrophages?
3. Is additional therapy indicated?

Data interpretation

1. The results shown in Table 59 were obtained from a 65-year-old man who presented with anaemia.

   a. What is the most likely diagnosis?
   b. What additional phenotypic markers might be helpful?

Table 59 Results for data interpretation question

Parameter	Value	Normal range
Haemoglobin (g/l)	85	130–180
Total white cell count (× 10⁹/l)	20	4–10
Platelets (× 10⁹/l)	150 000	150–450
Lymphocytes (× 10⁹/l)	15	1.5–3.5
Lymphocyte phenotype (%)		
CD3	55	62–69
CD4	35	37–64
CD8	20	11–36
CD19	45	3–13
Immunoglobulin subclass (g/l)		
IgG	8.0	7–16
IgA	1.2	0.8–4.7
IgM	0.5	0.5–3.0
Protein electrophoresis: no compact band detected		

Self-assessment: answers

Multiple choice answers

1. a. **True.** B cells are the most common cell type of origin in CLL.
   b. **False.**
   c. **False.**
   d. **False.**
   e. **False.** Although T-CLL does occur it is unusual.

2. a. **False.** Malignant paraproteins may be of any isotype.
   b. **True.** Paraprotein levels > 20 g/l are suggestive of a malignancy.
   c. **False.** Paraprotein levels < 10 g/l are more suggestive of monoclonal gammopathy of uncertain significance.
   d. **True.** 'Immunoparesis' is the term for low levels of the non-paraprotein isotype.
   e. **False.** See (d).

3. a. **False.** If there is low-level paraproteins, with no associated immunoparesis, negative Bence-Jones protein and no clinical features to suggest lymphoproliferation, bone marrow examination is not necessary.
   b. **False.** The figure is probably closer to 35%.
   c. **False.** Typical value is < 10 g/l.
   d. **True.** However, the assumption is that this is a very small clone and does not have malignant properties.
   e. **False.** By definition. The detection of Bence-Jones protein is suggestive of a malignant lymphoproliferative condition.

4. a. **False.** This occurs in mycosis fungoides.
   b. **False.** It is a condition of the elderly.
   c. **True.** The adhesion molecule CD11c is aberrantly expressed in this condition and is a useful diagnostic marker.
   d. **False.** The ratio is 4:1 for males to females.
   e. **True.** This is a clonal expansion of B cells.

5. a. **True.** Haemoglobin < 105 g/l is a poor prognostic factor.
   b. **True.** Male gender is a poor prognostic factor.
   c. **False.** Lymphocyte count < 0.6 is a poor prognostic factor.
   d. **False.** Age > 45 years is a poor prognostic factor.
   e. **False.**

Case history answers

History 1

1. a. This was not useful in that the history did not suggest localised, occult infection as the cause of symptoms.
   b. The history is not suggestive of an ANCA-associated vasculitis.
   c. The history is suggestive of Waldenstrom's macroglobulinaemia and bone marrow examination is essential.
   d. Plasma viscosity should be measured as he has a raised total IgM with a paraprotein detected. The history of recent confusion and loss of balance could reflect a hyperviscosity syndrome.
   e. The presence of leg ulceration might suggest cryoglobulinaemia; however, the normal serum C4 level makes cryoglobulinaemia very unlikely in this case and so the analysis would not help.

2. a. Alzheimer's disease is unlikely as the history is suggestive of other organic processes as potential causes of confusion.
   b. The patient's haemoglobin is slightly low but that should not by itself cause confusion and so anaemia can be excluded as a cause.
   c. Although urinary infection is a common cause of acute confusion in the elderly, in this case the history is more chronic.
   d. There is no evidence of significant hypoxia in the history.
   e. Hyperviscosity is the most likely diagnosis. It is a significant problem when total serum IgM is raised significantly. This causes slowing of the circulation and, therefore, of cerebration. Crucially, it responds to successful reduction of the paraprotein level.

History 2

1. The lymphocytes subset likely to predominate is CD19$^+$CD5$^+$. Lymphocyte phenotyping is a useful confirmatory test; a characteristic finding in B-CLL is that the abnormal B cells aberrantly express CD5, which is normally a pan-T antigen. Thus finding B cells carrying this pan-T marker (CD19$^+$CD5$^+$) is considered confirmatory evidence of B-CLL if there is the appropriate clinical presentation. Small numbers of CD19$^+$CD5$^+$ cells can be found in neonates and in some autoimmune disorders, but these are distinct from B-CLL cells.

2. Defective B cell function underlies the hypogammaglobulinaemia and recurrent infection.

3. The admission with bilateral pneumonia and additional history suggesting recurrent chest infection over the prior 6 months suggest that immunoglobulin replacement therapy (intravenous or subcutaneous) should be considered. CLL is an important cause of secondary immunodeficiency, and such therapy can improve quality of life immensely. It is, however, essential that all aspects of the patient's condition, care and prognosis should be considered prior to commencing additional therapy.

Data interpretation

1. a. The investigations indicate anaemia and leukocytosis in a man of this age. The differential white cells count indicates a significant increase in the lymphocyte count and the lymphocyte phenotype identifies that there is a much higher percentage of cells bearing the CD19 antigen (B cell marker). Taken together, these results suggest a B cell lymphoproliferative disorder. The serum immunoglobulin levels are normal so the differential does not include multiple myeloma at this stage. The most likely diagnosis is probably B cell chronic lymphatic leukaemia (B-CLL) although other more rare variants could explain the findings.

b. Additional markers that might be helpful would include CD5 (B cells in B-CLL are CD5+CD19+); if this is negative, one might proceed to look at markers associated with other B cell disorders such as CD11c (hairy cell leukemia). Non-Hodgkin's lymphoma in a leukaemic phase should also be considered and lymph node biopsy would be required for this.

12 Use of the immunology laboratory

Chapter overview

Clinical immunology laboratories provide a very wide range of tests useful in the diagnosis and monitoring of human disease. Most such laboratories will have subsections providing some or all of the following: autoimmune serology, immunochemistry, allergy, cellular immunology, and immunohistology. In the UK, clinical immunology laboratories are led by consultants trained in immunology. An important part of their role is to provide advice on the appropriate use of laboratory tests and the interpretation of results. The laboratory itself should be accredited and in the UK this means that the laboratory has undergone regular inspection by an accrediting body such as Clinical Pathology Accreditation (UK) Ltd (CPA-UK) and has satisfied all their standards of performance. The aim of this chapter is to help the reader to understand some important general principles regarding the use of laboratory tests and specialist laboratories and the spectrum of services provided by immunology laboratories in particular.

12.1 The immunology laboratory

Learning objectives

You should:
- understand that the laboratory tests are an aid to the diagnostic process and never a substitute for careful clinical history taking and physical examination
- be aware of the typical tests provided: autoimmune serology, immunochemistry, allergy and cellular immunology
- understand that some tests are used to assist in diagnosis and others are of value in monitoring disease activity, once a diagnosis is established
- know the importance of sensitivity, specificity, positive and negative predictive values, and pre- and post-test probability of diagnosis
- understand that external accreditation is an essential hallmark of a high-quality laboratory service.

The provision of laboratory immunology services in the UK is based on regional and subregional laboratories providing a broad range of immunological tests. Local hospitals may provide a limited repertoire of immunological tests but these should be developed in collaboration with the regional/subregional centre. Immunology laboratories are headed by consultant immunologists who work with a range of scientific staff to deliver the laboratory service, but who usually also provide direct clinical services in primary immunodeficiency, allergy and some aspects of autoimmune disease.

Major laboratory sections

The major sections of an immunology laboratory cover some or all of the following: autoimmune serology, immunochemistry, allergy, cellular immunology, immunohistology and tissue typing. Very few laboratories provide exactly the same test repertoires and the exact configuration of laboratories is usually shaped by local historical interests. All clinical laboratories must have rigorous quality control procedures to ensure that test results are accurate and reliable. In addition, clinical laboratories in the UK are subject to external accreditation procedures. These set standards for all aspects of laboratory practice from sample collection to result authorisation. This system is designed to ensure minimum acceptable standards are maintained in all laboratories.

Tests

Test requesting

Blood testing is an aid to clinical diagnosis and the decision to request blood tests should only be taken after careful clinical assessment and the establishment of a differential diagnosis. The results of laboratory investigations should then assist the clinician in prioritising the differential diagnosis and establishing a conclusive diagnosis for the patient.

What makes a good test?

A number of terms are used to describe the performance of tests. Predictive value theory is the most commonly used and describes a number of characteristics:

- *sensitivity*: the percentage of individuals with a condition that the test identifies
- *specificity*: the percentage of individuals who do not have the condition that the test excludes
- *positive predictive value*: the percentage of positive results that truly indicate the presence of the condition
- *negative predictive value*: the percentage of negative results that truly indicate that the condition is not present
- *diagnostic efficiency*: the percentage of individuals correctly classified by a test; in other words, what percentage of patients tested are correctly classified as positive or negative for the condition.

Ideally, one would expect all laboratory tests to have values approaching 100% for each of the criteria above; however, in practice, this is rare and it is, therefore, important to have some knowledge of the individual test's performance criteria before it is used. It is also important to realise that the person requesting the test influences its performance criteria. If a test is applied to a population with a very low prevalence of a disease (e.g. Wegener's granulomatosis in general practice), it is likely to have low specificity and a higher number of false-positives than if the same test were used in a population attending a renal unit in whom there would be a much higher prevalence of the condition.

What types of test are there?

Laboratory tests can be used for different purposes. The ideal laboratory test would identify all people with the condition in question and exclude all people without the condition. It would, therefore, have neither false-positives nor false-negatives. Unfortunately, very few laboratory tests approach these strict performance criteria. We, therefore, need to have an understanding of the diagnostic performance of an individual test before deciding how it could be used in practice.

Screening test

A screening test is one that if applied to a large unselected population will identify almost all people with the condition being sought. It is, however, also likely to detect people who do not have the condition (false-positives) but should not fail to identify people with the condition (false-negatives). It is said, therefore, to have a high sensitivity but does not require a high specificity.

Diagnostic test

A diagnostic test is one that should only be positive in people with the condition and rarely, if ever, have false-positives. It, therefore, must have high specificity (as closed to 100% as possible) and as high a sensitivity as possible.

If we accept that few blood tests are *perfect* in terms of having 100% specificity and sensitivity, it becomes clear that most blood tests are not truly *diagnostic* and different tests have very different performance characteristics.

How do we use laboratory tests?

After establishing the differential diagnosis for an individual patient, there is a **pre-test probability** of that being the correct diagnosis. This is influenced not only by the quality of history taking and examination but also by the prevalence of the disease in question. Once the test has been applied, that probability will change (either increased or decreased) to the **post-test probability**. The post-test probability is the likelihood of the disease now that the additional information (the test result) is known. A good test should demonstrate a significant difference between the pre- and post-test probability, but by definition a test result simply alters (increases/decreases) the likelihood of an underlying condition being present.

How should we interpret the results of tests?

Immunological blood tests vary considerably in whether they are suitable as screening or diagnostic tests or whether they need to be interpreted along with the results of other tests (e.g. in the investigation of immunodeficiency). The following sections briefly describe commonly available tests and indicate (where known) their approximate sensitivity and specificity for the conditions in question. If you are in doubt regarding the interpretation of the results of specialist tests, or indeed the appropriateness of requesting the tests, it is always wise to ask the laboratory in question for advice.

12.2 Autoimmune serology

Autoimmune serology involves the detection of both organ-specific and non-organ-specific autoantibodies in serum samples. The most common detection method used is indirect immunofluorescence (IIF) for serum antibodies (Fig. 62) and direct immunofluorescence (DIF) for antibodies in tissue sections (Fig. 63). Secondary testing methods (DIF on different substrates, enzyme-linked immunosorbent assay (ELISA), etc.) are often used to identify the fine specificity of such antibodies once they are initially detected. The majority of the autoimmune serology tests are detected in regional/subregional laboratories.

Indirect immunofluorescence

The most commonly used method for detection of serum autoantibodies is IIF. As indicated in Figure 62, a tissue

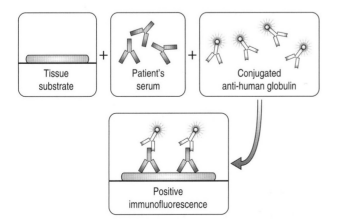

Fig. 62 Indirect immunofluorescent detection of serum autoantibodies.

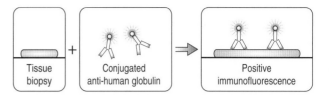

Fig. 63 Direct immunofluorescent examination of tissue sections.

substrate is applied to a glass slide and patient serum is incubated with this glass slide containing the tissue substrate. The choice of substrate varies between laboratories but is typically rat liver/kidney/stomach for those laboratories that offer **autoantibody screens**. Autoantibody screens on such composite tissue blocks detect antinuclear, anti-smooth muscle, anti-mitochondrial and anti-gastric parietal cell antibodies. Human epithelial cells (HEP2 cells) are used as substrate for the detection and characterisation of anti-nuclear antibodies. Autoantibodies are usually detected at a 'screening dilution' of serum, typically 1:80 and reported as the reciprocal of the weakest serum dilution at which the autoantibody is detectable (e.g. 1:320, 1:2560, etc.). Laboratories differ in both the techniques and dilutions used. It is, therefore, not possible to refer to 'normal ranges', but the local laboratory should provide this information for their own tests. Some of the following tests are only provided by specialist regional/supraregional laboratories and this is indicated by the note 'specialist laboratory test'.

Anti-nuclear antibodies

Anti-nuclear antibodies (ANA) are a range of autoantibodies that are found in serum that bind specifically to a range of nuclear antigens. Antibodies directed against different target antigens result in specific immunofluorescent patterns and these are associated with particular types of connective tissue disease. The pattern of ANA may, therefore, be diagnostically helpful and furthermore, specific secondary tests are used to confirm antibody binding to the target antigens (e.g. double-stranded DNA (dsDNA), ribonucleoprotein (RNP), Ro, La, etc.). The most common pattern of ANA is homogeneous, in which there is uniform staining across the whole of the nucleus. Homogeneous ANA are associated with a wide range of connective tissue disorders but may also occur as a non-specific finding after infection, trauma, surgery or in up to 10% of the healthy elderly. In order to assess the significance of an ANA, in addition to the clinical history, one should consider the following features:

- **class of antibody**: IgG ANA are more likely to be significant than IgM class (very few laboratories now measure IgM autoantibodies)

- **titre**: individual laboratories differ in their reported level of 'significance' but most would agree that a titre of less than 1:80 is unlikely to be significant
- **antigenic 'specificity**: homogeneous ANA may be associated with a range of nuclear target antigens, which are confirmed in the individual patient by secondary testing.

Patterns of anti-nuclear antibodies on indirect immunofluorescence

Anti-nuclear speckled antibody

An anti-nuclear speckled antibody pattern is found in some patients with systemic lupus erythematosus (SLE), mixed connective tissue disease, Sjögren's syndrome and scleroderma. This pattern is usually associated with antibodies to **extractable nuclear antigens** (ENA: see below).

Anti-nucleolar antibody

Anti-nucleolar antibody is typically found in patients with scleroderma, SLE and polymyositis.

Anti-centromere antibody

Anti-centromere antibody is detected in 60–70% of patients with the CREST variant of scleroderma (calcinosis, Raynaud's phenomenon, oesophageal dysfunction, sclerodactyly and telangectasia) and 20% of patients with generalised scleroderma. This antibody may also be found in patients with primary biliary cirrhosis

Anti-dsDNA antibody

Anti-dsDNA antibody is strongly suggestive of SLE although it is present in only 40–60% of patients with this disease.

Anti-extractable nuclear antigen antibodies

Antibodies to ENA are of use in the classification of clinical subsets of connective tissue diseases and in providing prognostic information. Antigenic specificities include RNP, Sm, Ro, La, Scl-70 (anti-topoisomerase-1) and Jo-1 (histidyl tRNA synthetase).

Anti-RNP antibody. Antibodies to RNP occur in patients with SLE and mixed connective tissue disease.
Anti-Sm antibody. Antibodies are very specific for a diagnosis of SLE but occur in only 25–30% of patients with this condition.
Anti-Ro antibody. Antibodies are found in patients with SLE (particularly with photosensitivity), cutaneous lupus erythematosus, Sjögren's syndrome, recurrent miscarriage, neonatal lupus and congenital heart block.
Anti-La antibody. Antibodies are detected in patients with SLE and Sjögren's syndrome.

Anti-Jo-1 antibody. Antibodies are found in 20-40% of patients with aggressive polymyositis usually in association with interstitial lung disease and arthralgia.
Anti-Scl-70 antibody. Antibodies are found in 20–40% of patients with scleroderma; they are more commonly found in the diffuse cutaneous form.

Non-nuclear autoantibodies

Non-nuclear autoantibodies are detected by IIF using a number of substrates including rat liver, kidney and stomach or specific organ tissue (adrenal gland or nervous tissue). Depending on the target antigen, they produce characteristic immunofluorescent patterns that are readily recognised by an experienced technician.

Anti-acetylcholine receptor antibody (specialist laboratory test)

Anti-acetylcholine receptor antibody is detected in 80–90% of patients with myasthenia gravis. It is a primary autoantibody that binds to the postsynaptic acetylcholine receptor, thus preventing acetylcholine binding and disrupting neuromuscular signalling.

Anti-adrenal antibody

Antibodies to the steroid-secreting cells of the adrenal cortex are detected in 60–70% of patients with idiopathic Addison's disease. They are useful in confirming the autoimmune nature of the condition

Anti-β_2-glycoprotein 1 antibody (specialist laboratory test)

Anti-β_2-glycoprotein 1 is an important cofactor in the clotting cascade. Antibodies against -β_2-glycoprotein 1 are found in a subset of patients with primary and secondary anti-phospholipid syndrome (see anti-cardiolipin antibody). Full assessment of suspected anti-phospholipid antibody syndrome should include measurement of anti-β_2-glycoprotein 1, anti-cardiolipin antibody as well as the lupus anticoagulant. Lupus anticoagulant measurement is a specialised test undertaken in coagulation laboratories. The use of these tests in combination is important because most patients will not be positive for all of them.

Anti-cardiac muscle antibody

Anti-cardiac muscle antibody is positive in some patients with Dressler's syndrome and postcardiotomy syndrome and may, therefore, be helpful in confirming the diagnosis.

Anti-cardiolipin antibody

Anti-cardiolipin antibody is found in the anti-phospholipid syndrome, which may be primary or occur as a secondary complication of SLE. The major features of anti-phospholipid syndrome are thromboses (arterial or venous), thrombocytopenia, recurrent spontaneous abortion and typical skin rash (livedo reticularis). Patients with anti-phospholipid syndrome may also have detectable lupus anticoagulant and all patients suspected of this condition should have a sample sent to the haematology laboratory for coagulation studies (see also anti-β_2-glycoprotein).

Anti-endomysial antibody

Anti-endomysial antibody is very specific (90–100%) for coeliac disease and is also detected in patients with dermatitis herpetiformis. Anti-endomysial, anti-gliadin and anti-tissue transglutaminase (anti-TTG) antibodies are used in combination as serological screening tests for coeliac disease. In most centres the use of coeliac disease-associated autoantibody testing means that patients have to undergo less-frequent jejunal biopsies as part of the diagnostic evaluation. In patients with coeliac disease who are on a gluten-free diet, anti-endomysial antibody often becomes negative. Therefore, it is essential to know if a patient is on a gluten-free diet before interpreting results.

Anti-glutamic acid decarboxylase antibody (specialist laboratory test)

Anti-glutamic acid decarboxylase antibody (anti-GAD) is detected in both the stiff man syndrome and type 1 diabetes mellitus (insulin-dependent diabetes; IDDM). Slightly different antigens are targeted in each condition; they are of diagnostic value in confirming stiff man syndrome.

Anti-gastric parietal cell antibody

Anti-gastric parietal cell antibody is present in 95% of patients with pernicious anaemia but is also detected in autoimmune type A gastritis, autoimmune thyroid disease, up to 30% of patients with iron-deficiency anaemia and 3% of the normal population (the incidence rising with increasing age).

Anti-ganglioside antibodies (specialist laboratory test)

Antibodies to gangliosides have been described in patients with peripheral neuropathies. These are only detected in specialist laboratories and, therefore, it usu-ally takes several weeks for results to be made available. Antibodies detected include:

- anti-membrane gangliosides (anti-GM1) in some patients with multifocal motor neuropathy and less frequently in Guillain–Barré syndrome
- anti-GD1 in patients with Guillain–Barré syndrome
- anti-GQ1b and anti-GT1a in > 90% patients with Miller–Fisher syndrome.

Anti-gliadin antibody

Anti-gliadin antibody is associated with coeliac disease and dermatitis herpetiformis with associated gluten enteropathy. Antibody levels reflect disease activity and can be useful in monitoring treatment. They are not as specific for coeliac disease as anti-endomysial antibody. Anti-gliadin antibodies are also detected in a wide range of other clinical conditions. The use of anti-gliadin antibodies as a screening test for coeliac disease is largely being superseded by the introduction of anti-TTG.

Anti-glomerular basement membrane antibody

Anti-glomerular basement membrane (GBM) antibody is a primary autoantibody found in patients with Goodpasture's syndrome (> 90% sensitivity). Binding of this autoantibody to glomerular and pulmonary basement membranes initiates a type II hypersensitivity reaction at those sites, with resultant organ-specific autoimmunity. The titre of autoantibody is often monitored to assess effectiveness of therapy (including plasmapheresis).

Anti-histone antibody

Anti-histone antibody is found in 18–50% of patients with SLE and in 95% of patients with drug-induced SLE.

Anti-IgA antibody (specialist laboratory test)

Anti-IgA antibody is detected in some patients with selective IgA deficiency. The vast majority of individuals suffer no adverse effects; however, they can cause blood product transfusion reactions (including reactions to intravenous immunoglobulin). It is rarely necessary to test for anti-IgA antibodies but is occasionally undertaken to investigate a serious transfusion reaction.

Anti-intrinsic factor antibody

Anti-intrinsic factor antibody is positive in > 75% of patients with pernicious anaemia. They are highly specific for pernicious anaemia if found in combination with gastric parietal cell antibody. Anti-intrinsic factor antibody may be detected before anaemia develops. The absence of anti-intrinsic factor antibodies does not exclude pernicious anaemia.

Anti-islet cell antibody (specialist laboratory test)

Anti-islet cell antibody is specific for type I diabetes mellitus and is detectable in the early (and preclinical) phase of the disorder. In clinical practice these tests are seldom required.

Anti-liver–kidney microsome antibody

Anti-liver–kidney microsome (LKM) antibody identifies a subgroup of patients with autoimmune (hepatitis B negative) chronic active hepatitis (type 2). This is the most common form of chronic active hepatitis in childhood and has a particularly poor prognosis. Anti-LKM antibody is also detected in hepatitis C infection.

Anti-mitochondrial antibody

Anti-mitochondrial antibody is detected at high titre in 95% of patients with primary biliary cirrhosis; low titres may also be found in chronic active hepatitis. A number of subtypes of mitochondrial antibodies have been described; each of these has slightly different IIF pattern. The important subtypes are:

- M1: associated with positive syphilis serology.
- M2a and M2b: associated with primary biliary cirrhosis.
- M5: associated with SLE and the anti-phospholipid syndrome.

Anti-neuronal cell antibody

Anti-neuronal cell (anti-Hu) autoantibody is found in paraneoplastic syndromes, typically in patients suffering from small cell carcinoma of the lung who develop sensory neuropathy or encephalomyelitis. The antibodies stain neuronal cell nuclei.

Anti-neutrophil cytoplasmic antibodies

Detection of anti-neutrophil cytoplasmic (ANCA) antibodies is indicated in the investigation of suspected primary systemic vasculitis. ANCA testing is not suitable as a screening test for all vasculitic syndromes. Use should be restricted to the investigation of patients suspected of primary systemic vasculitis affecting small- and medium-sized vessels (Ch. 8). Three main patterns are recognised:

- cytoplasmic (c-ANCA)
- perinuclear (p-ANCA)
- atypical ANCA.

The c-ANCA form has a high predictive value for active generalised Wegener's granulomatosis and can also be found in patients with microscopic polyangiitis. The specificity of this antibody is for proteinase 3 (PR3-ANCA).

Occurrence of p-ANCA with anti-myeloperoxidase (MPO) ANCA is specifically predictive for patients with active microscopic polyangiitis; some patients with Wegener's granulomatosis also have this antibody. The occurrence of p-ANCA with specificities other than MPO-ANCA occur in some patients with inflammatory bowel disease, sclerosing cholangitis, rheumatoid arthritis, SLE, chronic active hepatitis and other autoimmune diseases. In such patients, ANCA levels are often low and of uncertain significance. Atypical ANCA are found in some with drug-induced vasculitis but otherwise are of uncertain clinical significance.

Anti-myeloperoxidase antibody
Myeloperoxidase is the target antigen for the majority of p-ANCA and is associated with microscopic polyangiitis. The detection of p-ANCA and MPO-ANCA in combination with an appropriate clinical presentation has a high predictive value for microscopic polyangiitis.

Anti-proteinase 3 (PR3-ANCA) antibody
Proteinase 3 is the major target antigen for c-ANCA. The detection of PR3-ANCA in combination with c-ANCA has a high predictive value for Wegener's granulomatosis.

Anti-Purkinje cell antibody (anti-Yo)

Anti-Purkinje cell (anti-Yo) antibody is typically detected in women with gynaecological (most frequently ovarian, but rarely breast) cancer and a paraneoplastic cerebellar syndrome. It is occasionally detected in Hodgkin's disease. It is, therefore, an important test to perform in patients (especially postmenopausal women) presenting with unexplained cerebellar syndromes.

Anti-ribosomal antibody (ribosomal P antibody)

Anti-ribosomal antibody is found in 10–15% of patients with SLE, often in the absence of anti-dsDNA. The detection of these antibodies in individual patients is reported to be associated with an increased risk of neuropsychiatric symptoms and renal involvement.

Anti-skeletal (striated) muscle antibody

Anti-skeletal muscle antibody is characteristically detected in patients with myasthenia gravis who have a thymoma. They also occur in some patients with hepatitis, acute viral infections and polymyositis. Low titres may occur following viral infections, notably after Epstein–Barr virus and infectious hepatitis.

Anti-smooth muscle antibody

Anti-smooth muscle antibody occurs in high titres in patients with autoimmune (hepatitis B negative) chronic active hepatitis but may also be detected at low titre in patients with primary biliary cirrhosis or in healthy individuals following acute infection.

Anti-steroid cell antibody

Anti-steroid cell antibody is found in patients with type 1 autoimmune polyendocrinopathy syndrome and premature gonadal and ovarian failure. They react with the steroid-producing cells of the ovary or testis and usually the adrenal cortex. This antibody is only occasionally found in primary ovarian failure.

Anti-thyroid peroxidase antibody

Anti-thyroid peroxidase antibody is detected in patients with primary myxoedema, Hashimoto's thyroiditis and Graves' disease. Detection of this antibody in asymptomatic patients may be predictive of future autoimmune thyroid disease; in such circumstances, clinical follow up is advised with monitoring of thyroid function tests.

Anti-thyrotropin (TSH) receptor antibody

Antibodies to thyroid-stimulating hormone (TSH; also known as thyrotropin) receptor are detected in patients

with Graves' disease; however, the detection of this antibody is not essential to make the diagnosis.

Anti-tissue transglutaminase antibody (anti-TTG)

Tissue transglutaminase is the antigen against which anti-endomysial antibodies are directed. In most immunology laboratories, detection of anti-TTG antibodies has now superseded anti-gliadin antibody detection as the screening test for coeliac disease. In common with anti-endomysial antibody (detected by IIF), anti-TTG antibody titres fall when patients commence a gluten-free diet.

Anti-voltage-gated calcium channel antibody (specialist laboratory test)

Anti-voltage-gated calcium channel antibody is primary autoantibody found in the Lambert–Eaton myasthenic syndrome. It binds to the presynaptic membrane of the neuromuscular junction and prevents the release of acetylcholine into the synapse, thus preventing neuromuscular signalling and causing fatigability of muscles.

Anti-C3 nephritic factor

Anti-C3 nephritic factor (C3Nef) is an autoantibody detected in patients with membranoproliferative glomerulonephritis (type II) and partial lipodystrophy. The C3Nef binds to the alternate complement pathway C3 convertase (C3bBb) stabilising it and causing prolonged conversion of C3. Therefore, serum C3 levels are very low in this condition. A striking clinical feature of this condition is *partial lipodystrophy* (Fig. 64), in which there is loss of subcutaneous fat,

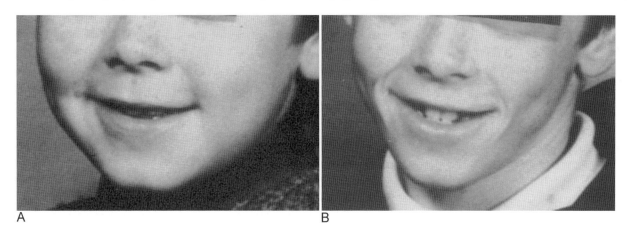

A   B

Fig. 64 Facial photographs of the same boy taken 2 years apart indicate the changes of partial lipodystrophy. Loss of subcutaneous fat associated with C3 nephritic factor positive, Type II membranoproliferative glomerulonephritis. This appearance is often mistakenly identified as cachexia.

typically affecting half or all of the face. This may be mistaken for cachexia or malnutrition but should alert the clinician to the possibility of underlying renal disease.

Rheumatoid factor

Rheumatoid factor measurement is indicated in the investigation of inflammatory arthropathies. High levels are associated with rheumatoid arthritis and patients with rheumatoid factor are more likely to have extra-articular manifestations such as vasculitis and nodules. Rheumatoid factor is not, however, of value in laboratory monitoring of disease activity; C-reactive protein (CRP) should be used. Low-titre rheumatoid factor may occur in other connective tissue/autoimmune diseases: SLE, chronic active hepatitis, scleroderma and in response to infection.

Skin reactive antibodies

In addition to the direct immunofluorescent detection of immune deposits in skin biopsies, IIF of serum can identify two circulating autoantibodies. *Anti-intercellular substance/desmosome antibody* is found in patients with all forms of pemphigus. The antibody level is related to disease activity and, therefore, is useful in monitoring treatment. *Anti-basement membrane zone antibody* is found in patients with bullous pemphigoid (Ch. 6).

12.3 Immunochemistry

Learning objectives

You should:

- understand the methods to measure normal and abnormal levels of serum immunoglobulins
- understand the role of C-reactive protein and complement in immune reactions and know when these should be measured
- know the significance of cryoglobulins
- know the significance of Bence-Jones proteins (free monoclonal light chains) in urine protein analysis.

The major elements of an immunochemistry section include the measurement of normal and abnormal serum immunoglobulins, allergen-specific IgE, acute phase protein measurement (e.g. CRP) and measurement of functional complement activity and individual complement components.

Table 60 Normal ranges for serum immunoglobulins

Age	IgG (g/l)	IgA (g/l)	IgM (g/l)
At birth (cord)	5.2–18.0	< 0.02	0.02–0.2
0–2 weeks	5.0–17.0	0.01–0.08	0.05–0.2
2–6 weeks	3.9–13.0	0.02–0.15	0.08–0.4
6–12 weeks	2.1–7.7	0.05–0.4	0.15–0.7
3–6 months	2.4–8.8	0.1–0.5	0.2–1.0
6–9 months	3.0–9.0	0.15–0.7	0.4–1.6
9–12 months	3.0–10.9	0.2–0.7	0.6–2.1
1–2 years	3.1–13.8	0.3–1.2	0.5–2.2
2–3 years	3.7–15.8	0.3–1.3	0.5–2.2
3–6 years	4.9–16.1	0.4–2.0	0.5–2.0
6–12 years	5.4–16.1	0.5–2.5	0.5–1.8
> 12 years	7.0–16.0	0.8–4.7	0.5–3.0

Serum immunoglobulin measurement

Assessment of IgG, IgM, IgA and serum proteins is essential in the investigation of suspected immunodeficiency and lymphoproliferative diseases.

Measurement of IgG, IgM, IgA and serum proteins by electrophoresis

Normal ranges for serum immunoglobulins vary with age and so it is important to know what is normal for the individual in question (Table 60). Total levels of serum immunoglobulins are usually measured by an automated technique called **rate nephelometry**. This provides numerical values for the concentration of immunoglobulin isotypes in serum but does not give qualitative information regarding the presence or absence of **paraproteins** (abnormal immunoglobulins). Abnormally elevated levels of immunoglobulin in the

Table 61 Elevations of serum immunoglobulins in disease

Isotype(s) increased	Associated conditions
IgG	Connective tissue diseases, Hashimoto's thyroiditis, chronic active hepatitis, sarcoid, acquired immuno-deficiency syndrome (AIDS)
IgA	Gastrointestinal/respiratory infection, Crohn's disease, coeliac disease, alcoholic liver disease, rheumatoid arthritis, ankylosing spondylitis
IgM	Acute viral infection, primary biliary cirrhosis, lymphoma, malaria, trypanosomiasis
IgG and IgA	Chronic respiratory infection (bronchiectasis/tuberculosis), cirrhosis, rheumatoid arthritis, AIDS
IgG and IgM	Systemic lupus erythematosus, leprosy, chronic active hepatitis
IgG, IgA and IgM	Chronic bacterial infection (endocarditis, osteomyelitis, deep abscess, empyema), sarcoid

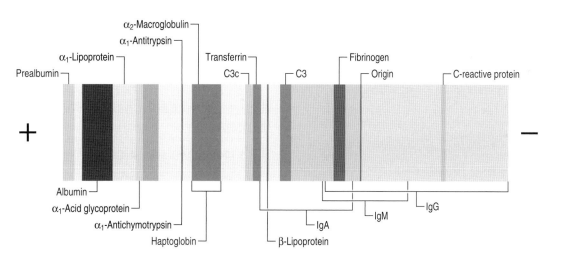

Fig. 65 Serum protein electrophoresis. An origin artefact is often weakly present; if a strong band occurs here, a cryoglobulin should be suspected.

absence of a paraprotein (i.e. polyclonal elevation) may occur in a number of disorders including chronic infections/inflammatory conditions, liver disease and autoimmune diseases. The pattern of isotype representation can give clues to underlying pathology (Table 61).

Serum protein electrophoresis is a different technique that separates serum proteins on the basis of their electrical charge. This produces an 'electrophoretic strip' in which the normal serum proteins migrate to specific positions (Fig. 65). Normal immunoglobulins usually occupy a spectrum of the β- and γ-regions; however, abnormal immunoglobulins (paraproteins) are seen as compact bands usually in the γ-region. It is, therefore, essential that both nephelometry and serum protein electrophoresis are performed together to ensure any abnormal proteins are identified. An example of an electrophoretic strip and the associated densitometry is shown in Figure 66.

Paraproteins

B cells normally secrete intact or fragmented immunoglobulin molecules, and monoclonal populations of B cells, therefore, have the potential to produce identical immunoglobulin molecules in very large quantities. This is important diagnostically as such identical molecules migrate characteristically as abnormal discrete bands (paraproteins) on electrophoresis of either serum or urine. Detection of a paraprotein will often be the first laboratory evidence of underlying B cell malignant disease. See Figure 61 for an example of a paraprotein identified on serum protein electrophoresis.

As discussed in Chapter 11, paraproteins are present in the majority of those with myeloma and Waldenstrom's macroglobulinaemia. In addition to the diagnostic value, monitoring the level of a paraprotein

is a sensitive marker of disease progression. However, not all paraproteins are associated with malignant disease and the distinct characteristics of monoclonal gammopathy of uncertain significance (MGUS) are indicated here and further discussed in Chapter 11.

Serum protein electrophoresis

Serum protein electrophoresis should be performed on all samples submitted for immunoglobulin analysis so that paraproteins may be identified. However, a number of other abnormalities may also be detected in such an analysis that can be helpful diagnostically. Figure 65 indicates the major bands seen on separation of normal serum. The strip is conventionally divided into α_1-, α_2, β_1-, β_2- and γ-regions and, as indicated, the immuno-

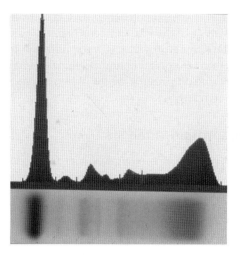

Fig. 66 Serum protein electrophoresis. The electrophoretic strip is at the bottom of the figure with the densitometric trace above it. There is a polyclonal increase in serum immunoglobulins in the gamma region.

globulins are chiefly found in the β- and γ-regions. However, normal polyclonal IgG can migrate as far as the α$_2$-region and, as paraproteins are by definition abnormal proteins, they may migrate to any position on the strip depending on their individual physical characteristics.

Paraprotein detection and measurement

Paraproteins may be considered as two basic types: those derived from a malignant clone of cells and those of uncertain origin (MGUS).

Malignant paraproteins. These are usually of high concentration (> 10 g/l) and associated with low levels of the non-paraprotein immunoglobulin (immunoparesis) and the presence of free monoclonal light chains in the urine (Bence-Jones protein). They occur in multiple myeloma and other lymphoproliferative diseases (e.g. Waldenstrom's macroglobulinaemia, chronic lymphocytic leukaemia and non-Hodgkin's lymphoma).

MGUS. This describes paraproteins that do not have the typical features described above. They tend to be < 10 g/l and are not associated with immunoparesis or urinary free light chains. They were previously known as **benign paraproteins**; however, long-term follow up of patients has shown that up to 25% of cases ultimately transform into malignant paraproteins. Many of the conditions that cause a polyclonal increase in immunoglobulins may also cause an MGUS (Table 61).

Measurement of paraprotein levels

Measurement of paraprotein levels is by visual inspection of the electrophoretic strip and usually software-based analysis of the size and density of the paraprotein band (**densitometry**). This is very different from the measurement of normal immunoglobulins by rate nephelometry and the results of the two analyses are not directly comparable.

Urine protein analysis

Urinary paraproteins of monoclonal free light chains are often referred to as Bence-Jones protein after the original laboratory technique used to identify them. Despite the redundancy of the laboratory technique, the name persists.

Urine electrophoresis

It is important to note that 'dipstick tests' for urinary protein do not reliably detect monoclonal free light chains. Normal urine contains very little protein (< 150 mg/24 hours for men and < 93 mg/24 hours for women) and urine samples must be concentrated prior to electrophoresis.

Urinary free light chains (Bence-Jones protein)

Early morning specimens are preferred for measurement of free light chains. A urine sample should accompany all serum samples submitted in cases of suspected paraproteinaemia. For disease monitoring, a 24-hour urine collection (no added preservative) is required.

IgG subclass and functional (specific) antibody testing

IgG subclass and functional (specific) antibody testing are used in the investigation of suspected primary immunodeficiency.

IgG subclasses

The measurement of IgG subclasses (1–4) is of limited value and should only be considered in the context of identifying primary immunodeficiency. Many would argue that IgG subclass measurement has been appropriately superseded by functional or specific antibody testing; however, most laboratories continue to provide the tests. The majority of serum IgG consists of IgG$_1$ and IgG$_2$, IgG$_3$ and IgG$_4$ being present at much lower levels. Deficiency of IgG$_2$ is associated with recurrent bacterial infections (Ch. 4).

Functional/specific antibodies

Functional antibody testing measures the amount of total IgG that binds specifically to individual antigens. The most frequent antigen studies are **tetanus toxoid** and **pneumococcal capsular polysaccharide**, the former being a protein (T dependent) antigen and the latter being polysaccharide (T independent) antigen. Thus two separate aspects of the immune response are assessed. Usual practice is to measure baseline levels of the functional antibodies and then immunise the patient with tetanus toxoid and Pneumovax II. A second blood sample is taken 4 weeks after immunisation for repeat testing. It is expected that there should be a fourfold rise in titre after immunisation; if this is demonstrated, it suggests that the antibody response is intact. Difficulties arise in the interpretation of immunisation responses because normal age-related ranges are not well defined. It is, therefore, advisable that this type of functional investigation is only undertaken in consultation with specialist immunologists.

Acute phase proteins and complement

C-reactive protein

CRP is an acute phase protein that is elevated in infections and other disorders associated with tissue damage and inflammation. It is of use in monitoring inflammatory disease activity and is particularly useful in monitoring response to therapy because it has a short serum half-life. Typical levels of CRP are:

- mild inflammation/viral infection: < 40 mg/l
- active inflammation/bacterial infection: 40–200 mg/l
- severe inflammation, invasive bacterial infection, some malignancies: up to 500 mg/l.

Complement components

Single point determinations of C3 and C4 are of limited value and serial measurements are recommended:

- raised levels of C3 and C4 levels are found in acute phase reactions and in chronic inflammation
- low C3 and C4 levels may occur in patients with SLE, particularly with renal involvement
- low C3 levels are found in patients with membranoproliferative glomerulonephritis or partial lipodystrophy associated with the presence of C3 nephritic factor
- low C3 levels, which return to normal in convalescence, are associated with acute poststreptococcal glomerulonephritis
- low C4 levels occur in patients with hereditary angioedema, cryoglobulinaemia or genetic deficiency of C4.

Other complement components are measured in specific conditions.

C3d. This degradation product of C3 will be elevated in conditions in which an acute phase response masks complement consumption. It is, therefore, of use in the interpretation of C3 and C4 levels and the long-term monitoring of connective tissue disorders. Elevated levels of C3d occur in those conditions associated with circulating immune complexes.

CH100. This is a screening test for complement function, indicated in the investigation of suspected immunodeficiency associated with recurrent pyogenic infections and atypical immune complex disorders. Values within the normal range indicate that the classical components (C1–C9) are present. Quantification of individual complement components should be undertaken in samples with subnormal CH100 levels.

C1 esterase inhibitor. Low levels (< 0.14 g/l) are found in 85% of patients with hereditary angioedema.

C1 esterase inhibitor (functional assay). This assay is used to establish C1 esterase inhibitor activity. Approximately 15% of patients with hereditary angioedema have normal antigenic levels of C1 esterase inhibitor but have a non-functional molecule. Both types of hereditary angioedema are associated with low/ absent serum C4 levels during an attack. The rare acquired form of C1 esterase inhibitor deficiency is associated with some lymphoproliferative disorders and SLE.

C1q. The primary indication for C1q measurement is in the differentiation of hereditary angioedema (normal C1q levels) from acquired C1 esterase deficiency (reduced C1q levels). Levels are also decreased in other conditions associated with immune complex-mediated complement activation.

Cryoprotein investigation

Cryoproteins include cryoglobulins and cryofibrinogens. Both are proteins that precipitate and form complexes at low temperatures. Cryofibrinogenaemia is thought to be very rare, while cryoglobulinaemia is not uncommon. Patients with cryoglobulinaemia may present with Raynaud's phenomenon, purpuric vasculitis, arthritis or nephritis (Ch. 8). An unexpectedly detected rheumatoid factor or low serum C4 may indicate the presence of a cryoglobulin.

Detection of cryoproteins is only possible if samples are collected carefully and appropriately and the laboratory is experienced in the necessary analyses. Submission of incorrectly collected samples prevents the detection of cryoproteins and may lead to the inappropriate exclusion of this from the differential diagnosis. Before blood is taken, syringes and collection bottles should be prewarmed to 37°C. For cryoglobulin detection, a clotted sample is required, collected in a plain tube. If cryofibrinogen is sought, a citrated sample is required and care should be taken to ensure that the sample does not become inadvertently heparinised (either through patient medication or sampling through a central venous line). Heparin causes cross-linking of cryofibrinogen and thus prevents complexing and detection as a precipitate. Once samples are drawn into the appropriate prewarmed bottles, they should be immediately immersed in water also at 37°C and maintained at that temperature during analysis. Classification of cryoglobulins is indicated in Table 42 (p. 131). Figure 67 shows a cryoprotein identified after appropriate collection, separation and storage of serum at 4°C.

Protein in cerebrospinal fluid

Analysis of protein production in cerebrospinal fluid (CSF) is useful in the investigation of suspected **multiple sclerosis**.

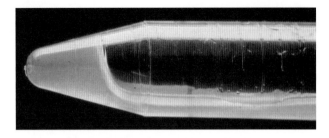

Fig. 67 Identification of a cryoprotein in serum that was collected and separated at 37°C and subsequently stored at 4°C. The gelatinous substance at the base of the test tube is the cryoprotein.

Paired CSF and serum samples are required and the purpose of the investigation is to look for evidence of abnormal immunoglobulin production within the central nervous system (CNS) that is not seen in serum. This occurs in multiple sclerosis and some other inflammatory neurological conditions. Levels of immunoglobulin in the CSF are very low and conventional electrophoresis is inadequate. However, use of special stains (including gold) or modified techniques including **isoelectric focusing** allows oligoclonal bands to be detected. These consist of two or more bands identified in the CSF but not in the serum. If oligoclonal bands are detected in both serum and CSF this is suggestive of a systemic inflammatory response and is not consistent with a localised process within the CNS.

Measurement of β₂-microglobulin

The light chain in MHC class I molecules is known as β_2-microglobulin; this low-molecular-weight protein is non-covalently linked to the heavy chains of the class I molecules. It is, therefore, expressed on the surface of all nucleated cells of the body. Raised serum levels are associated with clinical conditions characterised by a high rate of cellular (particularly lymphoid) cell death. Therefore, in myeloma and HIV-related disease, measurement of β_2-microglobulin has become one of the important laboratory parameters for assessing disease progression. It is important to note that β_2-microglobulin is normally filtered freely at the glomerulus and subsequently catabolised in the tubules. Poor renal function will, therefore, contribute to increased serum levels. The normal range for β_2-microglobulin quoted in our laboratory is 0.9–2.1 mg/l. Levels at presentation of > 20 mg/l are associated with a poor prognosis in myeloma.

Allergy assessments

Investigation in allergy is focused at confirming sensitisation to a suspected allergen as the cause of typic-ally allergic symptoms. These include allergic rhinitis and asthma as well as suspected food allergy. Food allergy is a controversial subject (Ch. 5) but it is worth re-emphasising that the symptoms expected in food allergy are urticaria, angioedema, acute gastrointestinal upset (vomiting/diarrhoea) or anaphylaxis. In contrast, symptoms of chronic fatigue, depression, joint pains, unexplained abdominal pain, etc. are *not* an indication for investigation of an allergic cause.

Total serum IgE

Measurement of total serum IgE is of limited value in the assessment of patients with allergic disease. A very wide range of IgE levels is found both in normal individuals and those with allergic diseases, and total serum IgE levels do not discriminate between these populations. IgE levels may be grossly elevated in some atopic patients and some with parasitic infection. Very high levels (> 2000 IU/l) may be detected in the rare hyper-IgE and recurrent infection syndrome.

Allergen-specific IgE

There are two main methods for confirmation of allergic sensitisation: skin prick tests (SPT) in vivo and detection of allergen-specific IgE in vitro. The SPT has the advantages of being a rapid, relatively cheap method of testing. It provides immediate answers for the patient and it is probably the more clinically informative method because it tests the functional integrity of the mast cell response in vivo. Problems with SPT have included standardisation of reagents and concerns regarding potential anaphylactic reactions (although the latter are very rarely reported).

In vitro allergen-specific IgE detection methods are semiquantitative and generally reported on a numerical scale (e.g. 0–6). The reported number does *not* have any correlation with the severity of clinical disease. In vitro testing is of value where SPT is difficult to perform or contraindicated:

- very young children
- patients with severe/extensive eczema or dermographism
- patients taking antihistamines that cannot be stopped
- patients in whom there is a significant risk of an anaphylactic reaction.

The use of allergen-specific IgE testing must be carefully considered and is not a substitute for careful clinical assessment. Detection of allergen-specific IgE by either in vivo or in vitro methods is of value in confirming allergic sensitisation suspected from the clinical history; however, neither should be used as a screening test for multiple allergens. Atopic individuals are likely to have multiple positive results, which can be very difficult to interpret meaningfully.

Anaphylaxis

Investigation can be helpful in clarifying suspected anaphylactic reactions, in particular reactions occurring during anaesthesia. Investigations are recommended for patients with grade II (cardiovascular reaction: tachycardia, hypotension), grade III (shock, life-threatening spasm of smooth muscles) and grade IV (cardiac and/or respiratory arrest) reactions.

Local practices will vary; however, some or all of the following are measured: mast cell tryptase; IgE and allergen-specific IgE (as appropriate); IgG, IgM and IgA; complement proteins C3, C4, C3d; CRP.

12.4 Cellular immunology

Learning objectives

You should:
- understand when to measure lymphocyte and neutrophil numbers and function
- be aware of the significance of such cellular abnormalities.

Investigation of the cellular immune system includes analysis of lymphocyte and neutrophil numbers and function. Cellular investigations are expensive to perform and complex to interpret, therefore, they should only be undertaken after consultation with specialist immunology staff. This section should be read with reference to the relevent conditions discussed in Chapter 4.

Lymphocyte phenotyping

The presence of specialised cells surface molecules, termed CD markers, on the surface of lymphocytes was discussed in Chapter 1, as was their value in the investigation of immunodeficiency (Ch. 4) and lymphoproliferative diseases (Ch. 11).

Lymphocyte phenotyping involves the use of a panel of monoclonal antibodies directed at the CD markers to analyse the various lymphocyte subpopulations present in peripheral blood (Table 62). Once the lymphocytes are stained with the fluorescently tagged monoclonal antibody, they are analysed using a flow cytometer, which identifies the percentages of cells bearing each monoclonal antibody. The panel of markers used should identify the major subpopulations of T cells as well as B cells and natural killer cells (Table 63); the panel will be varied depending on whether immunodeficiency or lymphoid malignancy is suspected. In general, laboratories need to receive the blood sample with ethylenediaminetetraacetic acid (EDTA) within a few hours of its being taken to allow analysis on the same day.

Serial CD4$^+$ cell measurements are of value in monitoring progression of HIV-related disease; however, measurement of CD4$^+$ cells has no place in the diagnosis of HIV infection until serological status is established. Requesting a CD4$^+$ cell count as a 'surrogate marker' of HIV infection is neither reliable nor ethical and would be refused by most laboratories.

Lymphocyte function

Lymphocyte function assessment is indicated in the investigation for primary immunodeficiency, particularly severe combined immunodeficiency. Blood is collected in heparinised tubes and incubated for 3 to 5 days with several mitogens. Lymphocyte growth is assessed by measurement of the incorporation of tritiated thymidine. Typical mitogens include

- phytohaemagglutinin (PHA)
- phorbol myristate acetate (PMA)
- anti-CD3.

Each of these stimulates lymphocyte proliferation by interacting with different target molecules either on the cell surface or in the cytoplasm; the results can, therefore, be very informative regarding the exact nature of

Table 62 Normal ranges for lymphocyte counts and subsets

Cell set	Cell count at varying ages ($\times 10^9$ cells/l (%))			
	<1 year	**1–6 years**	**7–17 years**	**> 18 years**
Total lymphocytes	2.7–5.4	2.9–5.1	2.0–2.7	1.6–2.4
CD3	1.7–3.6 (58–67)	1.8–3.0 (62–69)	1.4–2.0 (66–76)	0.7–2.4 (66–88)
CD4	1.7–2.8 (38–50)	1.0–1.8 (30–40)	0.7–1.1 (33–41)	0.5–1.6 (37–64)
CD8	0.8–1.2 (18–25)	0.8–1.5 (25–32)	0.6–0.9 (27–35)	0.2–0.7 (11–36)
CD19	0.5–1.5 (19–31)	0.7–1.3 (21–28)	0.3–0.5 (12–22)	0.03–0.3 (3–13)
Natural killer	0.3–0.7 (8–17)	0.2–0.6 (8–15)	0.2–0.3 (9–16)	0.2–0.4 (10–19)

Table 63 Typical lymphocyte phenotyping panel

CD marker	Corresponding lymphoid population
CD3	All T cells
CD4	Helper T cells
CD8	Cytotoxic T cells
CD19	B cells
CD16/56	Natural killer cells
CD25	Activated lymphocytes
HLA-DR	B cells and activated T cells

Table 64 Immunofluorescent findings on renal biopsy

Disease	Findings
Anti-glomerular basement membrane disease (Goodpasture's disease/syndrome)	Linear IgG, C3 and fibrin deposition along glomerular basement membrane
Henoch–Schönlein syndrome	Mesangial IgA, IgG, C3, fibrin
IgA nephropathy	Mesangial IgA, IgG, C3 and fibrin
Membranous glomerulonephritis	Granular IgG, IgA, IgM, C1q, C3 and C4
Mesangioproliferative glomerulonephritis	Variable IgM, C3, C4
Mesangiocapillary glomerulonephritis	Granular C3 ± immunoglobulin
Mesangiocapillary glomerulonephritis (type II)/dense deposit disease	Mesangial and basement membrane C3
Rapidly progressive glomerulonephritis	Granular IgG, IgM, C3 and fibrin
Scleroderma	Variable: IgG, C3, fibrin
Systemic lupus erythematosus	Granular IgG, IgA, IgM, C1q, C3, C4

any underlying defect. In addition to mitogens, antigens such as those from *Candida* sp. are used to identify specific defects (e.g. chronic mucocutaneous candidiasis).

Neutrophil function tests

Neutrophil defects may be suspected if there is a history of recurrent skin infections, chronic gingivitis and recurrent deep-seated bacterial and fungal infections. If the neutrophil count is normal the following functional tests may be considered:

- serial neutrophil counts every 3 days for a month to exclude cyclical neutropenia
- chemotaxis: may be defective in hyper-IgE and recurrent infection syndrome
- phagocytosis and killing: these two aspects are usually assessed together by measuring the uptake and killing of standard laboratory grown organisms
- nitroblue tetrazolium (NBT) test/respiratory oxidative burst: the nitroblue tetrazolium test was the original test for chronic granulomatous disease; this has largely been superseded by flow cytometric assessments of the respiratory oxidative burst
- adhesion molecules (CD15, CD18): absent in leukocyte adhesion deficiencies types 1 and 2.

12.5 Immunohistology

Learning objectives

You should:
- understand what tissues are used for immunohistology
- know when such tests would be done.

Examination of biopsy specimens by DIF can be extremely valuable in determining a diagnosis. The most common requests would be for examination of skin (Fig. 43) or renal biopsy (Table 64), although mucosal biopsies may also be examined. Tissue samples must be fresh and unfixed. Transport to the laboratory is best undertaken with tissue stored in liquid nitrogen.

Skin biopsy

Skin biopsy is indicated in the investigation of bullous skin diseases (pemphigoid/pemphigus), dermatitis herpetiformis, DLE/SLE and vasculitic disorders. Perilesional biopsies are suggested as lesional inflammatory changes may modify or alter the immunofluorescence appearances. The diagnosis of vasculitis is supported by the demonstration of immunoglobulin and complement components in dermal blood vessels, but these findings are not specific for any single form of vasculitis. Serum and plasma specimens for relevant autoantibody and complement studies as appropriate are indicated (see Table 65 for typical findings).

Renal biopsy

Examination of renal biopsy samples by DIF is helpful in identifying glomerular deposits of immunoglobulin and complementant (see Table 64 for typical findings).

Table 65 Index of diseases and the relevant investigations

Disease	Investigations
Addison's disease	Anti-adrenal antibody
Allergy	IgE, allergen-specific IgE
Anaphylaxis	Mast cell tryptase, IgE, allergen-specific IgE, immunoglobulins, C3, C4, C3d, C-reactive protein, urinary methylhistamine
Angioedema	C1 esterase inhibitor, C1q, C3, C4
Anti-phospholipid syndrome (APS)	Anti-cardiolipin antibody, anti-β_2-glycoprotein 1 antibody, lupus anticoagulant
Bullous skin disorders	Immunohistology, skin reactive antibodies, anti-gliadin antibody (in dermatitis herpetiformis), anti-endomysium antibody (in dermatitis herpetiformis)
Chronic active hepatitis	Anti-smooth muscle antibody, anti-liver kidney microsomal antibody, anti-mitochondrial antibody, anti-nuclear antibody
Chronic granulomatous disease	Neutrophil function test
Chronic lymphocytic leukaemia	Immunoglobulins, serum protein electrophoresis, lymphocyte phenotyping
Coeliac disease	Anti-endomysial antibody, anti-gliadin antibody, anti-transglutaminase antibody
Congenital heart block	Anti-Ro antibody
Connective tissue diseases	Anti-nuclear antibody, antibodies to extractable nuclear antigen (ENA)
CREST	Anti-centromere antibody
Cryoglobulinaemia	Cryoglobulins, C3, C4
Dermatitis herpetiformis	Immunohistology, anti-endomysial antibody, anti-gliadin antibody
Dermatomyositis	Anti-Jo-1 antibody
Diabetes mellitus	Anti-islet cell antibody
Discoid lupus erythematosus	Anti-nuclear antibody, immunohistology
Dressler's syndrome	Anti-cardiac muscle antibody
Fibrosing alveolitis	Anti-nuclear antibody
Glomerulonephritis	Anti-neutrophil cytoplasmic antibody, anti-myeloperoxidase antibody, anti-proteinase 3 antibody, anti-GBM antibody, C3/C4
Goodpasture's syndrome	Anti-GBM antibody
Graves' disease	Anti-thyroperoxidase antibody, anti-thyrotropin receptor antibody
Guillain–Barré syndrome	Anti-GM1 antibody, anti-GD1 antibody
Hashimoto's thyroiditis	Anti-thyroid antibody
HIV infection	Lymphocyte phenotyping, β_2-microglobulin
Immunodeficiency	Immunoglobulins, IgG subclasses, functional antibodies, CH100, C3, C4, C-reactive protein, cellular investigations
Infection	C-reactive protein, immunoglobulins, serum protein electrophoresis
Juvenile chronic arthritis	Rheumatoid factor, anti-nuclear antibody, C-reactive protein
Leukaemia/lymphoma	Cellular studies
Lymphoproliferative disorders	Serum protein electrophoresis, immunoglobulins, paraprotein detection and quantification, cellular studies, cryoglobulins
Myeloma	Immunoglobulins, serum protein electrophoresis, paraprotein detection and quantification, urinary Bence-Jones protein
Membranoproliferative glomerulonephritis (MPGN)	C3 nephritic factor, C3/C4
Microscopic polyangiitis	Anti-neutrophil cytoplasmic antibody, anti-myeloperoxidase antibody, anti-proteinase 3 antibody
Mixed connective tissue disease (MCTD)	Anti-nuclear antibody, anti-ENA antibody, anti-RNP antibody
Monoclonal gammopathy uncertain significance (MGUS)	Immunoglobulins, serum protein electrophoresis, paraprotein detection and quantification
Multiple sclerosis	Cerebrospinal fluid total protein, IgG ratio and index, oligoclonal bands
Myasthenia gravis	Anti-acetylcholine receptor antibody
Non-Hodgkin's lymphoma	Immunoglobulins, serum protein electrophoresis, cellular studies
Partial lipodystrophy	C3 nephritic factor, C3, C4
Pernicious anaemia	Anti-gastric parietal cell antibody, anti-intrinsic factor antibody
Pemphigus	Immunohistology, anti-intercellular substance/desmosome antibodies
Pemphigoid	Immunohistology, anti-basement membrane zone antibodies
Polymyositis	Anti-Jo-1 antibody
Premature ovarian failure	Anti-adrenal antibody, anti-steroid-producing cell antibodies
Primary biliary cirrhosis	Anti-mitochondrial antibody
Progressive systemic sclerosis	Anti-nucleolar antibody, anti-nuclear antibody, anti-Scl-70 antibody
Raynaud's phenomenon	Anti-centromere antibody
Rheumatoid arthritis	Rheumatoid factor, C-reactive protein, C3d, C3/C4
Sjögren's syndrome	Anti-nuclear antibody, anti-Ro antibody, anti-La antibody
Systemic lupus erythematosus	Anti-nuclear antibody, anti-dsDNA antibody, anti-ENA antibodies, anti-cardiolipin antibody, C3d, C3/C4
Vasculitis	Anti-neutrophil cytoplasmic antibody, anti-myeloperoxidase antibody, anti-proteinase 3 antibody, immunohistology, C-reactive protein
Waldenstrom's macroglobulinaemia	Immunoglobulins, serum protein electrophoresis, immunohistology
Wegener's granulomatosis	Anti-neutrophil cytoplasmic antibody (ANCA), anti-PR3-ANCA antibody

Self-assessment: questions

Multiple choice questions

1. Low serum C4 with normal serum C3 suggests:
   a. Mesangiocapillary glomerulonephritis type II
   b. Anaphylaxis
   c. C1 inhibitor deficiency
   d. Cryoglobulinaemia
   e. Hereditary deficiency

2. Which of the following antibodies is most likely to be associated with poor prognosis in systemic lupus erythematosus (SLE)?
   a. Anti-Sm (anti-Smith)
   b. Anti-cardiolipin
   c. Anti-ribonucleoprotein (anti-RNP)
   d. Anti-histone
   e. Anti-double-stranded DNA (anti-dsDNA)

3. The CD4⁺ lymphocyte count in peripheral blood:
   a. Can be a useful diagnostic test when HIV infection is suspected
   b. A value $< 400 \times 10^9/l$ is diagnostic of stage IV disease in the US Center for Disease Control and Prevention staging
   c. May be used to determine appropriate therapeutic options
   d. Is never $< 200 \times 10^9/l$ in a healthy adult
   e. Is the single most useful laboratory indicator of HIV disease progression

4. The detection of anti-nuclear autoantibodies in serum:
   a. Indicates an underlying autoimmune disease
   b. Indicates that the likely diagnosis is systemic lupus erythematosus
   c. May be normal
   d. Decreases with age
   e. May be a result of recent infection

5. Low serum C3 with normal serum C4 suggests:
   a. Mesangiocapillary glomerulonephritis type II
   b. Mixed connective tissue disease
   c. Systemic lupus erythematosus
   d. Cryoglobulinaemia
   e. Hereditary deficiency

6. The following statements are true:
   a. Anti-mitochondrial antibodies may predict the development of primary biliary cirrhosis in later life

b. The detection of low levels of IgG in an adult may indicate underlying malignancy
c. The detection of anti-Ro antibodies is associated with neonatal heart failure
d. A paraprotein of 1 g/l in a 70-year-old man is of no clinical significance
f. Angioedema is characterised by intense itching and epidermal spongiosis

Case history questions

History 1

A 25-year-old woman with heavy periods presents with tiredness. Her brother is on a gluten-free diet and her peripheral blood film shows Howell–Jolly bodies.

1. Which antibodies are likely to be detected?

   a. anti-nuclear antibodies
   b. anti-gliadin antibodies
   c. anti-GAD (anti-glutamatic acid decarboxylase) antibodies
   d. anti-tissue transglutaminase antibodies
   e. anti-islet cell antibodies.

History 2

A 45-year-old woman complains of fatigue, itch and non-specific joint pains. She is concerned about food allergy. On examination, she has periorbital xanthelasma but no joint deformity. Her haemoglobin is 12.5 g/l and her total white cell count is normal. Total IgE is normal but total serum IgM is significantly raised. Urinalysis is normal.

1. Which antibodies are most likely to be detected?

   a. anti-nuclear antibodies
   b. anti-mitochondrial antibodies
   c. anti-milk antibodies
   d. anti-smooth muscle antibodies
   e. anti-skeletal muscle antibodies.

History 3

A 40-year-old woman presents with unsteadiness of gait and double vision. Six months previously she had a total abdominal hysterectomy as treatment for endometrial cancer.

1. Which antibodies are likely to be detected?

    a. anti-voltage-gated calcium channel antibodies
    b. anti-acetylcholine receptor antibodies
    c. anti-GAD (anti-glutamic acid decarboxylase) antibodies
    d. anti-peripheral nerve antibodies
    e. anti-Purkinje cell antibodies.

History 4

A 68-year-old man is admitted to hospital with acute pneumonia. During his admission he complains of some weakness and double vision. His chest radiograph suggests an anterior mass lesion.

1. Which antibodies are likely to be detected:

    a. anti-smooth muscle antibodies
    b. anti-acetylcholine receptor antibodies
    c. anti-GAD (anti-glutamic acid decarboxylase) antibodies
    d. anti-skeletal muscle antibodies
    e. anti-Purkinje cell antibodies.

History 5

A 50-year-old woman presents with arthralgia of the hands and difficulty with swallowing. She reports that in the winter her hands become cold and painful.

1. Which one of the following autoantibodies is most specifically associated with her most likely diagnosis:

    a. anti-nucleolar antibodies
    b. anti-mitochondrial antibodies
    c. anti-Sm (anti-Smith) antibodies
    d. anti-centromere antibodies
    e. anti-smooth muscle antibodies.

Data interpretation

1. A 50-year-old nursing sister presented with a purpuric rash over the lower legs. There is a previous history of tonsillitis occurring 2 weeks prior to the development of the rash. A diagnosis of postviral thrombocytopenia is made and symptoms resolve over a 4-week period. Four months later she presented with numbness and weakness of her hands and feet with a recurrence of the purpuric rash.

    Chest radiograph showed normal lung fields. Urine microscopy showed no white cells/casts. Other results are shown in Table 66.

Which of the following is the most likely diagnosis:

    a. Henoch–Schönlein purpura
    b. polyarteritis nodosa
    c. Wegener's granulomatosis
    d. systemic lupus erythematosus
    e. microscopic polyangiitis.

Table 66 Results for data interpretation question

Parameter	Value	Normal range
Haemoglobin (g/l)	125	130–180
Total white cell count ($\times 10^9$/l)	8	4–10
Platelets ($\times 10^9$/l)	120	150–450
Erythrocyte sedimentation rate (mm/h)	80	—
C-reactive protein (mg/l)	145	0–10
Urea (mmol/l)	7.0	2.1–8.9
Creatinine (µmol/l)	105	53–133
Alanine aminotransferase (U/l)	17	< 45
Aspartate aminotransferase (U/l)	28	< 41
C3 (g/l)	1.7	0.7–1.7
C4 (g/l)	0.05	0.13–0.43
C4 allotyping	1 null allele	
Perinuclear antineutrophil cytoplasmic antibody (p-ANCA) (U/l)	Positive (1:160)	
Antineutrophil cytoplasmic antibody (MPO-ANCA) (U/l)	25	< 5

Self-assessment: answers

Multiple choice answers

1. a. **False.** Mesangiocapillary glomerulonephritis is associated with C3 nephritic factor and low levels of serum C3.
   b. **False.** Anaphylactic reactions are not characterised by low complement levels.
   c. **True.** Deficiency of C1 inhibitor causes failure of control of activation of the early components of the classical pathway.
   d. **True.** Cryoglobulinaemia causes inefficient (fluid phase) complement activation, which fails to efficiently convert C3.
   e. **True.** Hereditary deficiency of one or more alleles of C4 leads to this pattern of serum proteins.

2. a. **False.** Anti-Sm antibodies are important in establishing diagnosis but not prognosis.
   b. **True.** The detection of anti-cardiolipin antibodies is associated with thrombotic complications and, therefore, a worse prognosis in SLE.
   c. **False.**
   d. **False.**
   e. **False.** Anti-dsDNA antibodies are found in the majority of patients with SLE.

3. a. **False.** CD4$^+$ cell counts should never be used as a surrogate marker of HIV infection.
   b. **False.** At stage IV, CD4$^+$ cell counts would be $< 200 \times 10^9/l$.
   c. **True.** Serial monitoring of CD4$^+$ cell counts is used to inform the use of clinical algorithms for antimicrobial prophylactic regimens.
   d. **False.** CD4$^+$ cell lymphocyte counts may be low in otherwise healthy people or in those taking medication.
   e. **True.** CD4$^+$ cell counts indicate the progressive decline in immune function. Measurement of total plasma viral load now provides an effective means of monitoring the effect of antiviral therapy.

4. a. **False.** Anti-nuclear antibody production may be triggered by a number of a factors and auto-antibodies (particularly at low titre) are frequently detected in healthy individuals.
   b. **False.** Anti-nuclear antibodies are not specific for systemic lupus erythematosus.
   c. **True.**
   d. **False.** Detection of anti-nuclear antibodies is more common in the elderly.
   e. **True.**

5. a. **True.**
   b. **False.** This is not typically associated with complement consumption.
   c. **False.** Active systemic lupus erythematosus is usually associated with consumption of both C4 and C3.
   d. **False.** The reverse pattern is found in cryoglobulinaemia.
   e. **True.** Although very rare, hereditary deficiency of C3 does occur.

6. a. **True.** Longitudinal monitoring of liver biochemistry is, therefore, advised in asymptomatic patients in whom anti-mitochondrial antibodies are detected.
   b. **True.** This may be an indication of underlying lymphoproliferative disease.
   c. **True.** This may occur because of the development of heart block.
   d. **False.** It may not indicate underlying disease at the time of detection but should be followed up to ensure there is no evidence of malignant transformation.
   e. **False.** Angioedema is typically a non-itchy swelling that predominantly involves the dermis.

Case history answers

History 1

1. The history is suggestive of coeliac disease; anti-gliadin antibodies are sensitive but not specific indicators of this condition. Anti-tissue transglutaminase antibodies are more specific indicators of coeliac disease than anti-gliadin antibodies. Their sensitivity for the untreated condition is probably > 95%. Anti-GAD antibodies may be detected in stiff man syndrome or diabetes mellitus.

History 2

1. The history is suggestive of primary biliary cirrhosis and anti-mitochondrial antibodies are highly specific indicators of this condition. While anti-nuclear antibodies may be detected in such patients, they are not the most likely. The other antibodies would not be detected: anti-smooth muscle antibodies are found in acute hepatitis and after acute infection and anti-skeletal muscle antibodies are detected in a subset of patients with myasthenia gravis.

History 3

1. Anti-Purkinje antibodies are associated with cerebellar paraneoplastic syndromes, which most commonly occur in association with gynaecological malignancy. The other antibodies would not be expected: anti-voltage-gated calcium channel antibodies are detected in Lambert–Eaton myasthenic syndrome (a paraneoplastic syndrome usually associated with small cell carcinoma of the lung); anti-acetylcholine receptor antibodies are associated with classical myasthenia gravis; anti-GAD antibodies may be detected in stiff man syndrome or diabetes mellitus and anti-peripheral nerve antibodies would only occur in a peripheral neuropathy, which is not suggested by the history.

History 4

1. Anti-acetylcholine receptor antibodies are most likely, as the history is suggestive of myasthenia gravis, with anti-skeletal muscle antibodies, as these are associated with thymoma, which is suggested by the chest radiograph findings. The other antibodies would not be expected.

History 5

1. The history is suggestive of the CREST variant of scleroderma, which is associated with anti-centromere antibodies. The other antibodies are not as likely: anti-nucleolar antibodies may occur in systemic lupus erythematosus or scleroderma and anti-Sm antibodies are specific for systemic lupus erythematosus; anti-mitochondrial antibodies are specifically associated with primary biliary cirrhosis.

Data interpretation

1. The clinical history and physical findings are suggestive of a vasculitic condition, chiefly affecting the skin, but possibly also causing a neuropathy. The first episode may have been triggered by an upper respiratory tract infection. Investigations revealed a significantly raised erythrocyte sedimentation rate and C-reactive protein, consistent with a systemic inflammatory process. There was a low C4, which allotyping revealed as being caused by genetic deficiency rather than consumption. There were positive anti-neutrophil cytoplasmic antibodies (p-ANCA and MPO-ANCA). The physical distribution of the rash and the triggering by an upper respiratory tract infection could be consistent with Henoch–Schönlein purpura; however, that would be unusual at this woman's age and one would not expect positive ANCA serology. Polyarteritis nodosa may cause subcutaneous nodules but rarely if ever causes a purpuric rash. It is a vasculitis of medium-sized vessels and, therefore, is unlikely in this case where the clinical features are more suggestive of a small-vessel vasculitis. The history is not suggestive of Wegener's granulomatosis in that there are no respiratory or renal symptoms or signs. Systemic lupus erythematosus is also unlikely because the clinical features are not typical and the serology gives no indication of this. The most likely diagnosis is microscopic polyangiitis. This is a small-vessel vasculitis that may cause the clinical features described. The important confirmatory investigations are the very high C-reactive protein and positive p-ANCA and MPO-ANCA.

Index

Question and Answer sections are indicated in the form 63Q/67A